Oral Health Care: Pediatrics and Clinical Analysis

Oral Health Care:
Pediatrics and Clinical Analysis

Edited by **Regina Stuart**

hayle
medical

New York

Published by Hayle Medical,
30 West, 37th Street, Suite 612,
New York, NY 10018, USA
www.haylemedical.com

Oral Health Care: Pediatrics and Clinical Analysis
Edited by Regina Stuart

International Standard Book Number: 978-1-63241-307-9 (Hardback)

Printed in the United States of America.

Contents

Permissions

List of Contributors

Preface

This book deals with oral health care and its application in clinical and pediatric dentistry. Oral health care in pediatric dentistry is concerned with the entire oral health, covering preventive aspects for children right from their birth to adolescence, including all the spheres of dental care along with several distinct specialties. It also covers planning of a preventive program at individual and community levels. The recent research interests in oral health care encompass analyses about the role of tissue culture, stem cells, and other ground-breaking technologies available to the scientific community along with the conventional fields like physiology, anatomy, and pharmaceuticals, etc. of the oral cavity. Public health and epidemiology in oral health care is about the checking of the general oral health of a community, basic afflictions they are suffering from, and an all-inclusive approach for care and correction of the same. This book is a compilation of information contributed by internationally eminent and veteran specialists regarding the latest developments in several fields of oral health care.

This book is a comprehensive compilation of works of different researchers from varied parts of the world. It includes valuable experiences of the researchers with the sole objective of providing the readers (learners) with a proper knowledge of the concerned field. This book will be beneficial in evoking inspiration and enhancing the knowledge of the interested readers.

In the end, I would like to extend my heartiest thanks to the authors who worked with great determination on their chapters. I also appreciate the publisher's support in the course of the book. I would also like to deeply acknowledge my family who stood by me as a source of inspiration during the project.

Editor

Part 1

Pediatric and Preventive Dentistry

1

Pediatric Dentistry
– A Guide for General Practitioner

Mandeep S. Virdi

PDM Dental College and Research Institute, Bahadurgarh, Haryana
India

1. Introduction

Children a resource of the world are the promise of what our future is going to be. A healthy child is a better promise of a better world than an unhealthy child. Oral health is a very important aspect to ensure a healthy future therefore oral health for children is a worthy concern regardless of child's nationality, ethnicity or geographic location. Dentistry for children has come a long way from its humble beginning in 1924 with the publishing of first comprehensive text book on dentistry for children followed by formation of The American Academy of Pedodontics in the late forties, which was also recognized by council of dental education a part of the ADA to certify candidates to practice specialized dentistry for children. Mid eighties saw the present name American Academy of Pediatric Dentistry being adopted followed by defining pediatric dentistry which in the present day is defined as an age-defined specialty that provides both primary and comprehensive preventive and therapeutic oral health care for infants and children through adolescence, including those with special health care needs[1].

Pediatric Dentistry as the definition implies is a body of knowledge that is dependent upon curriculum of other dental subjects along with the latest development happening in various specialties of dentistry. To be able to give primary, comprehensive and preventive oral health care to children of all ages the pediatric dentist relies on preventive dentistry, pulpal therapy, instrumentation and restoration of teeth, dental material, oral surgery, preventive and interceptive orthodontics, and principals of prosthetics. Besides the dental knowledge, a working knowledge is also required of pediatric medicine, general and oral pathology along with growth and development. For the development of appropriate preventive strategy it is imperative that the pediatric dentist have knowledge of nutrition and systemic as well as topical effects of fluoride. To be able to deal effectively with children behavior management and a thorough knowledge of psychological development is imperative because child needs to be treated differently than the adult.

1.1 Prenatal stage

The prenatal period is a gestation of approximately nine months, beginning with the period of ovum that lasts for about two weeks and is marked by blast cyst getting attached to the wall of the uterus. This is followed by the period of embryo lasting for about next six weeks and is characterized by development of the organ systems. Following which the period of fetus lasting right up to the delivery of the child is the time when maturation of the newly formed organs takes place.

The role of pediatric dentist starts at pre natal stage in guiding the expecting parents to maintain oral health as the mouth is an obvious portal of entry to the body, and oral health reflects and influences general health and well being. Maternal oral health has significant implications for birth outcomes and infant oral health. Maternal periodontal disease, that is, a chronic infection of the gingiva and supporting tooth structures, has been associated with preterm birth, development of preeclampsia, and delivery of a small-for-gestational age infant. Prematurely born children have higher prevalence of enamel defects. In very low birth-weight children, the prevalence of enamel defects could be even higher. Both systemic and local factors contribute to the etiology of dental defects.

Low birth-weight children are often intubated at birth, and left-sided defects on maxillary anterior teeth occurred twice as frequently as right-sided defects, probably the result of trauma from left sided laryngoscopy.

Maternal oral flora is transmitted to the newborn infant, and increased cariogenic flora in the mother predisposes the infant to the development of caries. It is intriguing to consider preconception, pregnancy, or intrapartum treatment of oral health conditions as a mechanism to improve women's oral and general health, pregnancy outcomes, and their children's dental health. However, given the relationship between oral health and general health, oral health care should be a goal in its own right for all individuals. Regardless of the potential for improved oral health to improve pregnancy outcomes, public policies that support comprehensive dental services for vulnerable women of childbearing age should be expanded so that their own oral and general health is safeguarded and their children's risk of caries is reduced. Oral health promotion should include education of women and their health care providers' ways to prevent oral disease from occurring, and referral for dental services when disease is present [2].

2. Role of pediatric dentist at birth

Infant oral health, along with perinatal oral health, is one of the foundations upon which preventive education and dental care must be built to enhance the opportunity for a lifetime free from preventable oral disease. Caries is perhaps the most prevalent infectious disease in children. Almost half children have caries by the time they reach kindergarten. Early childhood caries (ECC) can be a particularly virulent form of caries, beginning soon after tooth eruption, developing on smooth surfaces, progressing rapidly, and having a lasting detrimental impact on the dentition. This disease affects the general population but is more likely to occur in infants who consume a diet high in sugar, and whose mothers have a low education level. Caries in primary teeth can affect children's growth, result in significant pain and potentially life-threatening infection, and diminish overall quality of life.

Caries is a disease that is, by and large, preventable. Early risk assessment allows for identification of parent-infant groups who are at risk for ECC and would benefit from early preventive intervention. The ultimate goal of early assessment is the timely delivery of educational information to populations at high risk for developing caries in order to prevent the need for later surgical intervention.

An oral health risk assessment for infants by 6 months of age allows for the institution of appropriate preventive strategies as the primary dentition begins to erupt. Caries risk assessment can be used to determine the patient's relative risk for caries. Even the most judiciously designed and implemented caries risk assessment tool, however, can fail to identify all infants at risk for developing ECC. In these cases, the mother may not be the colonization source of the child's oral flora, the dietary intake of simple carbohydrates may be extremely high, or other uncontrollable factors may combine to place the patient at risk for developing caries. Therefore, screening for risk of caries in the parent and patient coupled with oral health counseling, although a feasible and equitable approach to ECC control is not a substitute for the early establishment of the dental home. Whenever possible, the ideal approach to infant oral health care, including ECC prevention and management, is the early establishment of a dental home.

3. Anticipatory guidance

General anticipatory guidance given by AAPD for the mother (or other intimate caregiver) includes the following:
- Oral hygiene: Tooth-brushing and flossing by the mother on a daily basis are important to help dislodge food and reduce bacterial plaque levels.
- Diet: Important components of dietary education for the parents include the cariogenicity of certain foods and beverages, role of frequency of consumption of these substances, and the demineralization/remineralization process.
- Fluoride: Using a fluoridated toothpaste approved by the relevant Dental Association and rinsing every night with an alcohol-free, over-the-counter mouth rinse containing 0.05% sodium fluoride have been suggested to help reduce plaque levels and help enamel remineralization.
- Caries removal: Routine professional dental care for the mothers can help keep their oral health in optimal condition. Removal of active caries with subsequent restoration is important to suppress maternal MS reservoirs and has the potential to minimize the transfer of MS to the infant, thereby decreasing the infant's risk of developing ECC.
- Delay of colonization: Education of the parents, especially mothers, on avoiding saliva-sharing behaviors (eg. sharing spoons and other utensils, sharing cups, cleaning a dropped pacifier or toy with their mouth) can help prevent early colonization of MS in their infants.
- Xylitol chewing gums: Evidence demonstrates that mothers' use of xylitol chewing gum can prevent dental caries in their children by prohibiting the transmission of MS.

General anticipatory guidance for the young patient (0 to 3 years of age) includes the following:
- Oral hygiene: Oral hygiene measures should be implemented no later than the time of the eruption of the first primary tooth. Cleansing the infant's teeth as soon as they erupt with either a washcloth or soft toothbrush will help reduce bacterial colonization. Children's teeth should be brushed twice daily with fluoridated toothpaste and a soft, age-appropriate sized toothbrush. A "smear" of toothpaste is recommended for children less than 2 years of age, while a "pea-size" amount of paste is recommended

for children 2-5 years of age. Flossing should be initiated when adjacent tooth surfaces cannot be cleansed with a toothbrush.

- Diet: High-risk dietary practices appear to be established early, probably by 12 months of age, and are maintained throughout early childhood. Frequent night time bottle feeding, ad libitum breast-feeding, and extended and repeated use of a sippy or no-spill cup are associated with, but not consistently implicated in ECC. Likewise, frequent consumption of snacks or drinks containing fermentable carbohydrates (e.g., juice, milk, formula, soda) also can increase the child's caries risk.

- Fluoride: Optimal exposure to fluoride is important to all dentate infants and children. The use of fluoride for the prevention and control of caries is documented to be both safe and effective. Twice-daily brushing with fluoridated toothpaste is recommended for all children as a preventive procedure. Professionally-applied fluoride, as well as at home fluoride treatments, should be considered for children at high caries risk based upon caries risk assessment. Systemically-administered fluoride should be considered for all children drinking fluoride deficient water (<0.6 ppm).Caution is indicated in the use of all fluoride-containing products. Fluorosis has been associated with cumulative fluoride intake during enamel development, with the severity dependent on the dose, duration, and timing of intake. Decisions concerning the administration of additional fluoride are based on the unique needs of each patient.

- Injury prevention: Practitioners should provide age appropriate injury prevention counseling for orofacial trauma. Initially, discussions would include play objects, pacifiers, car seats, and electric cords.

- Non-nutritive habits: Non-nutritive oral habits (e.g., digit or pacifier sucking, bruxism, abnormal tongue thrust) may apply forces to teeth and dentoalveolar structures. It is important to discuss the need for early sucking and the need to wean infants from these habits before malocclusion or skeletal dysplasia's occur.

4. Birth to the eruption of first teeth

Besides the anticipatory guidelines some time conditions are present which require immediate attention these could include developmental anomalies such as

- **Partial ankyglosia (tongue tie)**

Tongue-tie is a condition in which the lingual frenulum is either too short or anteriorly placed limiting the mobility of the tongue.

Early in fetal development, the tongue is attached to the floor of the mouth. With cell death and atrophy, the only attachment is the frenulum. Tongue-tie results when the frenulum is short and this may limit the movement of the tongue. When there is an attempt to stick the tongue out, there may be a V shaped notch at the tip. The incidence is 0.5/1000 Physical exam will easily demonstrate the short or anteriorly placed lingual frenulum.

Years ago it was routine to clip the frenulum at the time of delivery. Midwives had a long sharp nail to cut the frenulum and obstetricians would inspect the mouth and cut the frenulum immediately after the delivery. Tongue-tie is associated with speech abnormalities especially lisping and inability to pronounce certain sounds.

Tongue-tie actually represents partial ankyloglossia and fusion represents complete ankyloglossia. Case reports indicate that squeals of ankyloglossia may include speech defects, difficulty in breastfeeding, or dental problems. However, controlled trials on ankyloglossia have not been appropriately studied, and therefore indications for therapy remain controversial. The tip of the tongue normally grows until 4 years of age, and initial restrictions of movement may improve as the child gets older. Therefore, frenulectomy should not be performed before 4 years of age [4].

MANAGEMENT
1. Physician education
2. Parental education and reassurance
3. Monitor for appropriate weight gain if exclusively breastfeeding
4. Complete fusion requires surgery

- **Paramedian lip pits (congenital lip pits)**

PITS OF THE LOWER lip (fistulas of lower lip, paramedian sinuses of lower lip, humps of lower lip, labial cysts, etc.) is a very rare congenital malformation, first described by Demarquay in 1845. This minimally deforming anomaly is remarkable chiefly for its association with facial clefts. The fact that clefts that occur in families with the lip pits anomaly have a stronger familial tendency than clefts in families without lip pits has attracted the attention of people dealing with cleft patients.

- **Bifid uvula**

A bifid or bifurcated uvula is a split or cleft uvula. Newborns with cleft palate also have a split uvula. The bifid uvula results from the incomplete fusion of the medial nasal and maxillary processes. Bifid uvulas have less muscle in them than a normal uvula, which may cause recurring problems with middle ear infections. While swallowing, the soft palate is pushed backwards, preventing food and drink from entering the nasal cavity. If the soft palate cannot touch the back of the throat while swallowing, food and drink can enter the nasal cavity. Splitting of the uvula occurs infrequently but is the most common form of mouth and nose area cleavage among newborns. Bifid uvula occurs in about 2% of the general population, although some populations may have a high incidence, such as Native Americans who have a 10% rate. Bifid uvula is a common symptom of the rare genetic syndrome Loeys-Dietz syndrome, which is associated with an increased risk of aortic aneurysm.

- **Hyperplastic labial frenum**
- **White Sponge Nevus**

White sponge nevus (WSN), also known as Cannon's disease, hereditary leukokeratosis of mucosa and White sponge nevus of Cannon, is an autosomal dominant skin condition. Although congenital in most cases, it can first occur in childhood or adolescence. It presents in the mouth, most frequently as a thick bilateral white plaque with a spongy texture, usually on the buccal mucosa, but sometimes on the labial mucosa, alveolar ridge or floor of the mouth. The gingival margin and dorsum of the tongue are almost never affected. Although this condition is perfectly benign, it is often mistaken for leukoplakia. There is no treatment, but because there are no serious clinical complications, the prognosis is excellent.

5. Normal teething and conditions associated with eruption of teeth

Teething is the process by which an infant's teeth erupt, or break through, the gums. Teething is also referred to as "cutting" of the teeth. Teething is medically termed odontiasis.

The onset of teething symptoms typically precedes the eruption of a tooth by several days. While a baby's first tooth can present between 4 and 10 months of age, the first tooth usually erupts at approximately 6 months of age. Some dentists have noted a family pattern of "early," "average," or "late" teethers.

A relatively rare condition, "natal" teeth, describes the presence of a tooth on the day of birth [7]. The incidence of such an event is one per 2,000-3,000 live births. Usually, this single and often somewhat malformed tooth is a unique event in an otherwise normal child. Rarely, the presence of a natal tooth is just one of several unusual physical findings which make up a syndrome. If the possibility of a syndrome exists, consultation with a pediatric dentist and/or geneticist can be helpful. The natal tooth is often loose and is commonly removed prior to the newborn's hospital discharge to lessen the risk of aspiration into the lungs.

Teething is generally associated with gum and jaw discomfort as the infant's tooth prepares to erupt through the gum surface. As the tooth moves beneath the surface of the gum tissue, the area may appear slightly red or swollen. Sometimes a fluid-filled area similar to a "blood blister" or eruption hematoma may be seen over the erupting tooth. Some teeth may be more sensitive than others when they erupt. The larger molars may cause more discomfort due to their larger surface area that can't "slice" through the gum tissue as an erupting incisor is capable of doing. With the exception of the eruption of the third molars (wisdom teeth), eruption of permanent teeth rarely cause the discomfort associated with eruption of "baby" (primary or deciduous) teeth.

Teething may cause the following symptoms:

- increased drooling, restless or decreased sleeping due to gum discomfort, refusal of food due to soreness of the gum region, fussiness that comes and goes, bringing hands to the mouth, mild rash around the mouth due to skin irritation secondary to excessive drooling, and rubbing the cheek or ear region as a consequence of referred pain during the eruption of the molars.

Importantly, teething is not associated with the following symptoms: fever (especially over 101 F), diarrhea, runny nose and cough, prolonged fussiness, or rashes over the body.

Sometime minimal intervention may be required during teething in the form of certain over-the-counter medicines can be placed directly on the gums to help relieve pain. They contain medications that temporarily numb the gum tissue. They may help for brief periods of time but have a taste and sensation that many children do not like. It is important not to let the medicine numb the throat because that may interfere with the normal gag reflex and may make it possible for food to enter the lungs. Medicines that are taken by mouth to help reduce the pain.

Acetaminophen (Tylenol) or ibuprofen (Advil or Motrin) can also help with pain. Ibuprofen should not be administered to infants younger than 6 months of age. Medications should be used only for the few times when other home-care methods do not help. Caution should be taken not to overmedicate for teething. The medicine may mask significant symptoms that could be important to know about.

Infant gums often feel better when gentle pressure is placed on the gums. For this reason, gently rubbing of the gums with a clean finger or having the child bite down on a clean washcloth. If the pain seems to be causing feeding problems, sometimes a different shaped nipple or use of a cup may reduce discomfort and improve feeding. Cold objects many help reduce inflammation as well, never put anything in a child's mouth that might enable the child to choke.

6. The primary dentition years

The first primary tooth emerges at around six months of age and by three years root development is complete. This is the preschool years and children are called pre schoolers and they are increasing their cognitive abilities but still in the preconceptual stage and should be considered unsophisticated in thinking. This sophistication only develops during the period of intuitive thought where in the child learns the skills of writing and classification after four years of age and can follow dental instructions given to him.

Another difference observed three years onwards is the development of self control where in these children can distract themselves for example when receiving anesthesia and can be tought to monitor there behavior and they may feel guilty if they are not following the expected norms. In clinical management terms the child is not emotionally mature but surely emotionally complex and will respond to praise and will hurt and respond to aggression and hostility.

6.1 Managing the developing occlusion

Guidance of eruption and development of the primary, mixed, and permanent dentitions is an integral component of comprehensive oral health care for all pediatric dental patients. Such guidance should contribute to the development of a permanent dentition that is in a stable, functional, and esthetically acceptable occlusion. Early diagnosis and successful treatment of developing malocclusions can have both short-term and long term benefits while achieving the goals of occlusal harmony and function and dentofacial esthetics.

Many factors can affect the management of the developing dental arches and minimize the overall success of any treatment. The variables associated with the treatment of the developing dentition that will affect the degree to which treatment is successful include, but are not limited to: chronological/mental/emotional age of the patient andthe patient's ability to understand and cooperate in the treatment; intensity, frequency, and duration of an oral habit; parental support for the treatment; compliance with clinician's instructions; craniofacial configuration; craniofacial growth; concomitant systemic disease or condition; accuracy of diagnosis; appropriateness of treatment.

Anomalies of primary teeth and eruption may not be evident/diagnosable prior to eruption, due to the child's not presenting for dental examination or to a radiographic examination not being possible in a young child. Evaluation, however, should be accomplished when feasible. The objectives of evaluation include identification of: all anomalies of tooth number and size (as previously noted); anterior and posterior crossbites; presence of habits along with their dental and skeletal sequelae.

Oral Habits and posterior crossbites should be diagnosed and addressed as early as feasible[8]. Parents should be informed about findings of adverse growth and developing malocclusions. Interventions/treatment can be recommended if diagnosis can be made, treatment is appropriate and possible, and parentsare supportive and desire to have treatment done.

Oral habits may apply forces to the teeth and dentoalveolar structures. The relationship between oral habits and unfavorable dental and facial development is associational rather than cause and effect. Habits of sufficient frequency, duration, and intensity may be associated with dentoalveolar or skeletal deformations such as increased overjet, reduced overbite, posterior crossbite, or long facial height. As preliminary evidence indicates that some changes resulting from sucking habits persist past the cessation of the habit, it has been suggested that early dental visits provide parents with anticipatory guidance to help their children stop sucking habits by age 36 months or younger.

6.2 Managing developing malocclusion in primary dentition

Anterior and posterior cross bites are malocclusions which involve one or more teeth in which the maxillary teeth occlude lingually with the antagonistic mandibular teeth. Dental crossbites result from the tipping or rotation of a tooth or teeth. The condition is localized and does not involve the basal bone. Skeletal cross bites involve disharmony of the craniofacial skeleton.

A simple anterior cross bite can be aligned as soon as the condition is noted, if there is sufficient space; otherwise, space needs to be created first. Such appliances as acrylic incline planes, acrylic retainers with lingual springs, or fixed appliances all have been effective. If space is needed, an expansion appliance also is required. Early correction of unilateral posterior crossbites has been shown to improve functional conditions significantly and largely eliminate morphological and positional asymmetries of the mandible.

Class II malocclusion (distocclusion) may be unilateral or bilateral and involves a distal relationship of the mandible to the maxilla or the mandibular teeth to maxillary teeth. This relationship may result from dental (malposition of the teeth in the arches), skeletal (mandibular retrusion and/or maxillary protrusion), or a combination of dental and skeletal factors. Early Class II treatment improves self-esteem and decreases negative social experiences. Incisor injury that is more severe than simple enamel fractures has been associated positively with increased overjet and prognathic position of the maxilla. Early treatment for Class II malocclusions can be initiated, depending upon patient cooperation and management this will result in an improved overbite, overjet, and intercuspation of posterior teeth and an esthetic appearance and profile compatible with the patient's skeletal morphology.

Class III malocclusion may be unilateral or bilateral and involves a mesial relationship of the mandible to the maxilla or mandibular teeth to maxillary teeth. This relationship may result from dental factors (malposition of the teeth in the arches), skeletal factors (asymmetry, mandibular prognathism, and/or maxillary retrognathism), or a combination of these factors. Treatment of Class III malocclusions is indicated to provide psychosocial benefits for the child patient by reducing or eliminating facial disfigurement and to reduce the severity of malocclusion by promoting compensating growth. Early Class III treatment in a growing patient will result in improved overbite, overjet, and intercuspation of posterior teeth and an esthetic appearance and profile compatible with the patient's skeletal morphology.

6.3 Local anesthesia for children

Local anesthetic administration is an important consideration in the behavior guidance of a pediatric patient[9]. Age-appropriate "nonthreatening" terminology, distraction, topical anesthetics, proper injection technique, can help the patient have a positive experience during administration of local anesthesia. In pediatric dentistry, the dental professional should be aware of proper dosage (based on weight) to minimize the chance of toxicity and the prolonged duration of anesthesia, which can lead to accidental lip or tongue trauma. Knowledge of the gross and neuroanatomy of the head and neck allows for proper placement of the anesthetic solution and helps minimize complications (eg, hematoma, trismus, intravascular injection). Familiarity with the patient's medical history is essential to decrease the risk of aggravating a medical condition while rendering dental care. Appropriate medical consultation should be obtained when needed.

The application of topical anesthetic may help minimize discomfort caused during administration of local anesthesia. Topical anesthetic is effective on surface tissues (2-3 mm in depth) to reduce painful needle penetration of the oral mucosa A variety of topical anesthetic agents are available in gel, liquid, ointment, patch, and aerosol forms.

Injectable anesthetic available for dental usage include lidocaine, mepivacaine, articaine, prilocaine, and bupivacaine. Absolute contraindications for local anesthetics include a documented local anesthetic allergy. Local anesthetics without vasoconstrictors should be used with caution due to rapid systemic absorption which may result in overdose. Epinephrine decreases bleeding in the area of injection. Epinephrine concentrations of 1:50,000 may be indicated for infiltration in small doses into a surgical site to achieve hemostasis but are not indicated in children to control pain.

6.4 Dental diseases in primary dentition years
6.4.1 Dental caries

Dental caries, also known as tooth decay or a cavity, is a disease where bacterial processes damage hard tooth structure (enamel, dentin, and cementum). These tissues progressively break down, producing dental caries (cavities, holes in the teeth). Two groups of bacteria are responsible for initiating caries: Streptococcus mutans and Lactobacillus. If left untreated, the disease can lead to pain, tooth loss, infection, and, in severe cases, even death. Today, caries remains one of the most common diseases throughout the world. Cariology is the study of dental caries. One particular condition that is seen in this age group is the Early Child hood Caries (ECC). The disease of early childhood caries (ECC) is the presence of 1 or more decayed (noncavitated or cavitated lesions), missing (due to caries), or filled tooth surfaces in any primary tooth in a child 71 months of age or younger. In children younger than 3 years of age, any sign of smooth-surface caries is indicative of severe early childhood caries (S-ECC). From ages 3 through 5, 1 or more cavitated, missing (due to caries), or filled smooth surfaces in primary maxillary anterior teeth or a decayed, missing, or filled score of ≥4 (age 3), ≥5 (age 4), or ≥6 (age 5) surfaces constitutes S-ECC[10].

The recommended method of preventing such a condition include

Reducing the mother's/primary caregiver's/sibling(s) MS levels (ideally during the prenatal period) to decrease transmission of cariogenic bacteria. Minimizing saliva-sharing activities (eg, sharing utensils) between an infant or toddler and his family/cohorts. Implementing oral hygiene measures no later than the time of eruption of the first primary tooth. If an infant falls asleep while feeding, the teeth should be cleaned before placing the child in bed. Tooth brushing of all dentate children should be performed twice daily with a fluoridated toothpaste and a soft, age-appropriate sized toothbrush. Parents should use a 'smear' of toothpaste to brush the teeth of a childless than 2 years of age. For the 2-5 year old, parents should dispense a 'pea-size' amount of toothpaste and perform or assist with their child's tooth brushing. Flossing should be initiated when adjacent tooth surfaces can not be cleansed by a toothbrush. Establishing a dental home within 6 months of eruption of the first tooth and no later than 12 months of age to conduct a caries risk assessment and provide parental education including anticipatory guidance for prevention of oral diseases. Avoiding caries-promoting feeding behaviors. In particular: Infants should not be put to sleep with a bottle containing fermentable carbohydrates. Ad labium breast-feeding should be avoided after the first primary tooth begins to erupt and other dietary carbohydrates are introduced. Parents should be encouraged to have infants drink from a cup as they approach their first birthday. Infants should be weaned from the bottle at 12 to 14 months of age. Repetitive consumption of any liquid containing fermentable carbohydrates from a bottle or no-spill training cup should be avoided. Between-meal snacks and prolonged exposures to foods and juice or other beverages containing fermentable carbohydrates should be avoided.

6.4.2 Behaviour management in dental clinic

Safe and effective treatment of dental diseases often requires modifying the child's behavior. Behavior guidance is a continuum of interaction involving the dentist and dental team, the patient, and the parent directed toward communication and education. Its goal is to ease fear and anxiety while promoting an understanding of the need for good oral health and the process by which that is achieved. For treating children a variety of behavior guidance approaches are used it is important to, assess accurately the child's developmental level, dental attitudes, and temperament and to predict the child's reaction to treatment. The child who presents with oral/dental pathology and noncompliance makes the management more challenging. The pediatric dental staff can play an important role in behavior guidance. Communication may be accomplished by a number of means but, in the dental setting, it is affected primarily through dialogue, tone of voice, facial expression, and body language. One should communicate with the child patient briefly at the beginning of a dental appointment to establish rapport and trust. However, once a procedure begins, the dentist's ability to control and shape behavior becomes paramount, and information sharing becomes secondary[11].

Various behavior management techniques such as Tell-show-do is used by many pediatric professionals. The technique involves verbal explanations of procedures in phrases appropriate to the developmental level of the patient (tell); demonstrations for the patient of the visual, auditory, olfactory, and tactile aspects of the procedure in a carefully defined, nonthreatening setting (show); and then, without deviating from the explanation and demonstration, completion of the procedure (do). The tell-show-do technique is used with communication skills (verbal and nonverbal) and positive reinforcement. Voice control is a controlled alteration of voice volume, tone, or pace to influence and direct the patient's behavior. Parents unfamiliar with this technique may benefit from an explanation prior to its use to prevent misunderstanding. Distraction is another technique involving diverting the patient's attention from what may be perceived as an unpleasant procedure. Giving the patient a short break during a stressful procedure can be an effective use of distraction prior to considering more advanced behavior guidance techniques.

Some children may require a more advanced behavior management techniques using pharmacological agents such as conscious sedation, deep sedation or general anesthesia. Nitrous oxide/oxygen inhalation is a safe and effective technique of giving conscious sedation to reduce anxiety and enhance effective communication. Its onset of action is rapid, the effects easily are titrated and reversible, and recovery is rapid and complete. Additionally, nitrous oxide/oxygen inhalation mediates a variable degree of analgesia, amnesia, and gag reflex reduction.

Some children and developmentally disabled patients require general anesthesia to receive comprehensive dental care in a safe and humane fashion. Many pediatric dentists (and others who treat children) have sought to provide for the administration of general anesthesia by properly-trained individuals in their offices or other facilities (eg, outpatient care clinics) outside of the traditional hospital setting. The Elective Use of Minimal, Moderate, and Deep Sedation and General Anesthesia in Pediatric Dental Patients practiced.

6.4.3 Preventing dental caries

Pit and fissure sealants has been described as a material placed into the pits and fissures of caries-susceptible teeth that micromechanically bonds to the tooth preventing access by cariogenic bacteria to their source of nutrients[12].

Fluoride application

Systemically-administered fluoride supplements

Fluoride supplements should be considered for all children drinking fluoride-deficient (<0.6 ppm) water. After determining the fluoride level of the water supply or supplies (either through contacting public health officials or water analysis), evaluating other dietary sources of fluoride, and assessing the child's caries risk, the daily fluoride supplement dosage can be determined using the Dietary Fluoride Supplementation Schedule.

Professionally-applied topical fluoride treatment

Professional topical fluoride treatments should be based on caries-risk assessment. A pumice prophylaxis is not an essential prerequisite to this treatment. Appropriate precautionary measures should be taken to prevent swallowing of any professionally-applied topical fluoride. Children at moderate caries risk should receive a professional fluoride treatment at least every 6 months; those with high caries risk should receive greater frequency of professional fluoride applications (ie, every 3-6 months). Ideally, this would occur as part of a comprehensive preventive program in a dental home.

Fluoride-containing products for home use

Therapeutic use of fluoride for children should focus on regimens that maximize topical contact, preferably in lower-dose, higher-frequency approaches. Fluoridated toothpaste should be used twice daily as a primary preventive procedure. Twice daily use has benefits greater than once daily brushing.

Additional at-home topical fluoride regimens utilizing increased concentrations of fluoride should be considered for children at high risk for caries.These may include overthe-counter or prescription strength formulations. Fluoride mouth rinses or brush-on gels may be incorporated into a caries-prevention program for a school-aged child at high risk.

6.4.4 Management of dental caries

Restorative treatment is based upon the results of an appropriate clinical examination and is ideally part of a comprehensive treatment plan. The treatment plan should take into consideration: developmental status of the dentition; caries-risk assessment, patient's oral hygiene, anticipated parental compliance and likelihood of timely recall,patient's ability to cooperate for treatment. The restorative treatment plan must be prepared in conjunction with an individually-tailored preventive program. Caries risk is greater for children who are poor, rural, or minority or who have limited access to care. Factors for high caries risk include decayed/missing/filled surfaces greater than the child's age, numerous white spot lesions, high levels of mutans streptococci, low socioeconomic status, high caries rate in siblings/parents, diet high in sugar, and/or presence of dental appliances. Studies have reported that maxillary primary anterior caries has a direct relationship with caries in primary molars, and caries in the primary dentition is highly predictive of caries occurring in the permanent dentition.

6.5 Pulp therapy for primary teeth

The primary objective of pulp therapy is to maintain the integrity and health of the teeth and their supporting tissues. It is a treatment objective to maintain the vitality of the pulp of a tooth affected by caries, traumatic injury, or other causes.

Vital pulp therapy for primary teeth diagnosed with a normal pulp or reversible pulpitis includes placement of a protective liner wich is a thinly-applied liquid placed on the pulpal surface of a deep cavity preparation, covering exposed dentin tubules, to act as a protective barrier between the restorative material or cement and the pulp. Placement of a thin protective liner such as calcium hydroxide, dentin bonding agent, or glass ionomer cement is at the discretion of the clinician. This placement in the deep area of the preparation is utilized to preserve the tooth's vitality, promote pulp tissue healing and tertiary dentin formation, and minimize bacterial microleakage.Adverse post-treatment clinical signs or symptoms such as sensitivity, pain, or swelling should not occur.

Indirect pulp treatment is a procedure performed in a tooth with a deep carious lesion approximating the pulp but without signs or symptoms of pulp degeneration. The caries surrounding the pulp is left in place to avoid pulp exposure and is covered with a biocompatible material. A radiopaque liner such as a dentin bonding agent, resin modified glass ionomer,calcium hydroxide, zinc oxide/eugenol,or glass ionomer cement is placed over the remaining carious dentin to stimulate healing and repair. Indirect pulp capping has been shown to have a higher success rate than pulpotomy in long term studies.It also allows for a normal exfoliation time. Therefore, indirect pulp treatment is preferable to a pulpotomy when the pulp is normal or has a diagnosis of reversible pulpitis.

Direct pulp cap can be done When a pinpoint mechanical exposure of the pulp is encountered during cavity preparation or following a traumatic injury, a biocompatible radiopaque base such as mineral trioxide aggregate (MTA)or calcium hydroxidemay be placed in contact with the exposed pulp tissue. The tooth is restored with a material that seals the tooth from microleakage.

A pulpotomy is performed in a primary tooth with extensive caries but without evidence of radicular pathology when caries removal results in a carious or mechanical pulp exposure. Thecoronal pulp is amputated, and the remaining vital radicularpulp tissue surface is treated with a long-term clinically successful medicament such as Buckley's Solution of formocresol or ferric sulfate. Electrosurgery also has demonstrated success. Gluteraldehyde and calcium hydroxide have been used but with less long-term success. MTA is a more recent material used for pulpotomies with a high rate of success.

Nonvital pulp treatment for primary teeth diagnosed with irreversible pulpitis or necrotic pulp include Pulpectomy Pulpectomy is a root canal procedure for pulp tissue that is irreversibly infected or necrotic due to caries or trauma. The root canals are debrided and shaped with hand or rotary files. Followed by obturation bye resorbable material such as nonreinforced zinc/oxideeugenol, iodoform-based paste (KRI), or a combination paste of iodoform and calcium hydroxide. The tooth then is restored with a restoration that seals the tooth from microleakage.

6.5.1 Expected outcome of pulp therapy

No post-treatment signs or symptoms such as sensitivity, pain, or swelling should be evident. There should be no radiographic evidence of pathologic external or internal root resorption or other pathologic changes. There should be no harm to the succedaneous tooth. A smooth transition from primary to permanent dentition should be afforded[13].

6.5.2 Acute dental trauma to primary teeth and management

The greatest incidence of trauma to the primary teeth occurs at 2 to 3 years of age, when motor coordination is developing. Dental injuries can have improved outcomes if the public is made aware of first-aid measures and the need to seek immediate treatment. Because optimal treatment results follow immediate assessment and care, dentists have an ethical obligation to ensure that reasonable arrangements for emergency dental care are available. The history, circumstances of the injury, pattern of trauma, and behavior of the child and/or caregiver are important in distinguishing nonabusive injuries from abuse.

After a primary tooth has been injured, the treatment strategy is dictated by the concern for the safety of the permanent dentition. If determined that the displaced primary tooth has encroached upon the developing permanent tooth germ, removal is indicated. In the primary dentition, the maxillary anterior region is at low risk for space loss unless the avulsion occurs prior to canine eruption or the dentition is crowded. Fixed or removable appliances, while not always necessary, can be fabricated to satisfy parental concerns for esthetics or to return a loss of oral or phonetic function.

When an injury to a primary tooth occurs, informing parents about possible pulpal complications, appearance of a vestibular sinus tract, or color change of the crown associated with a sinus tract can help assure timely intervention, minimizing complications for the developing succedaneous teeth. Also, it is important to caution parents that the primary tooth's displacement may result in any of several permanent tooth complications, including enamel hypoplasia, hypo calcification, crown/root dilacerations, or disruptions in eruption patterns or sequence. The risk of trauma-induced developmental disturbances in the permanent successors is greater in children whose enamel calcification is incomplete.

6.5.3 Managing premature loss of primary tooth

The premature loss of primary teeth due to caries, trauma, ectopic eruption, or other causes may lead to undesirable tooth movements of primary and/or permanent teeth including loss of arch length. Arch length deficiency can produce or increase the severity of malocclusions with crowding, rotations, ectopic eruption, crossbite, excessive overjet, excessive overbite, and unfavorable molar relationships. It is recommended that space maintainers be used to reduce the prevalence and severity of malocclusion following premature loss of primary teeth. Space maintenance may be a consideration in the primary dentition after early loss of a maxillary incisor when the child has an active digit habit. An intense habit may reduce the space for the erupting permanent incisor.

7. The transition from primary dentition to permanent dentition

This period is characterized by having distinctive need due to: a potentially high caries rate; increased risk for traumatic injury and periodontal disease; a tendency for poor nutritional habits; an increased esthetic desire and awareness; complexity of combined orthodontic and restorative care (eg, congenitally missing teeth); dental phobia; potential use of tobacco, alcohol, and other drugs; (8) pregnancy; (9) eating disorders; and (10) unique social and psychological needs.

The management of these patients can be multifaceted and complex. An accurate, comprehensive, and up-to-date medical history is necessary for correct diagnosis and effective treatment planning. Familiarity with the patient's medical history is essential to decreasing the risk of aggravating a medical condition while rendering dental care. If the parent is unable to provide adequate details regarding a patient's medical history, consultation with the medical health care provider may be indicated. The practitioner also may need to obtain additional information confidentially from an adolescent patient.

7.1 Management of dental caries during mixed dentition period

Immature permanent tooth enamel,a total increase in susceptible tooth surfaces, and environmental factors such as diet, independence to seek care or avoid it, a low priority for oral hygiene, and additional social factors also may contribute to the upward slope of caries during this period. It is important to emphasize the positive effects that fluoridation, routine professional care, patient education, and personal hygiene can have in counteracting the changing pattern of caries this population.

Fluoridation has proven to be the most economical and effective caries prevention measure. Both systemic benefit of fluoride incorporation into developing enamel and, topical benefits can be obtained through optimally-fluoridated water, professionally-applied and prescribed compounds, and fluoridated dentifrices.

Oral Hygine with a fluoridated dentifrice and flossing can provide benefit through the topical effect of the fluoride and plaque removal from tooth surfaces.This time of heightened caries activity and periodontal disease due to an increased intake of cariogenic substances and inattention to oral hygiene procedures warrant a good oral hygiene through daily plaque removal, including flossing, with the frequency and pattern based on the individual's disease pattern and oral hygiene needs

Diet management including diet analysis and modification can be very helpful to reduce the effect of carbohydrates, foods rich in sucrose and beverages with acidic Ph. A diet analysis should result in overall nutrient and energy needs calculation, psychosocial aspects of adolescent nutrition; dietary carbohydrate intake and frequency; intake and frequency of acid-containing beverages and wellness considerations.

Sealant placement is an effective caries-preventive technique that should be considered on an individual basis. Sealants have been recommended for any tooth, primary or permanent, that is judged to be at risk for pit and fissure caries. Caries risk may increase due to changes in patient habits, oral microflora, or physical condition, and unsealed teeth subsequently might benefit from sealant applications. Children at risk for caries should have sealants placed. An individual's caries risk may change over time; periodic reassessment for sealant need is indicated throughout this phase.

8. Restorative dentistry

In cases where remineralization of noncavitated, demineralized tooth surfaces is not successful, as demonstrated by progression of carious lesions, dental restorations are necessary. Preservation of tooth structure, esthetics, and each individual patient's needs must be considered when selecting a restorative material. Molars with extensive caries or malformed, hypoplastic enamel—for which traditional amalgam or composite resin restorations are not feasible—may require full coverage restorations. Each restoration must be evaluated on an individual basis. Preservation of noncarious tooth structure is desirable.

8.1 Periodontal disease

Gingivitis characterized by the presence of gingival inflammation without detectable loss of bone or clinical attachment is common in children. Normal and abnormal fluctuation in hormone levels, including changes in gonadotrophic hormone levels during the onset of puberty, can modify the gingival inflammatory response to dental plaque. Similarly, alterations in insulin levels in patients with diabetes can affect gingival health. In both situations, there is an increased inflammatory response to plaque. However, the gingival condition usually responds to thorough removal of bacterial deposits and improved daily oral hygiene.

Periodontitis aggressive periodontitis is more common in children and adolescents. Aggressive periodontitis can be localized or generalized. Localized aggressive periodontitis (LAgP) patients have interproximal attachment loss on at least two permanent first molars and incisors, with attachment loss on no more than two teeth other than first molars and incisors. Generalized aggressive periodontitis (GAgP) patients exhibit generalized interproximal attachment loss including at least three teeth that are not first molars and incisors. Successful treatment of aggressive periodontitis depends on early diagnosis, directing therapy against the infecting microorganisms and providing an environment for healing that is free of infection. a combination of surgical or non-surgical root debridement in conjunction with antimicrobial (antibiotic) therapy.

Necrotizing periodontal diseases The two most significant findings used in the diagnosis of NPD are the presence of interproximal necrosis and ulceration and the rapid onset of gingival pain. Patients with NPD can often be febrile. Necrotizing ulcerative gingivitis/periodontitis sites harbor high levels of spirochetes and P. intermedia, and invasion of the tissues by spirochetes has been shown to occur. Factors that predispose children to NPD include viral infections (including HIV), malnutrition, emotional stress, lack of sleep, and a variety of systemic diseases. Treatment involves mechanical debridement, oral hygiene instruction, and careful follow-up.Debridement with ultrasonics has been shown to be particularly effective and results in a rapid decrease in symptoms. If the patient is febrile, antibiotics may be an important adjunct to therapy. Metronidazole and penicillin have been suggested as drugs of choice.

8.2 Occlusal considerations

Malocclusion can be a significant treatment need in the transition period as both environmental and genetic factors come into play. Although the genetic basis of much malocclusion makes it unpreventable, numerous methods exist to treat the occlusal disharmonies, temporomandibular joint dysfunction, periodontal disease, and disfiguration which may be associated with malocclusion. Temporomandibular disorders require special attention to avoid long-termproblems. Congenitally missing teeth present complex problem and often require combined orthodontic and restorative care for satisfactory resolution.

Positional Malocclusion problems that present significant esthetic, functional, physiologic, or emotional dysfunction are potential difficulties in mixed dentition. These can include single or multiple tooth malpositions, tooth/jaw size discrepancies, and craniofacial disfigurements. Treatment of malocclusion should be based on professional diagnosis, available treatment options, patient motivation and readiness, and other factors to maximize progress. If need be an orthodontist should be included for treatment.

Congenitally missing permanent teeth can have a major impact on the developing dentition. When treating patients with congenitally missing teeth, many factors must be taken into consideration including, but not limited to, esthetics, patient age, and growth potential, as well as periodontal and oral surgical needs. Evaluation of congenitally missing permanent teeth should include both immediate and long-term management.

Abnormal or ectopic eruption patterns of the permanent teeth can contribute to root resorption, bone loss, gingival defects, space loss, and esthetic concerns. Early diagnosis and treatment of ectopically erupting teeth can result in a healthier and more esthetic dentition. Prevention and treatment may include extraction of deciduous teeth, surgical intervention, and/or endodontic, orthodontic, periodontal, and/or restorative care.

8.3 Traumatic injuries

The most common injuries to permanent teeth occur secondary to falls, followed by traffic accidents, violence, and sports. All sporting activities have an associated risk of orofacial injuries due to falls, collisions, and contact with hard surfaces. It has been demonstrated that dental and facial injuries can be reduced significantly by introducing mandatory protective equipment such as face guards and mouthguards. Additionally, participation in leisure activities such as skateboarding, rollerskating, and bicycling also benefit from appropriate protective equipment.

To efficiently determine the extent of injury and correctly diagnose injuries to the teeth, periodontium, and associated structures, a systematic approach to the traumatized child is essential. Assessment includes a thoroughmedical and dental history, clinical and radiographic examination, and additional tests such as palpation, percussion, sensitivity, and mobility evaluation. Intraoral radiography is useful for the evaluation of dentoalveolar trauma. If the area of concern extends beyond the dentoalveolar complex, extra oral imaging may be indicated. Treatment planning takes into consideration the patient's health status and developmental status, as well as extent of injuries. Advanced behavior guidance techniques or an appropriate referral may be necessary to ensure that proper diagnosis and care are given.

Management of traumatized tooth can vary from simple restoration or re attachment of a broken fragment in a tooth that does not involve pulp to advanced pulpal and periodontal management where these are involved.The objective of such management should be to maintain pulp vitality and restore normal esthetics and function.

Avulsion is the complete displacement of tooth out of socket. The periodontal ligament is severed and fracture of the alveolus may occur. The avulsed tooth should be replanted as soon as possible and then stabilized in its anatomically correct location to optimize healing of the periodontal ligament and neurovascular supply while maintaining esthetic and functional integrity. The tooth has the best prognosis if replanted immediately. If the tooth cannot be replanted within 5 minutes, it should be stored in a medium that will help maintain vitality of the periodontal ligament fibers. The best (ie, physiologic) transportation media for avulsed teeth include (in order of preference) Viaspan™, Hank's Balanced Salt Solution (tissue culture medium), and cold milk. Next best would be a non-physiologic medium such as saliva (buccal vestibule), physiologic saline, or water.

9. References

[1] American Dental Association Commission on Dental Accreditation. Accreditation standards for advanced specialty education programs in pediatric dentistry. Chicago, Ill; 2000

[2] Kim A. Boggess and Burton L. Edelstein. Oral Health in Women During Preconception and Pregnancy: Implications for Birth Outcomes and Infant Oral Health. Matern Child Health J. 2006 September; 10(Suppl 1): 169–174.

[3] Increased prevalence of developmental dental defects in low birth-weight, prematurely born children: a controlled study. W. Kim Seow, BDS, MDSc, FRACDS Carolyn Humphrys, BDSc David I. Tudehope, MBBS, FRACP. The American Academy of Pediatric Dentistry Volume 9 Number 3

[4] Levy, Paul Tongue-tie, Management of Short SubLingual Frenulum. Pediatrics in Review September 1995

[5] Shu, M.D., Jennifer (April 12, 2010). "Will a bifid uvula cause any problems?". CNN. Retrieved 2010-08-07

[6] Terrinoni A, Rugg EL, Lane EB, et al (Mar 2001). "A novel mutation in the keratin 13 gene causing oral white sponge nevus". J. Dent. Res. 80 (3): 919–923.

[7] Natal and neonatal teeth: a review.Adekoya-Sofowora CA.Niger Postgrad Med J. 2008 Mar;15(1):38-41

[8] Guideline on Management of the Developing Dentition and Occlusion in Pediatric Dentistry. Originating Committee Clinical Affairs Committee – Developing Dentition Subcommittee Review Council Council on Clinical Affairs Adopted 1990Revised 1991, 1998, 2001, 2005, 2009

[9] Malamed SF. Basic injection technique in local anesthesia. In: Handbook of Local Anesthesia. 5th ed. St. Louis, Mo: Mosby; 2004:159-69.

[10] Definition of Early Childhood Caries (ECC) Originating council on clinical affairs Review Adopted2003 AAPD Revised 2007, 2008

[11] American Academy of Pediatric Dentistry. Policy on interim therapeutic restorations. Pediatric Dent 2009;31 (special issue):38-9.

[12] Simonsen RJ. Chapter 2: Pit and fissure sealants. In: Clinical Applications of the Acid Etch Technique. 1st ed.Chicago, IL:Quint essence Publishing Co , Inc ;1978:19-42

[13] Guideline on Pulp Therapy for Primary and Immature Permanent Teeth, AAPD REFERENCE MANUAL V 3 3 /NO 611/12

Oral Health Care in Children – A Preventive Perspective

Agim Begzati[1], Kastriot Meqa[2], Mehmedali Azemi[3], Ajtene Begzati[1],
Teuta Kutllovci[1], Blerta Xhemajli[1] and Merita Berisha[4]

[1]*Department of Pedodontics and Preventive Dentistry, School of Dentistry,*
Medical Faculty, University of Prishtna, Prishtina,
[2]*Department of Periodontology and Oral Medicine, School of Dentistry,*
Medical Faculty,University of Prishtina, Prishtina,
[3]*Department of Paediatric, Medical Faculty, University of Prishtina, Prishtina,*
[4]*National Institute of Public Health of Kosovo, Department of Social Medicine,*
Medical Faculty, University of Prishtina, Prishtina
Republic of Kosovo

1. Introduction

Health has been described by the World Health Organization (WHO) as follows:"health comprise complete physical and social well-being and is not merely the absence of disease" (World Health Organization 1946).

According to World Health Organization, oral health is the overall health of teeth and tooth-supporting tissues, and oral soft tissues, with the aim of fulfilling physiological functioning of the masticatory organ for chewing, phonation and esthetics. The US the Department of Health defined the health as oral "standard of health of the oral and related tissues which enables an individual to eat, speak and socialize without active disease, discomfort or embarrassment and which contributes to general well-being" (US Department of Health, 2000). Oral health is integral to general health and should not be considered in isolation. Oral disease has detrimental effects on an individual's physical and psychological well-being and it reduces quality of life.

Oral health is not only important to person's appearance and sense of well-being, but also to person's overall health. Dental caries is the most common cause of the disturbances of normal functions in the oral cavity, respectively it is a lack of preventive and curative measures.

Gingivitis represents another serious problem for oral health. Data have shown a high prevalence of gingivitis among children. Gum disease is an inflammation of the gums, which may also affect the bone supporting the teeth, and may be followed with periodontitis. The role of dental plaque, respectively of the periopathogenic bacteria, has been considered as the most important factor in occurrence of caries and gum diseases. Plaque is a sticky colorless film of bacteria (biofilm) that constantly builds up, thickens and hardens on the teeth. If it is not removed by daily brushing and flossing, this plaque may harden into tartar and may contribute to inflammation and infections in the gums. Plaque is an important prerequisite in aethiology of caries because acid is generated within its substance to such an extent that enamel may be demineralised. Dietary sugars diffuse rapidly through plaque where they are converted to acids by bacterial metabolism. Mutans streptococci are now considered to be the major cariogenic bacteria species involved in the caries process. (Soames & Southam 1999; Norman & Franklin 1999).

Oral diseases may contribute in many serious conditions, such as heart disease and stroke, pneumonia and other respiratory diseases, diabetes. Untreated cavities can also be painful and lead to serious infections. Currently, studies have been examining whether there is a link between poor oral health and heart disease and between poor oral health and women delivering pre-term, low birth rate babies.

Caries and tooth supporting structures' diseases (gingivitis and periodontitis), as the most spreading diseases worldwide, do not disturb only the dental and oral functions, but due to the complications and consequences of non-prevention or lack of treatment they may seriously endanger the systemic health and influence directly the living quality. Thus these diseases should be characterized not only as medical, but also as social problem. These diseases have been studied and discussed also by the public health fields, such as: Dental public health, Oral public health, Community public health, etc.

Dental public health has been described by the American Board of Dental Health as the science and art of preventing and controlling dental disease and promoting dental health through organized community efforts (Winslow 1920).

The terms public health and community health are used synonymously, and both refer to the "effort that is organized by society to protect, promote and restore the health and quality of life of people" (Block 2003).

Since dental caries, as well as gingivitis and periodontitis, both have a high prevalence and etiological factor – the bacterial plaque, this chapter will be based on the explanation of the prevalence, ethiopathogenesis of the bacterial plaque and the role of the bacteria, favorizing factors for plaque accumulation (oral hygiene and feeding habits), and finally the role of the preventive measures from the educational perspective.

The explanation of these objectives will be done through scientific examinations conducted from the subjects regarding the dental caries in general and early childhood caries in particular, as well as through oral health promotion in children and mothers.

2. Dental caries

2.1 Definition, etiology and risk factors

Dental caries may be defined as a bacterial disease of the hard tissues of the teeth characterized by demineralization of the inorganic and destruction of the organic substance of tooth (Soames & Southam 1999).

Dental caries is one of the most prevalent diseases in children worldwide. The Centers for Disease Control and Prevention reports that dental caries is perhaps the most prevalent infectious diseases in children. Dental caries is five times more common than asthma and seven times more common than hay fever in children (US Department of Health and Human Services 2000).

Dental caries is a disease that affects all age groups, most commonly children.

The general opinion regarding the etiology of dental caries nowadays is that it is a very complex multifactorial disease, presented with high prevalence in all age groups. It has already been established that dental caries is a chronic infectious process with a multifactorial etiology. Dietary factors, oral microorganisms that can produce acids from sugars, and host susceptibility all need to coexist for caries to develop (Konig & Navia 1995).

Analyzing the etiology, prevalence, clinical specifics, consequences and complications, dental caries is estimated as a serious disease, which represents not only as a health problem, but also a great serious social and economic problem. Many studies, clinical, but mostly longitudinal epidemiological studies, have offered convincing facts on the multifactorial nature of this disease. The multitude of factors that influence in the dental caries occurrence, having in mind that they act together, not separately, contribute in the complexity of the pathogenesis of caries, making it more difficult to undertake efficient preventive measures.

There are some important factors that comprise the etiological circles of the dental caries: host or the tooth, dental or bacterial plaque, substrate – carbohydrates and saliva, and altogether co-react with the time factor. These circles are the *circulus viciosus* of the dental caries development. The hard dental structures, initially the enamel, undergo the demineralization process, respectively the caries. The caries development in the enamel surface is equally dependent from the inner hard dental structure and from the intensity of the extrinsic factors' action.

Newest concept in the field of dentistry gives an explanation how dental caries is caused as a result of the disturbance of the "Caries Balance" (Featherstone 2004). This misbalance may be manifested in the beginning of demineralization or during the process of remineralization. The theory of "Caries Balance" defines dental caries as a disease of hard dental tissues, and the destruction of the enamel surface as a result of the disruption of the balance of demineralization and remineralization. The defect in the enamel surface is a result of the domination of the demineralization process and such process has progressive course directed towards pulpar space. Which process will dominate depends on the proportions of the factors that constitute "Caries Balance", i.e. protetctive and pathological factors.

Pathological factors that include:
1. cariogenic bacteria,
2. frequent ingestion of fermentable carbohydrates, and
3. salivary dysfunction drive the caries process towards demineralization.

Protective factors that include:
1. salivary components,
2. fluoride and remineralization, and
3. antibacterial therapy drive the caries process towards remineralization.

Effective caries managment revolves around these principles.

In order to control dental caries, i.e. to prevent its occurrence or to start the remineralization process during initial stage, it is necessary that the proportions of these factors be kept in the direction of the protective factors. The level of risk for dental caries depends on the domination of the certain group of factors that participate in the "Caries Balance". If there is a domination of the pathological factors, the risk for dental caries will be higher and the treatment needs will require larger restorative interventions, as well as other consequences. If there is a domination of protective factors, then the invasive restorative dentistry will have fewer burdens, and concentrate in minimal restorations of superficial caries. Biological factors tend to be similar within all cultures and populations, although habit/environmental factors tend to be influenced specifically by the culture in place.

2.2 The epidemiology of dental caries

It has already been mentioned that dental caries is the mostly spread disease in the world. In a study carried out in Kosovo we have assessed the prevalence of dental caries in comparison with other countries. The data from this oral health assessment of children of Kosovo showed a very high caries experience in both the primary and permanent dentitions. Caries prevalence expressed via the DMFT index was very high. Epidemiological data (years 2002-2005) derived from our study showed a high prevalence of dental caries among children in Kosovo (89.2% among preschool children and 94.4% among school children). The mean dmft/DMFT index was 5.86 for preschool children (ages 2 to 6) and 4.86 for all school children (ages 7 to 14) (Begzati et al. 2011).

The results from the same previous study show that dental health of these children in Kosovo is worse than that of children in other European countries. Specifically, the mean dmft of five-year-olds at preschools in Kosovo (8.1) was found to be higher than the same value of preschool children in USA (1.7) and in many other European countries (1991-1995), including Ireland (0.9), Spain (1.0), Denmark (1.3), Norway (1.4), Finland (1.4), Netherlands (1.7), United Kingdom (2.0), France (2.5), and Germany (2.5). Our results are only comparable to the rates in Belarus (7.4), Sarajevo, Bosnia (7.53) (ages 5-7) and Albania (8.5), (Marthaler 1995; Kobaslia 2000). The low treatment rate of children in Kosovo (<2%) indicates a high treatment need. Also, the mean DMFT (5.8) of school children in Kosovo (age 12) was higher in comparison with school children (age 12) of the following developed countries: Netherlands (1.1), Finland (1.2), Denmark (1.3), USA (1.4), United Kingdom (1.4), Sweden (1.5), Norway (2.1), Ireland (2.1), Germany (2.6) and Croatia (2.6) (16). The mean DMFT of Kosovo's children (age 12) was similar to the mean values in Latvia (7.7), Poland (5.1) and a group of 12- to 14-year-olds in Sarajevo, Bosnia (7.18) (Marthaler 1995; Kobaslia 2000). As it was previously mentioned, the low treatment rate of the children in Kosovo is unfavorable and indicates a high treatment need.

2.3 Oral health assessment in school and preschool children – Epidemiological study

In order to assess the oral health of preschool and school children, the dental examination was carried out (Begzati et al. 2011). The sample in this study consisted of two groups derived from a multi-site examination: preschool and school children. From a total of 3,793 examined children, there were 1,237 preschool children (aged 2 to 6 years old) and 2,556 school children (aged 7 to 14 years old). This was a cross-sectional study conducted in randomly selected locations in Kosovo. The sample size was calculated with a confidence level of 95% and a confidence interval of 2.

The study was specifically based on the dmft/DMFT index, following the recommendations of the World Health Organization (WHO Oral Health Surveys 1997).

Preschool children were examined at various kindergartens in different locations of Kosovo. The examinations were done under natural light, using a dental mirror and a probe. It was performed by five dentists from the Prishtina University Dental Clinics, mainly from the Preventive Dentistry Department. The Study Group for Oral Health Promotion conducted the study, and the examiners received relevant training in advance. Diagnostic criteria were calibrated (Hunt 1986), with an inter-examiner reliability of kappa = 0.92 based on the examination of 30 children of different ages. For the caries assessments, all tooth surfaces were examined. Every defect in the tooth was tested with a probe, and every visual change in the enamel transparency in the early phases of demineralization was defined as a carious lesion. Decayed, filled and extracted/missing (due to caries) teeth were recorded in a modified WHO Oral Health Assessment Form.

DMFT (for permanent dentition) and dmft (for primary dentition) describe the number, or the prevalence, of caries in an individual. DMFT and dmft are methods to numerically express the caries experience and are obtained by calculating the number of decayed (D), missing (M), and filled (F) teeth (T).

2.3.1 The prevalence of caries of preschool children

In the sample, 28.6% of the children were with no observable clinical signs of caries (dmft =0) at the age of two. As expected, this percentage decreased with increasing age. Only 2.1% of six-year-old children were caries-free. The mean dmft in preschool children was 5.6. The lowest mean dmft was seen in two-year-old children (2.1), while the highest were in five- and six-year-olds (8.1 and 7.9, respectively). (Fig. 1)

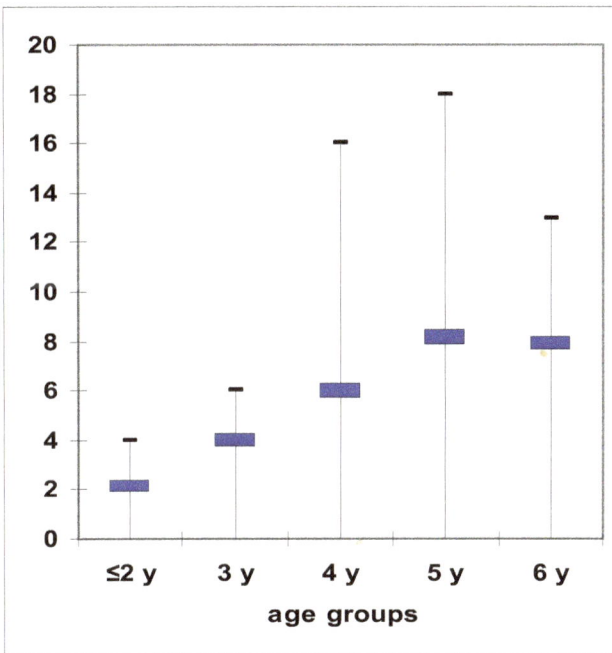

Fig. 1. Mean dmft of preschool children by age groups

As expected, the mean dmft among preschool children increased with age, with significant statistical differences between adjacent age groups (two-year-olds vs. three-year-olds, three-year-olds vs. four-year-olds, and four-year-olds vs. – $p<0.001$), except between five-year-olds and six-year-olds ($p>0.5$). An ANOVA test showed statistical differences between all of the age groups ($F=204.59$, $p<0.001$).

The greatest contribution to the dmft index was untreated caries, which varied from 2.04 for two-year-olds to 6.37 for five-year-olds. A slight decrease was showed among six-year-old children. Six-year-old children showed a slight decrease (6.09) (Fig. 1).

2.3.2 Caries prevalence of school children

The percentage of children with DMFT=0 at the age of six was 13.3%, and as expected, this decreased with age. At 14 years old, only 0.9% were with no observable clinical signs of caries. The mean DMFT index was 4.86 for all school children. The increase in the mean DMFT was related to age, increasing from 2.36 for 7-year-olds to 6.91 for 14-year-olds. There was no significant difference between the genders for any age group.

The mean DMFT of school children increased with age, with a statistically significant difference between the age groups tested with ANOVA (F=290.83, p<0.001).

The differences between adjacent age groups showed a difference for 7-year-olds vs. 8-year-olds, 9-year-olds vs. 10-year-olds, 10-year-olds vs. 11-year-olds, 11-year-olds vs. 12-year-olds, and 12-year-olds vs. 13-year-olds (p<0.0001). There was no difference for 8-year-olds vs. 9-year-olds (p>0.05) or 13-year-olds vs. 14-year-olds (p>0.05).

The greatest contribution to the DMFT index was untreated caries, which varied from 2.10 for 7-year-olds to 5.00 for 14-year-olds (Figure 2).

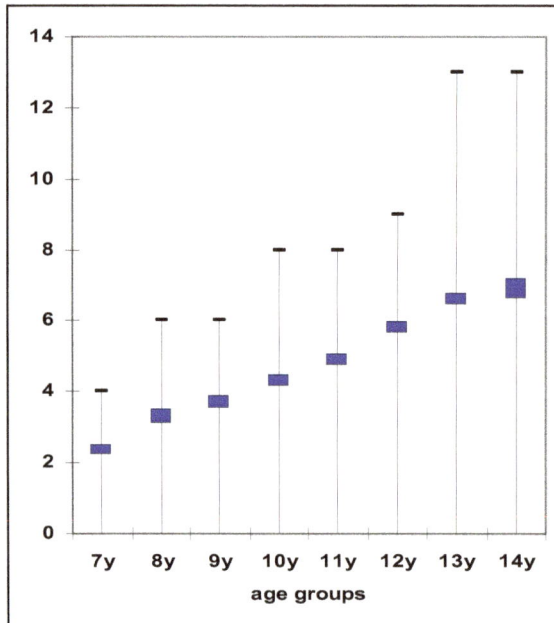

Fig. 2. Mean DMFT of school children by age groups

3. Early childhood caries

3.1 Definition of Early childhood caries (ECC)

The oral health of children is especially aggravated with the occurrence of the so-called early childhood caries. During the promotion of oral public health in urban kindergartens, the presence of extensive dental disease at children, known as early childhood caries (ECC), was recorded. ECC is an acute, rapidly developing dental disease occurring initially in the cervical third of the maxillary incisors, destroying the crown completely. Early onset and rampant clinical progression makes ECC a serious public health problem. Due to varying clinical, etiological, localization, and course features, this pathology is found under different names such as labial caries (LC), caries of incisors, nursing bottle mouth, rampant caries (RC), nursing bottle caries (NBC), nursing caries, baby bottle tooth decay (BBTD), early childhood caries (ECC), rampant infant and early childhood dental decay, and severe early childhood caries (SECC) (James 1957; Goose 1967; Fass 1962; Winter et al.1966; Derkson & Ponti 1982; Ripa 1988; Arkin 1986; Bruered et al. 1989; Kaste & Gift 1995; Tinanoff et al. 1998; Horowitz 1998; Drury et al. 1999).

According to Davis, the definition of this pathology has always been complex and "difficult to be described, but when it is seen, you know what it's about" (Davis 1998). Up to now there have been many proposals for definition and diagnostic criteria, described in detail by Ismail & Sohn 1999.

The preferred and most commonly used term today is early childhood caries (ECC), proposed by the Centers for Disease Control and Prevention (CDC) (Kaste et al. 1996).

Numerous biological, psychosocial, and behavioral risk factors are involved in the etiology of ECC, supporting the multifactorial character of the disease (Wyne 1999; Seow 1998). Based on this concept, dental caries can be defined as demineralization of tooth tissue consequent to a dental infection that is dependent on frequent exposure to fermentable carbohydrates and is influenced by saliva and fluoride and other trace elements (Drury et al. 1999). Dietary habits are also deeply implicated in the development of ECC, despite the fact that it is considered an infectious disease (Lopez 2000). Consumption of sweets with high concentrations of glucose, saccharine, or fructose, especially if taken in processed juices (Newbrun 1982), and their prolonged intake play an important role in caries development in children with ECC (Wendt 1991).

To evaluate the prevalence of ECC and various caries risk factors such as quantity of cariogenic *Streptococcus mutans* colonies, oral hygiene, sweets preference, bottle feeding in preschool children, and fluoride use, we have conducted a study at our preschool children (Begzati et al. 2010).

In this study we have included 1,008 children of both sexes, from 1 to 6 years of age, from 9 kindergartens of Prishtina, capital of Kosovo. The sample was random, representing 80% of all kindergarten children. The sample size was calculated with a confidence level of 95% and a confidence interval of 2.

3.2 Dental examination and diagnostic criteria of ECC

ECC was defined as "initial occurrence of caries in cervical region of at least two maxillary incisors." Using a careful lift-the-lip examination, the presence or absence of ECC was recorded depending on the presence of "noncavity caries/white spot lesions" or "cavity caries." With the aim of studying the clinical and etiological aspects of ECC, a sub-sample of children with ECC was included for further analysis. The latter part of the examination, which included the clinical study of ECC development (according to ECC stages), determination of bacterial colony sampling, oral hygiene index (OHI), and filling out of the questionnaire, was conducted in the Pediatric Dentistry Clinic of the School of Dentistry.

Children with ECC were examined using the light of the dental unit, with dental mirror and probe. All examinations were carried out by Prof Begzati, with intra-examiner reliability of kappa = 0.95 based on the examination of 15 children of different ages.

3.2.1 ECC prevalence

The prevalence of ECC varies in different countries, which may depend on the diagnostic criteria. While in some developed countries having advanced programs for oral health protection, the prevalence of ECC is around 5% (Derkson & Ponti 1982; Ripa 1988; Kaste et al. 1996; Davenport 1990; Hinds & Gregory 1995). In some countries of Southeastern Europe (Kosovo's neighbors), this prevalence reaches 20% (Bosnia) and 14% (Macedonia) (Huseinbegović 2001, Apostolova et al. 2003). Much higher ECC prevalence has been reported for such places as Quchan, Iran (59%) (Mazhari et al. 2007) and Alaska (66.8%) (Kelly & Bruerd 1987). At American Indian children the prevalence is 41.8% [23]. Similarly, in North American populations, the prevalence at high-risk children ranges from 11% to 72% (Berkowitz 2003).

In our study, from the total 1,008 examined children aged 1-6 years, the caries prevalence expressed in terms of the caries index per person, or dmft > 0, was 86.31%, with a mean dmft of 5.8. The prevalence of ECC was 17.36%, or 175 out of 1,008 examined children. The sub-sample of children with diagnosed ECC consisted of 150 children out of 175 invited for further analysis. Twenty-five children of this group from different kindergartens didn't show up in the Department. The mean age of children with ECC was 3.8 ± 1.2 years. The mean dmft in children with ECC was 11 ± 3.6. There was no statistical difference of ECC prevalence between genders (t test = 1.81, P = 0.07). As expected, the lowest mean dmft score was found at age 2 (6.47 ± 2.13), with an age-related increase in dmft of 12.8 at age 6 (Table 1). In comparing the mean dmft in ECC children with respect to age, there was a significant statistical difference between age 2 and ages 4, 5, and 6. (One-Way ANOVA test F = 16, P < 0.001).

Age (N)	dmft ± SD
2 (22)	5.5 ± 2.1
3 (42)	9.7 ± 3.4
4 (38)	12.8 ± 2.6
5 (36)	12.9 ± 2.7
6 (12)	12.8 ± 1.3
Total (150)	11 ± 3.6

Table 1. Mean dmft in children with ECC

3.2.2 Clinical course of ECC

In order to explain the clinical course of ECC, we propose the following stages in the occurrence and progression of carious lesions in ECC:

ECCi (initial stage)-white spot lesion or initial defect in enamel of cervix.

ECCc (circular stage)-lesion in the dentin and circular distribution of this lesion proximally.

ECCd (destructive stage)-destruction of more than half the crown without affecting the incisal edge.

ECCr (radix relicta stage)-total destruction of the crown.

The development of ECC on the maxillary incisors (at least 2) from its initial stage was monitored after a reexamination 1 year later (Table 2).

		Baseline	Reexamination
	N	27	25
	Mean dmft ± SD	5.1 ± 1.8	8.8 ± 0.7
ECC stages	Initial stage (N, %)	(27) 100%	(0) 0%
	Circular stage (N, %)	/	(7) 28%
	Destructive stage (N, %)	/	(5) 20%
	Radix relicta stage (N, %)	/	(9) 36%
	Extraction (N, %)	/	(4) 16%

Table 2. ECC progression from initial stage at 1-year follow-up

The clinical course /ECC stages were not equally distributed. The most commonly present stage was that of radix relicta (41.7%), while the stage that appeared least frequently was the initial stage (15.4%), or 27 out of 150 children with ECC. There was a significant difference between the stages of ECC (P < 0.0001). Twenty-five of the 27 children with ECC in the initial stage were reexamined 1 year after the baseline examination (2 children did not appear for reexamination due to address change). The 1-year reexamination showed that the initial stage had advanced to the circular stage in 28% of children, destructive stage in 20%, radix relicta stage in 36%, and having been extracted due to ECC in 16% of children. Mean age of subjects with initial stage of ECC was 2 ± 0.7. Mean dmft on reexamination showed an increase from 5.1 to 8.8 (P < 0.001).

3.2.3 Clinical consequences of ECC

Scientific research suggests that the development of ECC occurs in 3 stages. The first stage is characterized by a primary infection of the oral cavity with ECC. The second stage is the proliferation of these organisms to pathogenic levels as a consequence of frequent and prolonged exposure to cariogenic substrates. Finally, a rapid demineralization and cavitation of the enamel occurs, resulting in rampant dental caries (Berkowitz 2003).

A 1-year follow-up of ECC development from the initial stage, representing decay at the enamel level and its progression to more destructive stages, shows even development in all affected teeth. It is quite an acute development, because in 2/3 of the children, the ECC has progressed to more complicated stages destructive and radix relicta stages. Within 1 year, the dmft values have increased to 3.7. Consequently, these children commonly experience pain from pulpitis, gangrene, and apical periodontitis. Also, these conditions are often followed by abscesses and cellulitis, sometimes with phlegmona, seriously endangering the child's general health. De Grauwe, in describing the progression of ECC, has noticed that the development of caries from the enamel to the dentin level can occur within 6 months (De Grauwe 2004).

The rapid development of ECC and its clinical appearance, especially in primary incisors, identifies it in its initial stages as a risk factor for future caries in the primary and permanent dentitions (Al-Shalan et al. 1997).

Children with congenital heart anomalies are frequent patients in our departments, some of them exhibiting severe ECC. There is strong evidence that untreated dental disease is an important etiological factor in the pathogenesis of infective endocarditis, a condition that still carries a high risk of mortality (Child 1996).

3.3 Risk factors of caries in general and of ECC in particular
3.3.1 Contagious nature of ECC

There are many different types of microorganisms inhabiting the oral cavity, whose existence is maintained through ecological mechanism. This mechanism includes: saliva, crevicular gingival fluid, antimicrobial components of these fluids, intermicrobial synergism and antagonism, food, tooth, etc.

The presence of microorganisms in the dental plaque depends on the presence of cariogenic bacteria in saliva. Their amount in saliva depends on the secretion level, enzyme presence, as well as on mechanisms with synergistic or antagonistic action. The microorganisms initially present in saliva and afterwards adhering to the tooth surface cannot express their cariogenic action separately or in small amounts. Their cariogenic effect is higher as their affinity to create bacterial colonies increases. Of the great interest in the cariogenesis process are only two bacterial genera: mutant streptococci and lactobacills (Norman & Franklin 1999).

A very important role in occurrence of ECC is attributed to the bacterium *Streptococcus mutans*-called "the window of infection" (Caufield et al. 1993) in that it is responsible for the primary oral infection in the first phase of ECC (Berkowitz 1980; Berkowitz et al. 1996).

Mother is regarded as the so called "window of infection" of *S. mutans* transmission to the newborn.

As the data from the literature show, the role of S mutans in the etiology of ECC, especially in the initial phase, is very crucial (Berkowitz 1980, Caufield et al. 1993). These data also demonstrate the high prevalence of this bacterium in preschool children. *S. mutans* is found at the earliest ages, with the prevalence of 53% in 6- to 12-month-old children (Milgrom et al. 2000), 60% in 15-month-olds (Karn et al. 1988), 67% in 18-month-old Swedes (Hallonsten et al. 1995), and 94.7% in 3- to 4-year-old Chinese (Li et al. 1994).

Almost all preschool urban Icelandic children were found to carry S mutans (Holbrook 1993). According to the studies of Ge and Caufield, all S-ECC children were S mutanspositive (Ge et al. 2008). Borutta 2002, found that in 80% of children (3 years old) diagnosed with caries, the presence of *S. mutans* was demonstrated, while higher counts of this bacterium were found in children with ECC. The high prevalence of *S. mutans* was also demonstrated in our study: 98% of preschool children. Expressed in colony-forming units (CFU/mL saliva), 93% of the ECC children in our study had a high *S. mutans* counts (CFU > 105). Higher salivary counts of *S. mutans* have been correlated with high dmft values (11.5) in our study. This significant correlation between high dmft or caries experience and high *S. mutans* counts has been demonstrated in other studies (Köhler et al. 1988; Köhler et al. 1995; Twetman & Frostner 1991; Maciel et al. 2001).

3.3.2 *S. mutans* prevalence in children with ECC

In this study the presence of *S. mutans* was determined by using the CRT bacteria test (Ivoclar Vivadent, Liechtenstein) on the saliva previously stimulated by chewing paraffin. Bacterial counts were recorded as colony-forming units per milliliter (CFU/mL) of saliva. The number of bacterial colonies was graded as follows:

Class 0 and Class 1 (CFU < 10^5/mL saliva), and Class 2 and Class 3 (CFU $\geq$ 10^5/mL saliva), according to the manufacturers' scoring-card (Ivoclar-Vivadent, Lichtenstein).

In younger subjects, with less saliva collected, the modified spatula method was used.

The results showed that only a small number of children (2%) with ECC exhibited the absence of *S. mutans* (Class 0). In other words, *S. mutans* prevalence in children with ECC was 98%. The lowest class (Class 1) was recorded in 5% of the children with ECC, while classes that represent higher risk for caries (Classes 2 and 3) were present in 34% and 59%, respectively, of children with ECC (Table 3).

S. mutans	N	%	Mean dmft ± SD	Ttest
class				
Class 0	3	2%	3 ± 0	
Class 1	8	5%	5.4 ± 2.0	P<0.001
Class 2	51	34%	9.1 ± 3.0	
Class 3	88	59%	12.8 ± 2.5	
values in CFU/mL saliva				
< 10^5(0 and 1)	11	7%	4.7 ± 1.1	T=5.5
≥ 10^5(2 and 3)	139	93%	11.5 ± 3.2	P<0.001
Total	150	100%	11 ±3.6	

Table 3. S. mutans distribution in children with ECC

Only 11 children with ECC exhibited a low level of S. mutans colonies (CFU < 10^5), with the mean dmft of this group being 4.7. The groups with higher CFU of S. mutans (Classes 2 and 3), representing 93% of the children, had a mean dmft of 11.5 ±3. Comparing the mean dmft of children with ECC by S. mutans classes of CFU showed a significant difference between Class 1 and Classes 2 and 3 (t = 5.5, P < 0.001).

Considerable epidemiological studies have established a positive correlation between early childhood caries and S. mutans (Matee et al. 1992; Li et al. 2000; Berkowitz, 1996; Beighton et al. 2004).

3.3.3 Dietary habits in children with ECC

In a study, parents and kindergarten teachers were asked to fill out a questionnaire about child's dietary habits, including questions regarding frequency of sweets consumption throughout the day, as well as the type of sweets. Parents answered questions about bottle feeding: first use, duration, manner, and fluid content. They were also asked if they put their children to sleep with a bottle.

Sweets consumption in children with ECC

We found that the frequency of sweets consumption in approximately 93% of the children was 1–3 or more times a day. Sweets consumption between meals and during kindergarten hours was common. There was a statistical correlation between daily sweets consumption and dmft in children with ECC (F = 7.26, P < 0.001).

In our study, the frequency of sweets consumption of children with ECC was very high. It is of great concern that kindergartens as educational institutions do not have a more serious approach to a healthy diet and reduction of food containing sugar. On the contrary, at least once a day, sweet food (jam, chocolate, cream, biscuits, or cake) is served to children. Also, serving of this food is very common between meals. The literature shows the high caries values in children who have frequently used sweets (Holbrook et al. 1989), it also shows a high consumption of sweets between meals (Ölmez et al. 2003).

Bottle feeding in children with ECC

Another important factor in the etiology of ECC is bottle feeding, which is accompanied by high salivary counts of S. *mutans*. The relationship between bottle usage and salivary counts of S. *mutans* has been reported (Mohan et al. 1998). In our children, the duration of bottle feeding with sweetened milk or juice is very long, wherein nearly 4/5 of children are bottle fed from 1 to 3 and more years. Most of the children with ECC represent subjects who are bottle fed up to age 2 (48%) and 3 and up (39%). Of the children with ECC, 6% were not bottle fed and 7% were bottle fed up to age 1. Comparing the dmft of children with ECC with regard to duration of bottle feeding shows statistical correlation (F = 20.83, $P < 0.001$).

Another harmful practice is putting children to sleep with a juice-filled bottle, which is practiced in 2/3 of children with ECC, although Johnsen (1982) has reported that 78% of parents of children with ECC had attempted to substitute water for a cariogenic liquid (e.g., apple juice, formula) in the bedtime nursing bottle. A review of the literature from the etiological point of view of ECC shows that "the use of a bottle at night" is not the only cause of ECC (Plat & Cebazas 2000).

3.3.4 Tooth brushing and the OHI in children with ECC

Regarding tooth brushing parents and kindergarten teachers were asked to fill out a questionnaire about the: frequency, parents' participation during brushing, how it was controlled, and use of fluoride-containing toothpaste and fluoride tablets.

The OHI was determined by using the Plaque Test (Ivoclar Vivadent) according to the Greene-Vermilion index.

There is a high level of negligence in the oral hygiene of our children. More than half do not brush their teeth at all, exhibiting a very high OHI (1.52). No child recorded OHI-1. Although a dmft of 13 was found in children with OHI-3, no significant difference was found when comparing the dmft with respect to OHI (F = 2.52, $P = 0.085$).

The importance of the primary dentition of oral health promotion must be focused on the education of mothers to motivate their children for oral hygiene. Unfortunately, we found "bad conviction" of mothers regarding primary teeth that they will be replaced, thus neglecting the care for children's teeth. Data from the literature show that cooperation of mothers is very important in overcoming the belief that the deciduous dentition can be neglected (Rasmund & Tracy 2003).

Regarding the frequency of tooth brushing, around 52% of the children did not brush at all, but there was no statistical difference in dmft in terms of frequency of brushing (F = 2.10, $P = 0.106$).

Oral hygiene habits established at the age of 1 can be maintained throughout early childhood (Wendet 1995).

3.3.5 Fluoride use

From the answers of mothers regarding fluoride use, we ascertained a considerable lack of knowledge about the benefits of this agent in maintaining healthy tooth structure. This information gap can be inferred from their answers. When asked, "Do you give fluoride tablets to your child?" their answers were stated as if they have been asked about some medication: "I give those tablets to my child as needed." The absence of fluoride in

Kosovo's municipal drinking water may highly influence caries prevalence rates in children.

Nutritional counseling, fluoride therapy, and oral hygiene may be required to prevent development of carious lesions in children. In the case of high-risk patients such as children with ECC with a predominance of high salivary counts of *S. mutans*, the use of either the antibacterial rinse chlorhexidine gluconate or the oral health care gel chlorhexidine has been suggested (Featherstone 2004).

3.3.6 Social factors

The oral health promotion and preventive measures are also influenced by social and economical factors. Statistical data from our country such as: large families (with average size of 6.5 members), high unemployment rate (in 2008 it marked 45.4%, for female 56.4%), high birth rate (16%) and the lowest economical growth in the region (Statistical Office of Kosovo 2008), represent some of the aggravating factors when dealing with the health issues of the population, including oral health issues. Given the complexity of factors associated with ECC, it is unfortunate that most of the interest has only been from dental organizations. The critical change needed to accomplish the necessary research for the prevention of ECC should be expanding our network by involving other health professionals, community leaders, national organizations serving children, and political leaders (Ismail 1998).

3.4 Preventive measures for ECC

Early childhood caries (ECC) is a health problem with biological, social and behavioral determinants. Intervention treatment does not resolve this problem. It is difficult, sometimes impossible and expensive.

The only safest way is prevention of this complex pathology. European Academy of Pediatric Dentistry (2008) has recommended general strategies for ECC prevention:

- Oral health assessments with counseling at regularly scheduled visits during the first year of life are an important strategy to prevent ECC.
- Children's teeth should be brushed daily with a smear of fluoride toothpaste as soon as they erupt.
- Professional applications of fluoride varnish are recommended at least twice yearly in groups or individuals at risk.
- Parents of infants and toddlers should be encouraged to reduce behaviours that promote the early transmission of mutans streptococci.

Based on these recommendations, we will describe detailed preventive measures: primary prevention – prenatal and postnatal care; and secondary prevention – parents' and dental professionals' role.

3.4.1 Primary prevention

- It should begin during prenatal period and it consists of pregnant woman's needs' fulfillment with necessary and healthy products;
- Proper quality of food for the newborn during the enamel maturation phase;
- Fluoridation of newly-erupted teeth;
- Antimicrobial therapy with chlorhexidine.

3.4.2 Secondary prevention

- Mothers' education on recognizing the first signs of ECC using "lift-the-lip" technique. The aim of this measure is early detection of the so-called **"white spot"**.
- Parents should be encouraged to avoid bad feeding habits of their children and give effort for proper feeding:
  - breast-feeding of the baby;
  - the use of cup instead of the bottle as early as possible;
  - not sleeping with bottle in mouth;
  - avoid the use of fabricated juices or soda;
  - the use of natural, a little sweetened, juice or tea, or just water;
  - avoid the discontinuation of bottle use by the method "bottle is gone";
  - reduce the liquid in the bottle, gradually by night,
  - reduce sweets as much as possible;
  - no sweets between meals;
  - daily tooth brushing, at least twice a day, obligatory before going to bed.
- Necessary consultations with the dentist -
  Professional educational activities targeting primary health care providers (pediatricians, internists, family physicians, obstetricians, mid-level medical practitioners):
  - early identification of disease,
  - fluoride supplements as appropriate,
  - healthful feeding practices,
  - snacking behaviors that promote good oral health, and
  - referral to the dentist by 12 months of age.

4. Gingivitis and periodontitis

The periodontium, also known as "the supporting structures of the teeth", comprises a developmental, biologic, and functional unit, which undergoes certain changes with age and is subjected to morphologic changes related to functional alterations.

The attachment of the tooth to the bone tissue of the jaws and maintenance of the oral cavity masticatory mucosa surface's integrity are the main functions of the periodontium.

The periodontium (περι = around, οδονσ = tooth) comprises the following tissues 1) the gingiva, 2) the periodontal ligament, 3) the root cementum, and 4) the alveolar bone.

4.1 Normal anatomy
4.1.1 Gingiva

In the coronal direction the coral pink gingiva terminates in the free gingival margin, which has a scalloped outline. In the apical direction the gingiva is continuous with the loose, darker red alveolar mucosa (lining mucosa) from which the gingiva is separated by a, usually, easily recognizable borderline called either the mucogingival junction (arrows) or the mucogingival line. Since the hard palate and the maxillary alveolar process are covered by the same type of masticatory mucosa, there is no mucogingival line present in the palate. Two parts of the gingiva can be differentiated: 1) the *free gingiva* and 2) the *attached gingiva*.

4.1.2 Periodontal ligament

The soft, richly vascular and cellular connective tissue which joins the root cementum with socket wall and surrounds the roots of the teeth is the periodontal ligament. The periodontal ligament is situated in the space between the roots of the teeth and the lamina dura or the alveolar bone proper. The alveolar bone surrounds the tooth to a level approximately 1mm apical to the cemento-enamel junction.

The portions of the principal fibers of the periodontal ligament which are embedded in the root cementum and in the alveolar bone proper are called *Sharpey's fibers*.

4.1.3 Root cementum

The cementum is a special mineralized tissue covering the root surfaces. It has many features in common with bone tissue. It contains no blood or lymph vessels, has no innervation, does not undergo physiologic resorption or remodeling, but is characterized by continuing deposition throughout life. It attaches the periodontal ligament fibers to the root and contributes to the process of repair after damage to the root surface.

Different forms of cementum have been described, such as acellular, extrinsic fiber cementum; cellular, mixed stratified cementum; and cellular, intrinsic fiber cementum.

4.1.4 Alveolar bone

The alveolar process is defined as the parts of the maxilla and the mandible that form and support the sockets of the teeth.

Together with the root cementum and the periodontal membrane, the alveolar bone constitutes the attachment apparatus of the teeth, the main function of which is to distribute and resorb forces generated by, for example, mastication and other tooth contacts.

4.2 Classification of periodontal diseases

The classification of periodontal diseases (Flemmig 1999) was revised in a workshop (AAP classification of periodontal diseases) that took place in 1999. This classification includes eight main categories:

- Gingival diseases
- Chronic periodontitis
- Aggressive periodontitis
- Periodontitis as a manifestation of systemic diseases
- Necrotizing periodontal diseases
- Abscesses of the periodontium
- Periodontitis associated with endodontic lesions
- Developmental or acquired deformities and conditions.

4.3 Prevalence of periodontal diseases

Inflammatory alterations of gingiva are found among the majority of children in the primary dentition. The prevalence of gingivitis reaches its maximum at around 11 years among girls, whereas among boys 2 years later (Massler et al. 1952)

Studies from 24 European countries from 1982 to 1992 (Sheiham et al. 2002) using Community Periodontal Index of Treatment Needs (CPITN) showed these results:

- the mean prevalence of shallow pockets (CPITN-3) is 36% in West Europe and 45% in East Europe
- the mean prevalence of deep pockets (CPITN-4) is 9% in West Europe and 23% in East Europe

-    the average of periodontitis affected sextants was 0.2-2.4 for CPITN-3 and 0-0.8 for CPITN-4.

The Third National Health and Nutrition Examination Survey (NHANES III) as the largest population-based study during 1988-1994 showed that periodontitis affected at least 35% of US population between 30 and 90 years of age, with mild form in 22% and advanced form in 13%. The severe forms of periodontitis affected more men than women, and more African-Americans and Hispanics than Caucasians.

Tooth loss may be the definitive consequence of destructive periodontal disease. Teeth lost due to periodontal disease's consequences are evidently not in agreement with registration in epidemiological surveys. The prevalence and the severity of the disease may, thus, be underestimated.

The so-called histologically healthy gingiva is possible only under experimental conditions and is attained by prolonged and overall nonexistence of microbial plaque. Thus, the more appropriate term used to express the health of gingiva is clinically normal gingiva, which almost always is followed by a polymorphonuclear granulocyte and lymphocyte infiltrate.

The form of periodontal disease that affects the primary dentition, the condition formerly called prepubertal periodontitis, has been reported to appear in both a generalized and a localized form (Page et al. 1983).

4.4 Risk factors for periodontitis

There is an abundance of both empirical evidence and substantial theoretical justification for accepting the widespread belief that many diseases have more than one cause, i.e. that they are of multifactorial etiology (Kleinbaum et al. 1982).

In a relatively large number of cross-sectional studies, multiple risk putative risk factors for periodontal disease have been examined (Beck et al. 1990, Grossi et al. 1994, Horning et al. 1992, Ismali & Szpunar 1990).

4.4.1 Tobacco smoking

The biological possibility of a connection between tobacco smoking and periodontitis was found on the potential effects of several tobacco-related substances, notably nicotine, carbon monoxide and hydrogen cyanide. Data from the NHANES III study (Tomar & Asma 2000) suggested that 42% of periodontitis cases in the USA can be attributed to current smoking, and 11% to former smoking.

4.4.2 Diabetes mellitus

Diabetes as a risk factor for periodontitis has been addressed and debated for several years (Genco & Loe 1993), but recently, a number of biological mechanisms have been identified, by which the disease may contribute to impaired periodontal conditions. Examiners showed that diabetics were three times more likely to suffer from periodontal disease than non-diabetics (Emrich et al. 1991).

4.5 Periodontal disease and risk for systemic disease

Besides the risk from periodontitis deriving from the systemic diseases, it has been suggested that periodontal diseases may represent a possible risk factor for systemic diseases. Emerging facts show that periodontal diseases, in fact, have systemic consequences.

DeStefano et al (1993) in a prospective group of 9760 subjects found a nearly two-fold higher risk of **coronary heart disease** for patients with periodontal infection. But other studies have failed to document this association, indicating that this association is more complex and conditional (Hujoel et al. 2000).

Another systemic consequence that may be attributed to the periodontal disease is **preterm low birth-weight**. It has been hypothesized that women with preterm labor may be indirectly affected through remote infections, one of which is periodontal disease (McGregor et al. 1988). In a pioneer study conducted by Offenbacher et al. (1996) with 124 subjects it was found that periodontitis, defined as 60% and more sites with attachment loss of 3 and more millimeters, conferred 7.9 fold risk for preterm low birth weight cases. A study in Kosovo with 200 parturients has acquired results of lower odd ratio (more than 3 fold), but significantly higher with women with periododntitis compared with women with no periodontitis (Meqa 2007).

5. Oral Health promotion

Good health is a major resource for social, economic and personal development. Political, economic, social, cultural, environmental, behavioral and biological factors can enhance or impair health. Health promotion action aims at making these conditions conducive to health. Health promotion therefore goes beyond health care. It puts health on the agenda of policy makers in all sectors and at all levels, directing them to be aware of the health consequences of their decisions and to accept their responsibilities for health.

An important role in the oral health promotion activities, besides dental professionals, belongs to the kindergarten and school teachers, as well as mothers at home. Surely, mother's role is very important and decisive in child's education, not only from the aspect of oral health.

Health care for children cannot be designed without understanding their vulnerability and essential link to parents. Health professionals, educators, and researchers must partner with parents in all activities related to children's health, from clinical care to community programs to policy planning. Parental oral disease, attitudes, and past experiences with dental care have a direct impact on their own and their developing child's oral health. Disease transmission, the practice of oral home care, and development of healthy attitudes towards oral health are all impacted by family factors. (Wendy & Mouradian 2001).

5.1 Mother's knowledge regarding oral health care

It is of the greatest interest to maintain mother's oral health during pregnancy. In our studies we have found that oral health problems among pregnant women are as common as among children. Oral health should be an integral part of prenatal care. Improving oral health during pregnancy not only enhances the overall health of women, but also contributes to improving the oral health of their children.

Because of the complexity of factors related to dental caries, the role of oral health education is believed to be very important, especially for mothers.

In order to explain the mother's importance, respectively her knowledge related to oral health promotion, we have conducted a study in our country. Mothers who accompanied their children to the University Dentistry School of Kosovo, Pedodontics Department, were interviewed. The aim of our study was to determine the caries experience and parental knowledge regarding primary preventive measures for dental caries in children, mainly from the educational perspective of mothers in Kosovo. Data related to the following information was collected: social (mother's age, economic status, mother's level of education, employment, number of children in the family), dental experiences (dental visits, reasons of the visits), oral hygiene (daily frequency, knowledge of tooth brushing techniques, tooth brushing duration), feeding habits (sugar consumption, bottle feeding), fluoride and antimicrobial agents use, knowledge on their role in dental health, and pregnancy (prenatal control, premature birth).

There is no doubt of the importance of the maternal role in maintaining good oral health among their children. The mother's level of education is quite important, especially in our country, where women do not have a sufficient level of education. According to the official data, nearly half of all women completed only their primary education (44.9%) while only 7.2% finished high school or obtained a university degree. Unfortunately, even in this century, illiteracy exists in Kosovo, with the level ranging from 2% to 4%. The number of illiterate women is almost three times higher than that of men. Demographic data are characterized by a high birth rate (15.7%), equivalent to an average of three children per mother. Social data show low employment rates among women. The unemployment rate is approximately 62% for women and 35% for men. Even though female presence is very high in trade and services such as health or education, oral health education has been mostly neglected (Kosovo Statistical Office 2008).

The results of our examination have shown that maternal effort, as well as their knowledge of oral health protection for their children, is largely inadequate. This inadequacy also has been reflected in the dental status of the children, with a mean dmft 6.3. The highest mean dmft was recorded among children whose mothers finished primary and secondary school while a lower mean dmft (4.5) was recorded among children whose mothers finished high school or obtained a university degree. Although mothers with higher educational levels had more knowledge, as evidenced by the lower mean dmft, it was still high according to WHO standards. When the dmft index structure was analyzed, 78% of the teeth were decayed, 16% were extracted, and only 6% were filled. The children's dental health status was even worse given the high prevalence of ECC (above 21%), with a mean dmft of 11 for these cases.

The dental experiences of our children, for nearly two-thirds of all respondents, unfortunately involved visits to the dentist only when the pain appeared.

Our examination was based on maternal levels of knowledge regarding oral health (over 600 interviewed mothers), especially since they play crucial roles in educating their children. However, we made an attempt to raise the attention of not only mothers, but also of health professionals regarding the importance of the early prevention of dental and oral diseases in children through pre- and postnatal health education.

5.2 Prenatal health education

Health education ought to start during the prenatal period. It consists of regular OB/GYN visits and adequate access to necessary medical advice for both maternal and pediatric health. Unfortunately, only 8% of the mothers sought advice from their obstetrician regarding oral health protection measures for their future child. Nearly three-quarters of the mothers neglected their own oral health by not visiting the dentist during their pregnancies. Even though mothers reported occasional discomfort regarding their oral health, such as gingival bleeding or toothaches, their visits to the dentist were very rare, with only 21% seeking help from the dentist. Another factor driving maternal negligence towards their own oral health was the inadequate level of preparedness among healthcare personnel, as well as their hesitant attitudes. Pregnant mothers who neglect to address their oral health issues may face consequences in their general health status, as well as in oral health status, with frequent dental caries, erosions, and periodontal disease. According to the U.S. Department of Health and Human Services, improving oral health during pregnancy not only enhances the overall health of women, but also contributes to improved oral health for their children. Oral health should be an integral part of prenatal care.

Pregnancy and early childhood are particularly important times to access oral health care because the consequences of poor oral health can have a lifelong impact (US Department of Health and Human Services, 2000)

Dental problems such as caries, erosion, epulis, periodontal infection, loose teeth, and ill-fitting crowns, bridges, and dentures may have special significance during pregnancy (Casassimo 1996, Gajendra 2004).

The bacteria responsible for periodontal disease are capable of producing a variety of chemical inflammatory mediators such as prostaglandins, interleukins and tumor necrosis factor that can directly affect the pregnant woman (Romero et al. 2004).

Data from the literature have shown that oral health problems are common in pregnant women and in young children (Crall 2005). Untreated cavities in mothers may be associated with the risk of caries in children. Finally, untreated oral infections may become systemic problems during pregnancy and may even contribute to preterm birth (Lewit & Monheit 1992).

Periodontal disease is caused by gram-negative anaerobic bacteria. Studies have suggested that periodontal infections may contribute to the birth of preterm/low birth weight babies (Geopfert et al. 2004).

In our study, the prevalence of premature births is 9%, and it has been reported that children born prematurely have a higher prevalence of ECC.

Improving the oral health of pregnant women prevents complications of dental diseases during pregnancy, has the potential to decrease early childhood caries and may reduce preterm and low birth weight deliveries. Assessment of oral health risks in infants and young children, along with anticipatory guidance, has the potential to prevent early childhood caries.

5.3 Postnatal health education
5.3.1 First dental visit

Regarding the issue of parental effort on seeking professional advice from the dentist, the data from the literature do not show satisfactory levels in other countries. Even in the developed nations, there is a dominant perception that children do not need early dental visits because they will subsequently lose their baby teeth.

For instance, Dr. Horowitz has stated that *"it is pretty hard for the parent to believe that the child should be sent to the dentist after the first tooth has erupted, and maybe earlier. A mistake that I made by myself, relying in my dentist's advice not sending my child to the dentist before he turns three. Later I realized that it was a mistake"* Reagan continues to cite authors Horowitz and Hale, who think that an important attention should be paid to the first dental visit and suggest that "the dental community needs to step forward and encourage these early visits" (Regan 2002).

We found that 18% of the mothers had no idea when their children should visit a dentist, while more than half believed that their children should first visit a dentist when they are three years old. Unfortunately, a considerable portion of mothers (18%) believe that the first visit to the dentist should occur only when the child is in pain.

While the common perception 30 years ago was that the first dental visit should occur at the age of three, today it is preferred that the first visit occur before the child's first birthday, specifically between 6 and 12 months of age.

5.3.2 Mother's knowledge about contagious nature of dental caries

It is already understood that dental caries is a contagious disease. There are many ways of transmission from the mother's mouth to the child's mouth, such as by kissing or when mothers "clean" their children's pacifiers or taste their children's juice or food (Berkowitz 1983). This bad habit was also recorded in our study. When mothers were asked whether they cleaned their baby's pacifiers or tasted the fluid from their baby's bottle, 35% confirmed such behaviors. According to the results of our study, mothers were not aware of this bacterium and the ways of it's transmission in the child's mouth.

Previously, it was believed that mutans streptococci were not present in a child's mouth until the eruption of the first tooth. However, some recent examinations have proven that high *S. mutans* levels may be observed in some children before their first birthday (Plotzitza et al. 2002). *S. mutans* was also found in the dental plaque of 12-month-old babies (Habibian et al. 2002).

Data from the literature have confirmed such a correlation; if the mother's SM count is low, the child's count is low as well, and vice versa (Köhler & Andreen 1984). Nevertheless, this hypothesis needs further clarification.

5.3.3 Mother's knowledge regarding feeding habits

Bottle feeding – It has been demonstrated that bottle feeding may contribute to dental caries, especially early childhood caries (ECC). The relationship between bottle usage and high salivary levels of the cariogenic bacteria *S. mutans* has been reported (Mohan et al. 1998). Surprisingly, even though a considerable number of mothers in our study were unemployed and did not send their children to kindergarten, they fed their children with bottles (65%). Unfortunately, maternal knowledge regarding the role of bottle feeding in the occurrence of ECC was generally low (12%). An unfavourable practice involves mothers' putting their children to sleep with milk- or juice-filled bottles, which was practiced for 74% of the children. Other authors have also reported on this bad practice (Jonsen 1988). Several studies have reported that the majority of the U.S. preschool population take, or have taken, a bottle to bed (Kaste & Gift 1995).

In one study of children in the U.S. Head Start programs, a surprisingly high proportion (69%) of the children without maxillary anterior caries reported taking a bottle to bed, while 86% of the children with maxillary anterior caries reported taking a bottle to bed (O'Sullivan & Tinanoff 1993).

In another study, 90% of the children in a population with and without caries were bottle-fed between 12 and 18 months of age, although the prevalence of nursing caries was only 20% (Serwint et al. 1993).

The importance of bottle feeding with the occurrence of caries (especially in early and rampant occurrence in very young children) is reflected in the terminology of this pathology. The term 'baby bottle tooth decay' was proposed by the Healthy Mothers - Healthy Babies Coalition as an alternative that would be more appropriate for patient acceptance and focus increased attention on the potential harms of using a nursing bottle (Arkin 1986).

More recent evidence suggests that taking a bottle to bed may be a stronger predictor of frontal tooth ECC patterns than previously believed (Douglass et al. 2001).

Sweets consumption – There was a high percentage of sweets consumption among our children. Unfortunately, even though over 70% of mothers are aware that sweets can damage the children's teeth, they do not give efforts to reduce this habit. Nearly 90% of the children consumed sweets at least once a day. Another serious factor is that sweets were consumed in between meals among 2/3 of children. In developed countries, advanced preventive programs focused on reducing the consumption of sweets. Data from the literature indicate that only 21% and 45% of children in Finland and Denmark, respectively, consumed sweets once a week (Matilla et al. 2000). The consumption of sweets containing sucrose constituents may be considered an important factor in the occurrence of caries (Marthaler 1990). The association between the intake of sucrose and dental caries has been well established in numerous studies, conducted mainly in northern and western European countries and in North America (Rugg-Gunn 1993). On the other hand, authors have reported that with the correct implementation of preventive and educational measures, there was a reduction in the development of caries, despite continued consumption of sucrose containing foods (Marthaler 1990).

Kosovar cuisine is similar to that in the Middle and Near East, especially regarding sweets, with relatively frequent and high amounts of starch. The mechanism by which the starch added to sucrose increases the cariogenic potential of foods could be that the presence of starch increases the retention time of the food in the mouth (Lingstrom et al. 1993). Additionally, there are some indications that starch can increase acid production from sucrose when both nutrients are present together (Glor et al. 1988).

Studies in the literature have reported a correlation between the consumption of sweets and *S. mutans* colonies, especially associated with high counts. It is obvious that there could be a threshold for the number of oral *S. mutans* colonies that eventually allow fermentable carbohydrates to exert harmful effects on teeth (Garsia-Closas et al. 1997).

5.3.4 Mother knowledge regarding oral hygiene

Whether the child will start tooth brushing at an early age depends on maternal habits. Cleansing of the baby teeth should be started by the time of eruption of the first primary tooth. A small piece of clean gauze or a small toothbrush can be used. The child imitates parental behaviours, including oral hygiene habits. In a study in England, Witlle (1988) reported that 60% of children started brushing their teeth from the age of one; presumably, their teeth were initially brushed by their parents.

Another study in England reported that in 80% of cases, mothers brushed the teeth of their children (Holt RD et al. 1996).

A study conducted in Bosnia, a country that is geographically close to Kosovo, concluded that only 3% of the parents assisted their children with their first tooth brushing efforts (Huseinbegović 2001).

In our study, 38% of the mothers stated that their children did not brush their teeth at all. Over 90% had no knowledge regarding proper tooth brushing techniques. Mothers rarely assisted their children during tooth brushing (5%). Studies in the literature show a strong relationship between the poor maternal oral health and the prevalence of caries in their children (Dye et al. 2011).

5.3.5 Fluoride and antimicrobial agent utilization

Fluoride, the key agent in battling caries, works primarily by topical action: inhibition of demineralization and enhancement of re-mineralization. Fluoride incorporated during tooth development is insufficient to play significant role in caries protection. Fluoride is needed regularly throughout life to protect teeth against caries. It is now realized that the most important action mechanism of fluoride takes place on the enamel surface of the tooth. Fluoride inhibits the loss of minerals and promotes the re-mineralization process. The data from literature demonstrated the importance of fluoridation on the prevention of dental caries. Preschool children from Ireland showed a very low mean dmft (0.9), largely because their drinking water was regularly fluoridated (Marthaler et al. 1996).

A study in Tennessee, USA, reported a mean dmft of 4.15 for the fluoridated communities and a mean dmft of 7.49 for the non-fluoridated communities (David et al. 2001).

Recommendations for fluoride supplementation can be made based on the fluoride content of the water, the child's age, and the child's caries risk. Among all endogenous and exogenous methods, the most effective method is water fluoridation. The drinking water in Kosovo is insufficient and has a fluoride level of less than 0.3 mg/l; however, the optimal range is between 0.8 and 1.5 mg/l.

In the absence of fluoridated water, fluoride tablets may be used. Weintraub (1999) claims that "before you think of any preventive measure, *put fluoride salts on the teeth*".

The systemic and topical use of fluoride is the most effective measure to prevent dental caries. Exposure to topical fluoride via fluoridated toothpaste twice a day is a major component of caries prevention therapy. Fluoride varnish may be applied with a soft brush, and reapplication is recommended every 3 to 6 months.

Antimicrobial treatment of caries is based on the use of two well-known agents (fluoride and chlorhexidine) for achieving selective antimicrobial control of carious microflora. Fluoride and chlorhexidine have an antimicrobial action against M. Streptococci that is significantly higher than that which they have against other non-cariogenic bacterial species. A combination of fluoride varnish and chlorhexidine application is used to lower the mutans streptococci count. Another successful antibacterial therapy against cariogenic bacteria is treatment with a chlorhexidine gluconate rinse or gel.

Mothers from our study had not used fluoride and any antimicrobial agents (e.g., chlorhexidine), nor did they have any knowledge regarding their utilization. The data from literature have confirmed the positive antibacterial role of chlorhexidine in *S. mutans* colonies' destruction. Antimicrobial treatment strategy has become a real concern for many dental professionals. A multitude of clinical trials confirms the caries-inhibiting effect of chlorhexidine (Zhang at al. 2006).

6. Oral health strategies

The initiatives undertaken by WHO, have global impact on the national and international policy development, one of which is the WHO Global Oral Health Program.

High prevalence of oral diseases, such as dental caries, is not only individual preoccupation, but also a serious public health problem. WHO is continuously developing strategies and objectives on prevention of oral disease through oral health promotion. Thus, it may be of a great interest for the readers to get familiar with these WHO strategies and objectives.

6.1 The objectives of the WHO Global Oral Health Program (ORH) (www.who.int/oral_health/strategies_2010)

The objectives of the WHO Global Oral Health Program (ORH), one of the technical programs within the Department of Chronic Diseases and Health Promotion (CHP), have been reoriented according to the new strategy of disease prevention and promotion of health. Greater emphasis is put on developing global policies in oral health promotion and oral disease prevention, coordinated more effectively with other priority programs of CHP and other clusters and with external partners.

Several principles form the basis for the carried out work. The WHO Oral Health Program works on building oral health policies towards effective control of risks to oral health, based on the common risk factors approach. The focus is on modifiable risk behaviors related to diet, nutrition, use of tobacco and excessive consumption of alcohol, and hygiene.

Oral health is part of total health and essential to quality of life and WHO projects intend to translate the evidence into action programs. The Oral Health Program therefore gives priority to integration of oral health with general health programs before community or national levels. The WHO Oral Health Program works from the life-course perspective, currently the community programs for improved oral health of the elderly and of children is given high priority. The implementation of school oral health programs within the framework of the WHO Health Promoting Schools Initiative is supported and guidelines are developed. Oral health systems reorientation towards prevention and health promotion is recommended in light of the Ottawa Charter, the primary health care concept and the Jakarta Declaration on leading Health Promotion into the 21st Century. In addition, global goals for oral health by the year 2020 strive for development of quality of oral health systems. The Program works on application of evidence-based strategies in oral health promotion, prevention and treatment of oral diseases worldwide, health systems research and development. Emphasis is also given on prevention and care of oral mucosal lesions, including oral cancer and oral manifestations of HIV/AIDS, cranio-facial disorders, trauma and injuries.

6.2 Oral health within WHO strategic directions

WHO's goals are to build healthy populations and communities and to combat ill health. Four strategic directions provide the broad framework for focusing WHO's technical work, which also have implications for the Oral Health Program.

- Reducing oral disease burden and disability, especially in poor and marginalized populations.
- Promoting healthy lifestyles and reducing risk factors to oral health that arise from environmental, economic, social and behavioral causes.
- Developing oral health systems that equitably improve oral health outcomes, respond to people's legitimate demands, and are financially fair.
- Framing policies in oral health, based on integration of oral health into national and community health programs, and promoting oral health as an effective dimension for development policy of society.

In accordance with WHO overall priorities, the Global Oral Health Program has adopted the following priorities and strategic orientations.

6.3 Strategies and approaches in oral disease prevention and health promotion

Priority is given to diseases linked by common, preventable and lifestyle related risk factors (e.g. unhealthy diet, tobacco use), including oral health.

High relative risk of oral disease relates to socio-cultural determinants such as poor living conditions; low education; lack of traditions, beliefs and culture in support of oral health. Communities and countries with inappropriate exposure to fluorides imply higher risk of dental caries and settings with poor access to safe water or sanitary facilities are environmental risk factors to oral health as well as general health.

6.4 Health promotion and oral health

The WHO Oral Health Program applies the philosophy "think globally - act locally". The development of program for oral health promotion in targeted countries focuses on:

- Identification of health determinants; mechanisms in place to improve capacity to design and implement interventions that promote oral health.
- Implementation of community-based demonstration projects for oral health promotion, with special reference to poor and disadvantaged population groups.
- Building capacity in planning and evaluation of national program for oral health promotion and evaluation of oral health promotion interventions in operation.
- Development of methods and tools to analyze the processes and outcomes of oral health promotion interventions as part of national health program.
- Establishment of networks and alliances to strengthen national and international actions for oral health promotion. Emphasis is also given to the development of networks for exchange of experiences within the context of the WHO Mega Country Program.

7. Conclusion

Oral health is integral to general health and should not be considered in isolation. Oral diseases have detrimental effects on an individual's physical and psychological well-being and reduce quality of life. The commonest disease is dental caries. Other important conditions are gum (periodontal) disease. Dental caries is one of the most prevalent diseases among children worldwide. Its lack of treatment and complications that may occur can endanger general health. The development of dental caries is a dynamic process. Caries progression or reversal is determined by the balance between protective and pathological factors in the mouth. The most important component in the treatment of the caries disease is prevention. Understanding the balance between pathological factors and protective factors is the key to successful prevention of caries. Analyzing the etiology, prevalence, clinical specifics, consequences and complications, caries in general and ECC in particular are estimated as serious diseases, which represent not only health problem, but also a great serious social and economic problem. A well-recognized association exists between socio-economic status and oral health, and trends suggest that disease is increasingly concentrated in the lower income groups. However, oral diseases are largely preventable. In underdeveloped countries, oral health consequences due to dental caries also represent a serious public health problem. The presence of dental caries, especially of ECC, may reflect on the oral health status of children in countries with insufficient health system and inefficient primary dentistry. Early Childhood Caries (ECC) is a public health problem with biological, social and behavioral determinants. The preventive activities must start at an early age. Home-care methods are more than necessary. Primary prevention must start in the prenatal stage to fulfill the needs of pregnancy. Parents should be encouraged to avoid bad feeding habits and to instruct and supervise their children in tooth brushing. Mothers should be instructed to use the lift-the-lip technique to spot the white-spot lesions as first signs of dental caries. Newly erupted teeth must be treated with fluoride agents, and, as needed, antimicrobial agents containing chlorhexidine and thymol. Further investigation is needed to assess the effectiveness of new intervention strategies beyond traditional measures that are not strictly dependent on access to dental professional providers.

Education is the essential pillar of the preventive measures. The main role in this pillar plays mother's education, respectively her knowledge regarding the oral health. Unfortunately, an overall preventive program in oral health promotion, including oral health education, is absent in many underdeveloped countries. There are some negative indicators that contribute to the low levels of oral health knowledge, such as the lack of curriculum subjects on oral health, the lack of training and seminars on the issue, insufficient print materials for educational purposes, the lack of information for pregnant women, and negligence by dentists regarding measures for mothers to educate their children. Although some mothers with higher educational levels were highly motivated to improve their children's oral health, much more needs to be accomplished. Institutional efforts towards maternal and pediatric oral health education must be implemented immediately. Permanent and sustained oral health promotion organized with the participation of the entire civil society, with the mandatory presence of key stakeholders in the areas of education and healthcare, represent one of the highest priorities. The WHO strategies and objectives implementation regarding oral health promotion should be understood in the right manner and should be implemented continuously.

8. References

AAP Workshop on the Classification of Periodontal Diseases 1999. In: Flemmig, T.M. (1999). Periodontitis. *Ann Periodontol,* Vol. 4, pp. 32-37.

Apostolova, D., Asprovsa, V. & Simovska N (2003). Circular caries-ECC-a problem at the earliest age. *8th Congress of the Balkan Stomatological Society,* (Abstract Book) Tirana, 2003.

Arkin, E.B. (1986). The Healthy Mothers, Healthy Babies Coalition: four years of progress. *Public Health Repository,* Vol. 101, pp. 147-156.

Beck, J.D., Koch, G.G., Rozier, R.G. & Tudor, G.E. (1990). Prevalence and risk indicators for periodontal attachment loss in a population of older community-dwelling blacks and whites. Journal of Periodontology Vol. 61, pp. 521-528.

Beighton, D., Brailsford, S., Samaranayake, L.P., Brown, J.P., Ping, F.X., Grant-Mills, D., Harris, R., Lo, E.C., Naidoo, S., Ramos-Gomez, F., Soo, T.C., Burnside, G. & Pine, C.M. (2004). A multi-country comparison of caries-associated microflora in demographically diverse children. *Community Dental Health,* Vol. 21, pp. 96–101.

Begzati, A., Berisha, M. & Meqa, K. (2010). Early childhood caries in preschool children of Kosovo - a serious public health problem. *BMC Public Health*, Vol. 10, pp. 788.

Begzati, A., Meqa, K., Siegenthaler, D., Berisha, M. & Mautsch, W. (2011). Dental health evaluation of children in Kosovo. *European Journal of Dentistry*, Vol. 5, pp. 32-39.

Berkowitz. R.J., Turner, J. & Green, P. (1980). Primary oral infection of infants with Streptococcus mutans. *Archives of Oral Biology*, Vol. 25, pp. 221-224.

Berkowitz, R.J. (1996). Etiology of nursing caries; a microbiologic perspective. Journal of Public Health *Dentistry*, Vol. 56, No. 1, pp. 51-54.

Berkowitz, R.J. (2003). Causes, Treatment and Prevention of Early Childhood Caries: A Microbiologic Perspective. *Journal of the Canadian Dental Association*, Vol. 69, No. 5, pp. 304-307.

Block, L.E. (2003). Dental public health: An Overview. In Gluck GM, Morganstein WM eds: *Jong's Community Dental Health*, 5th ed., St. Louis, Mosby.

Borutta, A., Kneist, S. & Eherler, D.P. (2002). Oral health and Occurrence of Salivary S. mutans in Small Children, *Journal of Dental and Oral Medicine*, Vol. 4, No. 3, Poster 128.

Bruered, B., Kinney, M.B. & Bothwell, E. (1989). Preventing baby bottle tooth decay in American Indian and Alaska native communities: a model for planning. *Public Health Repository*, Vol. 104, No. 6, pp. 631-640.

Casassimo, P. (1996). Bright Futures in Practice: Oral Health. Arlington, VA: *National Center for Education in Maternal and Child Health*.

Caufield, P.W., Cutter, G.R. & Dasanayake, A.P. (1993). Initial acquisition of mutans streptococci by infants: evidence for a discrete window of infectivity. *Journal of Dental Research*, Vol. 72, No. 1, pp. 37-45.

Centers for Disease Control and Prevention (CDCP), conference. Atlanta, GA, September 1994.

Child, J.S. (1996). Risks for and prevention of infective endocarditis. In: Child JS, ed. *Cardiology Clinics – Diagnosis and Management of Infective Endocarditis*. Philadelphia, Pa: WB Saunders Co, Vol. 14, pp. 327-343.

Constitution of the World Health Organization. Geneva, World Health Organization, 1946, p 3.

Crall, J.J. (2005). Opportunities for improving maternal and infant health through prenatal oral health care. In: McCormick MC, Siegal JE, editors. *Prenatal Care*. Cambridge: University Press pp. 261-270.

Davenport, E.S. (1990). Caries in preschool child: Aetiology. *Journal of Dentistry*, Vol. 18, pp. 300-303.

David, E.B., Rebecca, W.H., James, A.G., Jennifer, U.B. & William, W.W. (2001). Successful Implementation of Community Water Fluoridation via the Community Diagnosis Process. *Journal of Public Health Dentistry*, Vol. 61, No. 1, pp. 28-33.

Davis, G.N. (1998). Early childhood caries-a synopsis. *Community Dentistry and Oral Epidemiology*, Vol. 26, No. 1, pp. 106-116.

De Grauwe, A., Aps, J.K. & Martens, L.C. (2004). Early Childhood Caries (ECC): What's in a name? *European Journal of Pediatric Dentistry*, Vol. 5, No. 2, pp. 62-70.

Derkson, G.D. & Ponti, P. (1999). Nursing bottle syndrome: prevalence end etiology in a non fluorided city. *Journal of the Canadian Dental Association*, Vol. 6, pp. 389-393.

DeStefano, F., Anda, R.F., Kahn, H.S., Williamson, D.F. & Russell, C.M. (1993). Dental disease and risk of coronary heart disease and mortality. British Medical Journal Vol. 306, pp. 688-691.

Douglass, J.M., Tinanoff, N., Tang, J.M.W. & Altman, D.S. (2001). Dental caries patterns and oral health behaviours in Arizona infants and toddlers. *Community Dentistry and Oral Epidemiology,* Vol. 29, pp. 14–22.

Drury, Th.F., Horowitz, A.M., Ismail, A.I., Maertens, M.P., Rozier, R.G. & Selwitz, R.H. (1999). Diagnosing and reporting Early Childhood Caries for Research Purposes. *Journal of Public Health Dentistry,* Vol. 59, pp. 192-197.

Dye, B.A., Vargas, C.M., Lee, J.J., Magder, L. & Tinanoff, N. (2011). Assessing the relationship between children's oral health status and that of their mothers. *Journal of American Dental Association,* Vol. 142, No. 2, pp. 173-183.

Emrich, L.J., Shlossman, M. & Genco, R.J. (1991). Periodontal disease in non-insulin-dependent diabetes mellitus. Journal of Periodontology Vol. 62, pp. 123-131

Fass, E.N. (1962). Is bottle feeding of milk a factor in dental caries? *Journal of Dentistry for Children,* Vol. 29, pp. 245-251.

Featherstone, J.D.B. (2004). The Caries Balance: The Basis for Caries Management by Risk Assessment. *Oral Health and Preventive Dentistry,* Vol. 2, No 1, pp. 259-264.

Gajendra, S. & Kumar, J.V. (2004). Oral health and pregnancy: a review. *New York State Dental Journal,* Vol. 70, No. 1, pp. 40-44.

Garcia-Closas, R., GarcIa-Closas, M. & Serra-Majem, L. (1997). A cross-sectional study of dental caries, intake of confectionery and foods rich in starch and sugars, and salivary counts of streptococcus mutans in children in Spain. *American Journal of Clinical Nutrition,* Vol, 66, pp. 1257-1263.

Ge, Y., Caufield, P.W., Fisch, G.S. & Li, Y. (2008). Streptococcus mutans and Streptococcus sanguinis Colonization Correlated with Caries Experience in Children. *Caries Research,* Vol. 42, pp. 444–448.

Genco, R.J. & Loe, H. (1993). The role of systemic conditions and disorders in periodontal disease. Periodontology 2000 Vol. 2, pp. 98-116

Glor, E.B., Miller, C.H. & Spandau, D.F. (1988). Degradation of starch and its hydrolytic products by oral bacteria. *Journal of Dental Research,* Vol. 67, pp. 75-81.

Goepfert, A.R., Jeffcoat, M.K., Andrews, W.W., Faye-Petersen, O., Cliver, S.P. & Goldenberg, R.L. et al. (2004). Periodontal disease and upper genital tract inflammation in early spontaneous preterm birth. *Obstetrics and Gynecology,* Vol. 104, No. 4, pp. 777-783.

Goose, D.H. (1967). Infant Feeding and Caries of the Incisors: an Epidemiological Approach, *Caries Research,* Vol. 1, pp. 167-173.

Grossi, S.G., Zambon, J.J., Ho, A.W., Koch, G., Dunford, R.G., Machtei, E.E., Norderyd, O.M. & Genco, R.J. (1994). Assessment of risk for periodontal disease. I. Risk indicators for attachment loss. Journal of Periodontology Vol. 65, pp. 260-267

Guidelines on Prevention of Early Childhood Caries (2008). *An EAPD Policy Document Approved by the EAPD Board November 2008.*

Habibian, M., Beighton, D., Stefenson, R. & Lawson, M. (2002). Relationship between dietary behaviors, oral hygiene and mutans streptococci in dental plaque of group of infants in southern England. *Archives of Oral Biology,* Vol. 6, pp. 491-498.

Hallonsten, A.L., Wendt, L.K., Mejar, I., Birkhed, D., Hakansson, C., Lindwall, A.M., Edwardsson, S. & Koch, G. (1995). Dental Caries and prolonged breast-feeding in

18-month- old. Swedish children. *International Journal of Pediatric Dentistry*, Vol. 5, No. 3, pp. 149-155.

Hinds, K. & Gregory, J.R. (1995). National diet and nutritional survey: Children aged 1-1/2 to 4-1/2 years. Vol.2: *Report of the dental survey*. London: HMSO.

Holbrook, W.P., Kristinsson, M.J., Gunnarsdóttir, S. & Briem, B. (1989). Caries prevalence, Streptococcus mutans and sugar intake among 4-year-old urban children in Iceland. *Community Dentistry and Oral Epidemiology*, Vol. 17, No. 6, pp. 292-295.

Holbrook, W.P. (1993). Dental caries and cariogenic factors in pre-school urban Icelandic children. Caries Research, Vol. 27, No. 5, pp. 431-437.

Holt, R.D., Winter, G.B., Downer, M.C. & Bellis, W.J. (1996). Caries in pre-school children in Camden 1993/94. *British Dental Journal*, Vol. 181, pp. 405-410.

Horning, G.M., Hatch, C.L. & Cohen, M.E. (1992). Risk indicators for periodontitis in a military treatment population. Journal of Periodontology Vol. 63, pp. 297-302.

Horowitz, H.S. (1998). Research issues in early childhood caries. *Community Dentistry and Oral Epidemiology*, Vol. 26, No. 1, pp. 67-81.

Hujoel, PP., Drangsholt, M., Spiekerman, C. & DeRouen, T.A. (2000). Periodontal disease and coronary heart disease risk. JAMA Vol. 284, pp. 1406-1410.

Hunt, R.J. (1986). Percent agreement, Pearson's correlation, and kappa as measures of inter-examiner reliability. *Journal of Dental Research*, Vol. 65, pp. 128-130.

Huseinbegović, A. (2001). Social and medical aspects of primary dentition caries in urban conditions. Master degree- Sarajevo.

Ismail, A.I. & Szpunar, S.M. (1990). Oral health status of Mexican-Americans with low and high acculturation status: findings from southwestern HHANES, 1982-84. Journal of Public Health Dentistry Vol. 50, pp. 24-31.

Ismail, A.I. (1998). Prevention of early childhood caries. *Community Dentistry and Oral Epidemiology*, Vol. 26, No. 1, pp. 49-61.

Ismail, A.I. & Sohn, W. (1999). A Systematic Review of Clinical Diagnostic Criteria of Early Childhood Caries. *Journal of Public Health Dentistry*, Vol. 59, No. 3, pp. 171-191.

James, P.M.C., Parfitt, G.J. & Falkner, F. (1957). A study of the aetiology of labial caries of the deciduous incisor teeth in small children. *British Dental Journal*, Vol. 103, No. 2, pp. 37–40.

Johnsen, D.C. (1982). Characteristics and backgrounds of children with "nursing caries." *Pediatric Dentistry*, Vol. 4, No. 3, pp. 218–224.

Jonsen, D. (1988). Pediatric Dentistry, Total Patient Care Philadelphia, Lee & Febiger.

Karn, T.A., O'Sullivan, D.M. & Tinannoff, N. (1988). Colonization of mutans streptococci in 8- to 15- month-old children. *Journal of Public Health Dentistry*, Vol. 58, No. 3, pp. 248-249.

Kaste, L.M. & Gift, H.C. (1995). Inappropriate infant bottle feeding. Status of the Healthy People 2000 Objective. *Archives of Pediatric and Adolescence Medicine*, Vol. 149, pp. 786-791.

Kaste, L.M., Selwitz, R.H., Oldakowski, R.J., Brunelle, J.A., Win, D.M. & Brown, L.J. (1996). Coronal Caries in the Primary and Permanent Dentition of Children and Adolescents 1-17 Years of Age: United States, 1988-1991, *Journal of Dental Research*, Vol. 75, Special No., pp. 631-641.

Kelly, M. & Bruerd, B. (1987). The prevalence of baby bottle tooth decay among two native American populations. *Journal of Public Health Dentistry*, Vol. 47, No. 2, pp. 94–97.

Kleinbaum, D.G., Kupper, L.L. & Morgenstern, H. (1982). Epidemiologic Research. Principles and quantitative methods, 1st ed. New York: Van Nostrand Reinhold.

Kneist, S., Laurisch, L. & Heinrich-Weltzein, R. (1999). Der neue CRT-Mikrobiologischer hintergrund zum nachweis von S. mutans. *Oralprophylaxe*, Vol. 21, pp. 180-185.

Kobaslia, S., Maglaic, N. & Begovic, A. (2000). Caries prevalence of Sarajevo children. *Acta Stomatologica Croatica*, Vol. 34, pp. 83-85.

Konig, K.G. & Navia, E.M. (1995). Nutritional role of sugars in oral health. *American Journal of Clinical Nutrition* Vol. 62, Suppl. pp. 275S-83S.

Kosovo Statistical Office. (2008). Women and men in Kosovo. Available at http://esk.rks-gov.net/publikimet/cat_view/8-statistikat-e-popullsise.html, Accessed 20 July 2011.

Köhler, B. & Andreen, I. (1984). Influence of caries-preventive measures in mothers on cariogenic bacteria and caries experience in their children. *Archives of Oral Biology*, Vol. 39, pp. 907-911.

Köhler, B., Andreen, I. & Jonsson, B. (1988). The earlier the colonization by mutans streptococci, the higher the caries prevalence at 4 years of age. *Oral Microbiology and Immunology*, Vol. 3, pp. 14-17.

Köhler, B., Bjarnason, S., Care, R., Mackevica, I. & Rence, I. (1995). Mutans streptococci and dental caries prevalence in a group of Latvian preschool children. *European Journal of Oral Sciences*, Vol. 103, No. 4, pp. 264-266.

Lewit, E.M. & Monheit, A.C. (1992). Expenditures on Health Care for Children and Pregnant Women. *Future Child*, Vol. 2, No. 2, pp. 95-114.

Li, Y., Navia, J.M. & Caufield, P.W. (1994). Colonization by mutans streptococci in mouths of 3- and 4- year -old Chinese children with or without enamel hypoplasia. *Archives of Oral Biology*, Vol. 39. No. 12, pp. 1057-1062.

Li, Y., Wang, W. & Caufield, P.W. (2000). The fidelity of mutans streptococci transmission and caries status correlate with breast-feeding experience among chinese families. *Caries Research*, Vol. 34, pp. 123–132.

Lingstrom, P., Birkhed, D., Granfeldt, Y. & Björck, I. (1993). pH measurements of human dental plaque after consumption of starchy foods using the micro-touch and the sampling method. *Caries Research*, Vol. 27, pp. 394-401.

Lopez, L., Berkowitz, R.J., Moss, M.E. & Weinstein, P. (2000). Mutans streptotocci prevalence in Puerto Rican babies with cariogenic feeding behaviors. *Pediatric Dentistry*, Vol. 22, No. 4, pp. 299–301.

Maciel, S.M., Marcenes, W. & Sheiham, A. (2001). The relationship between sweetness preference, levels of salivary mutans streptococci and caries experience in Brazilian pre-school children. *International Journal of Paediatric Dentistry*, Vol. 11, pp. 123-130.

Marthaler, T.M. (1990). Changes in the prevalence of dental caries: how much can be attributed to changes in diet? Diet, nutrition and dental caries. *Caries Research*, Vol. 24, Suppl. l, pp. 3-15.

Marthaler, M., O'Mullane, M. & Vrbic, V. (1996). The prevalence of dental caries in Europe 1990-1995. *Caries Research*, Vol. 30, pp. 237-255.

Massler M, Cohen A, Shour I (1952). Epidemiology of gingivitis in children. J Am Dent Assoc , Vol. 45, pp. 319-324.

Matee, M.I., Mikx, F.H., Maselle, S.Y. & Van Palenstein-Helderman, W.H. (1992). Mutans streptococci and lactobacilli in breast-fed children with rampant caries. *Caries Research*, Vol. 26, pp. 183–187.

Matilla, M.L., Rautava, P., Sillanpaa, M. & Paunio, P. (2000). Caries in Five-year-old Children and Associations with Family-related Factors. *Journal of Dental Research* Vol. 79, No. 3, pp. 875-881.

Mazhari, F., Talebi, M. & Zoghi, M. (2007). Prevalence of Early Childhood Caries and its Risk Factors in 6-60 months old Children in Quchan, *Dental Research Journal*, Vol. 4, No. 2, pp. 96-101.

McGregor, J.A., French, J.I., Lawellin, D. & Todd, J.K. (1988). Preterm birth and infection: pathogenic possibilities. *American Journal of Reproductive Immunology* Vol. 16, pp. 123-132.

Meqa, K. (2007). Relationship between periodontal disease and preterm low birth weight. Masters degree, University of Prishtina Dentistry School.

Milgrom, P., Riedy, C.A., Weinstein, P., Tanner, A.C., Manibusan, L. & Bruss, J. (2000). Dental caries and its relationship to bacterial infection, hypoplasia, diet, and oral hygiene in 6- to 36-month-old children. *Community Dentistry and Oral Epidemiology*, Vol. 28, No. 4, pp. 295-306.

Ministry of Public Administration. Statistical Office of Kosovo. (http://esk.rks-gov.net/eng/index.php?option=com_docman&task=doc_download&gid=870&Itemid=8). Accessed on October 20th, 2010.

Mohan, A.M., O'Sallivan, D.M. & Tinanoff, N. (1998). The relationship between bottle usage/content, age and number of teeth with mutans streptococci colonization in 6-24 – month-old children. *Community Dentistry and Oral Epidemiology* Vol. 26, Suppl. 1, pp. 12-20.

Newbrun, E. (1982). Sugar and dental caries: a review of human studies. *Science*, Vol. 217, No. 4558, pp. 418–423.

Norman, O.H. & Franklin, G. (1999). *Primary Preventive Dentistry*. Appleton & Lange, Stamford, Connecticut.

Offenbacher, S., Katz, V., Fertik, G., Collins, J., Boyd, D., Maynor, G., McKaig, R. & Beck, J. (1996). Periodontal infection as a possible risk factor for preterm low birth weight. *Journal of Periodontology* Vol. 67, pp. 1103-1113.

O'Sullivan, D.M. & Tinanoff, N. (1993). Social and biological factors contributing to caries of the maxillary anterior teeth. *Pediatr Dent Vol.* 15, pp. 41-44.

Ölmez, S., Uzamis, M. & Erdem, G. (2003). Association between early childhood caries and clinical, microbiological, oral hygiene and dietary variables in rural Turkish children. *The Turkish Journal of Pediatrics*, Vol. 45, pp. 231-236.

Page, R.C., Bowen, T., Altman, L., Vandesteen, E., Ochs, H., Mackenzie, P., Osterberg, S., Engel, L.D. & Williams, B.L. (1983). Prepubertal periodontitis. I. Definition of a clinical disease entity. *Journal of Periodontology* Vol. 54, pp. 257-271.

Plat, L. & Cebazas, M.C. (2000). Early childhood dental caries. Building community system for young children. Los Angeles, CA: University of California-Los Angeles Center for Healthier Children, Families and Communities, Vol. 32, exec. summ. (4 pp.).

Plotziza, B., Kneist, S., Berger, J. & Hetzer, G. (2002). Occurrence of salivary S. mutans in one-year old children: Poster ORCA.

Reagan, L. (2002). Big Bad Cavities: Breastfeeding Is Not the Cause. *Mothering* Vol. 113 (July/August).

Reisine, S. & Douglass, J.M. (1998). Psychosocial and behavioral issues in early childhood caries. *Community Dentistry and Oral Epidemiolology*, Vol. 26, No. 1, pp. 32-44.

Ripa, L.W. (1988). Nursing caries: a comprehensive review. *Pediatric Dentistry*, Vol. 10, pp. 268-282.

Romero, R., Chaiworapongsa, T., Kuivaniemi, H. & Tromp, G. (2004). Bacterial vaginosis, the inflammatory response and the risk of preterm birth: a role for genetic epidemiology in the prevention of preterm birth. *American Journal of Obstetrics and Gynecology*, Vol. 190, No. 6, pp. 1509-1519.

Rosamund, L.H. & Tracy, W. (2003). An oral health promotion program for an urban minority population of preschool children. *Community Dentistry and Oral Epidemiolology*, Vol. 31, No. 5, pp. 392-399.

Rugg-Gunn, A.J. (1993). *Nutrition and dental health.* Oxford, United Kingdom: Oxford University Press.

Seow, W.K. (1998). Biological mechanisms of early childhood caries. *Community Dentistry and Oral Epidemiolology*, Vol. 26, No. 1, pp. 8-27.

Serwint, J.R., Mungo, R., Negrete, V.F., Duggan, A.K. & Korsch, B.M. (1993). Child-rearing practices and nursing caries. *Pediatrics*, Vol. 92, pp. 233-237.

Sheiham, A. & Netuveli, G. (2002). Periodontal diseases in Europe. *Periodontol 2000*, Vol. 29, pp. 104-121.

Soames, J.V. & Southam, J.C. (1999). *Oral Pathology.* 3rd ed. Oxford.

Tinanoff, N., Kaste, L.M. & Corbin, S.B. (1998). Early childhood caries: a positive beginning. *Community Dentistry and Oral Epidemiolology*, Vol. 26, No. 1, pp. 117-119.

Thakib, A., et al. (1997). Primary incisor decay before age 4 as a risk factor for future dental caries. *Paediatric Dentistry*, Vol. 9, pp. 37-41.

Tomar, S.L. & Asma, S. (2000). Smoking-attributable periodontitis in the United States: findings from NHANES III. National Health and Nutrition Examination Survey. *Journal of Periodontology* Vol. 71, pp. 743-751.

Twetman, S. & Frostner, N. (1991). Salivary mutans streptococci and caries prevalence in 8-year-old Swedish schoolchildren. *Swedish Dental Journal*, Vol. 15, No. 3, pp. 145-151.

US Department of Health and Human Services. (2000). *Oral Health in America*: A Report of the Surgeon General. Rockville, MD: US Department of Health and Human Services, National Institute of Dental and Craniofacial Research, National Institutes of Health.

Weintraub, J.A. (1999). Prevention of early childhood caries: a public health perspective. *Community Dentistry and Oral Epidemiolology*, Vol. 26, Suppl. 1, pp. 62-66.

Wendt, L.K., Hallonstein, A.L. & Koch, G. (1991). Dental caries in one- and two-year-old children living in Sweden. Part I – A longitudinal study. *Swedish Dental Journal*, Vol. 15, No. 1, pp. 1–6.

Wendt, L.K. (1995). On oral health in infants and toddlers. *Swedish Dental Journal*, Vol. 19, Suppl., pp. 106:1-62.

Wendy, E. & Mouradian, M.D. (2001). The Face of a Child: Children's Oral Health and Dental Education. *Journal of Dental Education.* Volume 65, No. 9, pp. 821-831.

Winslow, C.E. (1920). The untitled fields of public health. *Modern Medicine* Vol. 2, p. 183.

Winter, G.B., Hamilton, M.C. & James, P.M.C. (1966). Role of comforter as en etiological factor in rampant caries of deciduous dentition. *Archives of Diseases in Children*, Vol. 417, pp. 207 212.

Whittle, J.G. & Whittle, K.W. (1988). Household income in relation to dental health and dental health behaviors: the use of super profiles. *Community Dental Health*, Vol. 15, pp. 150-154.

World Health Organization (1997). *Oral Health surveys.* Basic Methods (4th ed.), World Health Organization, Geneva.

World Health Organization (2008). *The World Oral Health Report 2003.* Continuous improvement of oral health in the 21st century – the approach of the WHO Global Oral Health Programme, http://www.who.int/oral_health/media/en/orh_report03_en.pdf. Accessed October 15th, 2010.

World Health Organization (2010). http://www.who.int/oral_health/strategies/hp/en/index.html. Accessed October 15th, 2010.

Wyne, A.H. (1999). Early childhood caries: nomenclature and case definition. *Community Dentistry and Oral Epidemiology*, Vol. 7, pp. 313-315.

Zhang, Q., van't Hof, M.A. & Truin, G.J. (2006). Caries-inhibiting effect of chlorhexidine varnish in pits and fissures. *Journal of Dental Research*, Vol. 85, pp.469–472.

Early Childhood Caries: Parent's Knowledge, Attitude and Practice Towards Its Prevention in Malaysia

Shani Ann Mani[1], Jacob John[3], Wei Yen Ping[2] and Noorliza Mastura Ismail[4]
[1]Universiti Sains Malaysia,
[2]Formerly Universiti Sains Malaysia,
[3]University of Malaya,
[4]Melaka Manipal Medical College
Malaysia

1. Introduction

Early childhood caries (ECC) is defined as the presence of 1 or more decayed, missing or filled tooth surfaces in any primary tooth in a child 71 months or younger (Drury et al., 1999). ECC is the most common chronic disease in young children and may develop as soon as teeth erupt (Douglass et al., 2004). It is a significant public health problem and certain segments of society, such as the socially disadvantaged have the highest burden of disease (Vargas & Ronzio, 2006). In the US, although prevalence of caries was decreasing overall, the severity was increasing in these groups of people (Douglass et al., 2002).

A number of risk factors are associated with ECC, which can be broadly classified into biological and social risk factors (Berg & Slayton, 2009). Biological risk factors include nutritional variables, feeding habits and early colonization of cariogenic micro-organisms. Social risk factors comprise low parental education, low socio-economic status and lack of awareness about dental disease (Hallett & O'Rourke, 2003). ECC affects the quality of life of families and their affected children due to dental pain and subsequent tooth loss resulting in difficulty in eating, speaking, sleeping and socializing (Edelstein et al., 2006; Pahel et al., 2007). Treatment of ECC has numerous inherent difficulties. It is costly (Casamassimo et al., 2009; Kanellis et al., 2000) and takes up time of the child and caretaker (Casamassimo et al., 2009; Vargas & Ronzio, 2006). Not all dentists are trained to handle children and many general practitioners are not keen to treat young children (Vargas & Ronzio, 2006). Treatment necessitates extensive rehabilitation under general anaesthesia and recurrence rates of caries are high thus requiring retreatment (Almeida et al., 2000; Tate et al., 2002). Hence the dental profession favours a preventive approach towards management of ECC (Ismail, 2003; Vargas & Ronzio, 2006). The earliest form of prevention can be achieved by educating parents and primary caregivers about ECC. Preventive guidelines towards ECC are found in many countries and most have their own individualized programs which aim at training parents to recognize ECC early and seek treatment. Anticipatory guidance is one of the approaches used at antenatal visits and for new mothers (Meyer et al.; Plutzer & Spencer,

2008). Age-one dental visit (Savage et al., 2004) and "Lift-the-lip" training are undertaken in some countries as an approach to identify ECC at its earlier stages (Alexander & Mazza).

Establishing good oral health in the early years is important for a lifetime of good oral health (Clarke et al., 2001). Tooth brushing activity fell far short of professional expectations in parents and toddlers when observed using home-based videotaped sessions, although parents thought the sessions were effective in achieving clean teeth (Zeedyk et al., 2005). Hence, improving oral hygiene in early childhood requires that mothers' own tooth brushing habits and their infant oral cleaning skills are improved (Mohebbi et al., 2008). Infant feeding practices were also found to be poor in South East-Asian countries like Taiwan (Tsai et al., 2006), Myanmar (van Palenstein Helderman et al., 2006) and Korea (Jin et al., 2003) with increased indulgence to between-meal snacks, sweetened solution in nursing bottle, sweets and prechewed rice. Many studies have concluded that parents are in definite need of advice on feeding and oral hygiene practices (Singh & King, 2003). Prevention is the key for ECC, and can be achieved successfully by knowledgeable and efficacious caregivers (Finlayson et al., 2005). It is suggested that other models for disease initiation and progression needs to be explored besides known risk factors such as poor oral hygiene and diet control (Hallett, 2000). Children living in stressful environments or without parental support could be at a higher risk for developing ailments such as dental caries (Mattila et al., 2000). The family dynamics can play a major role in the oral health of children (Da Silva, 2007).

Oral health literacy is the degree to which individuals have the capacity to obtain, process, and understand basic oral health information and services needed to make appropriate health decisions (Berg & Slayton, 2009). Parents' literacy in oral health is an important factor contributing to the overall health of children (Da Silva, 2007). Caregivers of children with ECC were more likely to believe that caries could not affect a child's health while those who believed primary teeth are important had children with significantly less decay (Schroth et al., 2007). Parental knowledge about infant oral health was found to be lacking in many studies (Blinkhorn et al., 2001; Gussy et al., 2008; Hoeft et al., 2010; Orenuga & Sofola, 2005; Singh & King, 2003). The factors associated with decreased knowledge and poor attitudes among primary caregivers of children include low socioeconomic status (Dykes et al., 2002; Finlayson et al., 2007), living in deprived areas (Silver, 1992; Williams et al., 2002), ethnicity or immigrant status (Skaret et al., 2008; Williams et al., 2002), lack of further education (Szatko et al., 2004; Williams et al., 2002), high caries status in the children (Szatko et al., 2004) and difficult past dental experience (Tickle et al., 2003) among others. However, oral health specific self efficacy and knowledge measures are potentially modifiable cognitions and interventions can lead to healthy dental habits (Finlayson et al., 2007).

Oral health surveys of 5 year-old and 6-year-old pre-school children in Malaysia showed a high caries prevalence of 76.2% and 74.5% in 2005 and 2007 respectively (Oral Health Division, 2007, 2009). With the existence of the preschool program since 1984 (Oral Health Division, 2003) and the program for antenatal mothers since early 1970's (Oral Health Division, 2004) among other strategies, Malaysia aims to achieve its objective of 50% caries-free 6-year-old's by 2020 (Talib, 2010). Since infants and toddlers are not in control of their oral health, the parental role is of utmost importance. We hypothesize that the problem of high prevalence of ECC in Malaysia may to be due to poor knowledge, attitudes and practice towards factors associated with ECC. So far, one study done in Serdang, Malaysia found that parents of children with early childhood caries had adequate knowledge and positive attitude towards maintaining satisfactory dental care in their pre-school children

(Syahrial et al., 1995). However, practice among these parents was not evaluated. The aim of this study was to assess the existing knowledge, attitude and practice of early childhood oral health related factors among parents of infants and toddlers in Kelantan, Malaysia.

2. Materials and methods

A thirty-item close-ended questionnaire, consisting of ten items each addressing knowledge, attitudes and practice of early childhood oral health related factors was designed jointly by the research group which included a pediatric dentist and community dental health specialist. All aspects of early childhood oral health including oral development, diet, nursing habits, oral hygiene habits, fluoride, transmissibility of oral bacteria, importance of primary teeth and attitude towards acquiring new knowledge were addressed in the questionnaire. The scoring in the knowledge domain included true/false/don't know component, while the attitude and practice domain used a 5 point and 4 point Likert scale respectively. Some items in the practice domain did not follow the likert scale. A section for socio demographic data was included at the beginning of the questionnaire to assess the socioeconomic status, educational level and occupation of the primary caretakers. The questionnaire was constructed in English and later translated into Bahasa Malaysia, the local language and back-translated to English. The instrument was pretested on 5 randomly selected subjects before the conduct of the study.

In this cross sectional study, 120 parents of infants and toddlers aged 6 months-2 years attending four public Maternal and child health care clinics in the state of Kelantan, Malaysia were randomly selected and invited to participate in the study. Children are usually brought by parents to these centers for immunization. Inclusion criteria were parents of normal healthy children aged between 6 months and 2 years who were the primary caretakers of their children. Parents who were not the primary caretakers of the children or who had children with medical problems were excluded. After obtaining written consent from the participants, the self administered questionnaires were given out. The participants were requested to return the questionnaires immediately upon completion. The subjects who required help in reading were assisted. The ethical clearance was obtained from the Human Ethics Committee of Universiti Sains Malaysia. The data was entered into SPSS software, version 12.0 (SPSS Inc, Chicago, 2001) for analysis.

3. Results

A total of 102 out of 120 questionnaires were returned (response rate of 85%). The demographic data of the respondents is presented in Table 1. The majority of the respondents were female (92%), Malay (99%), and homemakers (71%). Sixty nine percent had secondary education and 45% were in the moderate income group.

Table 2 shows the response of the participants to ten knowledge questions. While majority of parents (92%) knew when the first tooth erupted in the mouth, not that many (62%) were sure of when all the 20 teeth should be present in their child's mouth. About half of the parents knew (49%) that caries can affect infants below 2 years old. Almost all respondents knew the types of food causing dental caries and the importance of brushing children's teeth. Fewer parents (81%) knew that children's mouth should be cleaned before teeth erupted. About 78% of the parents knew that weaning from the bottle should start at 1 year of age. Most parents (85%) knew that fluoride is important for preventing tooth decay and about half of them (52%) knew that they should start using toothpaste with fluoride for cleaning their child's teeth when the child learns to spit. Sixty four percent knew that it is necessary to do fillings in their baby's teeth.

Variables			n	(%)
Sex	Male		10	(9.8)
	Female		92	(90.2)
Ethnicity	Malay		99	(97.1)
	Chinese		3	(2.9)
Age in years	Range -	19-42		
	Mean -	31.8		
	Mode -	34		
Marital Status	Married		101	(99)
	Single		1	(1)
Occupation	Male	working outside the home	10	(9.8)
	Female-	Homemaker	72	(70.6)
		Working outside the home	18	(19.6)
Household income*	Low income (<RM 699)		38	(37.3)
	Moderate income (RM 700-1611)		46	(45.1)
	High income (> RM1612)		18	(17.6)
Educational level	Primary		12	(11.8)
	Secondary		70	(68.6)
	Tertiary		20	(19.6)

* Income group classification based on The 8th Malaysian Plan
  RM- Ringgit Malaysia

Table 1. Demographic data of the participants

Table 3 shows the attitude of the respondents to early childhood oral health related factors. The responses 'strongly agree' and 'agree' & 'disagree' and 'strongly disagree' were grouped together. About 22% and 43% of the parents thought that children should visit the dentist at 1 year and 3 years respectively, while 25% thought that it is sufficient to visit the dentist when there is a problem such as pain (data not shown). Almost all parents also agreed that a balanced diet is important for healthy teeth. Most parents (73%) thought that tooth decay is not caused by bacteria that are transmitted by sharing feeding utensils and 49% of them thought that night time bottle/breast feeding cannot cause tooth decay. More than half of them (64%) thought that frequent and prolonged breast/bottle feeding in the day time cannot cause tooth decay. Fifty two percent thought that effective cleaning of teeth can be achieved by the child him/herself. Many (46%) were not aware that swallowing of toothpaste can be harmful to a child's health. Seventy percent of parents agreed that pacifier use can affect the normal development of children's teeth.

Knowledge items	True (T) n(%)		Don't know(N) n(%)		False (F) n(%)	
Tooth decay can affect infants below 2 years of age	50	(49.0)	11	(10.5)	41	(40.2)
When does the first baby tooth appear the child's mouth?	94	(92.2)	4	(3.9)	4	(3.9)
Your child will have a complete set of 20 milk teeth by the age of…	62	(62.0)	11	(10.8)	29	(28.4)
The main types of food that can cause tooth decay are..	101	(99.0)	1	(1.0)	0	(00.0)
Weaning from a baby bottle to a sipping cup should be planned when the child is …	80	(78.4)	6	(5.9)	16	(15.7)
Cleaning your baby's mouth after each should begin even before teeth erupt.	83	(81.4)	6	(5.9)	13	(12.7)
Brushing your baby's teeth is important for oral health.	102	(100)	0	(00.0)	0	(00.0)
Fluoride in toothpaste is important for preventing tooth decay.	87	(85.3)	11	(10.8)	4	(3.9)
You should start using toothpaste with fluoride for cleaning your child's teeth:…	53	(52.0)	12	(11.8)	37	(36.3)
It is not necessary to do fillings in baby's teeth.	24	(23.5)	13	(12.7)	65	(63.7)

Table 2. Knowledge of the respondents

Attitude items	Strongly disagree /Disagree n (%)		Don't know n (%)		Strongly agree/Agree n (%)	
Tooth decay is caused by bacteria that are transmitted by sharing feeding utensils (eg: spoon)	74	(72.6)	9	(8.8)	19	(18.6)
When do you think you should take your baby for a dental check up after the teeth erupt?	25	(24.5)	11	(10.8)	66	(64.7)
A balance diet is essential for the healthy growth of a baby's teeth	1	(1.00)	3	(2.9)	98	(96.1)
Night time bottle/breast feeding can cause tooth decay	50	(49.0)	18	(17.6)	34	(33.3)
Frequent and prolonged breast/bottle feeding in the day time can cause tooth decay	65	(63.7)	17	(16.7)	20	(19.6)
A child`s teeth should be cleaned/brushed as soon as the teeth erupt	8	(7.9)	4	(3.9)	90	(88.3)
Effective cleaning of teeth can be achieved by the child him/herself	45	(44.2)	4	(3.9)	53	(51.9)
Swallowing of fluoride toothpaste can be harmful to a child's health	47	(46.1)	32	(31.4)	23	(22.5)
It is important for a child to visit the dentist before 2 years old.	24	(23.5)	16	(15.7)	62	(60.8)
Prolonged used of pacifier can affect the normal development of a child's teeth.	14	(13.7)	17	(16.7)	71	(69.6)

Table 3. Attitude of the respondents

Table 4 summarizes the practice of early childhood oral health related behaviors among parents. Fourteen percent of parents never examined their children's mouth. A considerable number of parents (67.6%) practiced biting food into small pieces before giving the child. There were only 11.8% of the parents who never bought sweetened food for their baby. About half of the parents (45%) gave sweetened liquid or juice in the bottle to their children.

About 47% of the parents always practiced giving plain water after feeding the child. Semisolid food was started at one year of age in 38% of the children. Sixty percent of parents regularly brushed their children's' teeth and 11% used full brush length amount of toothpaste to brush their child's teeth.

Practice items	Never n (%)		Sometimes n (%)		Often n (%)		Always n (%)	
Do you bite the food into small pieces before giving to your child?	33	(32.4)	44	(43.1)	12	(11.8)	13	(12.7)
How often do you examine the mouth of your baby?	14	(13.7)	47	(46.1)	17	(16.7)	24	(23.5)
How often do you buy sweetened food for your child?	12	(11.8)	80	(78.4)	7	(6.9)	3	(2.9)
How often do you give sweetened liquid/juice to baby in bottle?	56	(54.9)	35	(34.3)	7	(6.9)	4	(3.9)
How often do you give plain water after each feed?	5	(4.9)	16	(15.7)	33	(32.4)	48	(47.1)
When did you start semisolid food for your child?	16	(15.7)	16	(15.7)	39	(38.2)	31	(30.4)
How often do you brush your baby's teeth?	2	(2.00)	12	(11.8)	27	(26.5)	61	(59.8)
How much toothpaste do you use to brush your child`s teeth?	3	(2.90)	11	(10.8)	46	(45.1)	42	(41.2)
Do you use pacifier dipped into sweet liquid for your child?	100	(98.0)	0	(00.0)	1	(1.00)	1	(1.00)
Do you take the effort to improve your dental health knowledge?	13	(12.7)	37	(36.3)	8	(7.8)	44	(43.1)

Table 4. Practice of the respondents

4. Discussion

Oral disease, predominantly caries in young children can be prevented to a great extent if parents are sufficiently educated and motivated. Oral health literacy is one of the important factors affecting oral health. Poor health literacy is associated with poorer perceptions of health, decreased utilization of services and poorer understanding of verbal and written instructions of self-care (Jackson, 2006; Yin et al., 2009). Maternal attitude is significantly correlated to the oral health of their children (Abiola Adeniyi et al., 2009; Wigen et al.,2011). Parents of caries-free children had more positive beliefs and attitudes than those with caries when studied over a period of time (Skaret et al., 2008). Hence the assessment of knowledge, attitude and practice among primary caretakers of young children can indicate knowledge areas that are deficient and attitudes and practices that are erroneous.

In this study, 99% of parents knew the types of food that can cause tooth decay, yet, 45% of parents gave sweetened liquid in the bottle. In addition, about 49% parents disagreed that nighttime bottle/breastfeeding can cause dental caries and 64 % did not think that frequent daytime bottle/breast feeding caused tooth decay. It is apparent that parents knew that sugars in the diet can cause dental caries, but were not aware of hidden sugars and their effects. In other studies, urban Mexican American and immigrant Latino mothers rarely recognized cariogenic food beyond candy and demonstrated uncertainty as to how exactly bottle feeding is detrimental to oral health (Hoeft et al., 2010; Horton & Barker, 2008). In another study, ninety eight percent of children had juice in bottles or sippy cups (Southward et al., 2006). In Hong Kong, 60% gave fruit juices in bottles, some consuming non-diary products more than six times per day (Chan et al., 2002). Bottle feeding was also highly prevalent in the above study, with majority having the bottle at naptime. Generally, parents of children with ECC were significantly more likely to disagree that nighttime nursing was safe, proving that knowledge among parents is high, but not reflected in the dental health of their children (Schroth et al., 2007). In another study, parents had good knowledge of diet related risk factors, but half the children where given bottle at bedtime (Gussy et al., 2008). However, poor knowledge was noted in Wu-Han, China (Petersen & Esheng, 1998) where only 42% of mothers knew that dental caries is caused by sugar while only 39% of mothers in Romania (Petersen et al., 1995) knew that dental caries is caused by sugar. In most studies, few could identify the diet with hidden sugars (Hoeft et al., 2010; Horton & Barker, 2008; Petersen et al., 1995).

Prolonged duration of bottle use put a population of low income Latino preschool children at increased risk for ECC (Hoeft et al., 2010). In our study, almost one–third (32%) of mothers initiated semisolid food after 1 and half years of age and 15.7% thought that bottle should be stopped after two and half years, indicating prolonged bottle/breast feeding beyond the recommended 1 year of age. Hence, this population is clearly at risk for ECC, but this could not be confirmed since no clinical examination was done. Similar findings of prolonged bottle feeding up to 2 years in 73% of the children were also reported from Hong Kong (Chan et al., 2002). Yet in another study, the children were weaned from the bottle during the day, but continued nighttime bottle feeding (Riedy et al., 2001). Another Asian study showed an increased risk for ECC due to prolonged duration of breast-feeding (van Palenstein Helderman et al., 2006). In some studies, mothers indicated that other caregivers encourage use of the bottle/sugar in diet when the mothers were away at work, even though mothers were not in favor of such practices (Amin & Harrison, 2009; Riedy et al., 2001).

Customarily, oral health education messages refer to kissing and sharing of utensils as the primary method of vertical transmission of oral bacteria. Knowledge of transmissibility of oral bacteria is minimal in this study population since 72.6% disagreed that bacteria can be transmitted by sharing feeding utensils. In addition, 67.6% of parents practiced biting hard food into small pieces before giving it to the child. Tasting food before giving it to the child was practiced at least sometimes by most respondents in rural Australia (Gussy et al., 2008). Mothers also did not mention the role of bacteria in other studies (Gussy et al., 2008; Hoeft et al., 2010). On the other hand, mother's of children who underwent treatment of ECC under GA showed better knowledge of oral bacteria in the etiology of ECC (Amin & Harrison, 2009).

Cleaning a child's mouth should begin before teeth erupt and tooth brushing is recommended when the first tooth erupts at least once daily till 2 years and subsequently twice daily (Berg & Slayton, 2009). Generally, mothers with higher confidence in brushing their children's teeth and with higher frequency of brushing themselves had children with cleaner teeth (Gussy et al., 2008; Mohebbi et al., 2008). Those children who started tooth brushing earlier also have less caries (Chan et al., 2002). In this study, it was very encouraging to note that all parents in this study knew that brushing is important for baby's teeth, 81.4% parents knew that a baby's mouth should be cleaned even before the teeth erupt, 88% agreed that they should brush their baby's teeth as soon as it erupted. About 60% and 27% of the parents reported brushing their child's teeth twice and once daily respectively. However, 52% thought that effective cleaning can be achieved by the children themselves. Similar results were seen in other studies (Gussy et al., 2008). Most children aged 3 years and below in another study were allowed to brush their own teeth (Chan et al., 2002). Many studies have revealed that most mothers are aware that poor oral hygiene is a cause for caries (Blinkhorn et al., 2001; Gussy et al., 2008; Hoeft et al., 2010; Szatko et al., 2004), while other studies discovered that mothers did not place enough emphasis on tooth cleaning (Hood et al., 1998). Tooth brushing was reportedly delayed in some instances, where child temperament did not allow the parent clean teeth (Blinkhorn et al., 2001; Hoeft et al., 2010; Riedy et al., 2001).

Generally, the use of fluoridated toothpastes was known by mothers as useful in preventing tooth decay (Gussy et al., 2008; Schroth et al., 2007; Szatko et al., 2004). Studies have shown that many parents are not clear as to whether fluoride should be used in young children and how much should be used (Blinkhorn et al., 2001; Gussy et al., 2008). Our study showed that 85.3% of parents knew that fluoride in toothpaste is important for preventing caries in teeth, however, 46% disagreed that swallowing of fluoride toothpaste is harmful to the health and 31% were not sure of its harmful effects. Forty one percent and 45% used smear and pea-size amount of toothpaste respectively, while 11% used full length toothpaste. Hence, majority of the parents were familiar with the correct amount of toothpaste to be used. This could be due to the fact that most fluoridated toothpaste tubes have printed instructions on the cover which are easy to follow, but the rationale behind the guidelines are not apparent to the parents, since they were not aware of the harmful effect of the fluoride. Majority of the respondents used the correct amount to toothpaste in other studies also (Gussy et al., 2008), while only 41% used pea-size amount in another study (Blinkhorn et al., 2001). In Wu-Han China, only 43% of mothers knew that dental caries can be prevented by fluoride (Petersen & Esheng, 1998).

Attitudes towards importance of primary teeth vary among parents. In rural Australia (Gussy et al., 2008), all parents agreed that their child's teeth were important, while in Manitoba (Schroth et al., 2007), 4.2% disagreed that primary teeth are important. In our study, 63.7% of parents knew that it is necessary to do fillings in baby's teeth, similarly, almost half of the mothers (47%) wanted their child's decayed teeth to be filled in the UK (Blinkhorn et al., 2001). On the other hand, another study in the UK revealed that only 6% of mothers wanted their child's asymptomatic primary tooth to be filled (Tickle et al., 2003), and two-thirds of mothers in Poland opined that care of deciduous teeth was unnecessary (Szatko et al., 2004).

In Malaysia, community programs to promote oral health instituted by the Ministry of Health are in place for a number of years, for example: school dental service (started from 1950) and oral health care for antenatal mothers program (since 1970s) (Oral Health Division, 2004). All subjects (ages range from 19-41) in this study should have undergone at least one dental health program at some time or the other and this explained the higher levels of knowledge when compared to some other studies. In July 2008, the Oral health division of the Ministry of health Malaysia launched the Early Childhood Oral Healthcare program with the slogan 'Never too early to start' (Oral Health Division, 2008). The primary target group was primary health care providers with the aim of educating parents attending the public health clinics, childcare providers and health personnel about early childhood oral health. The objective of this program was to create awareness of various preventive aspects of early childhood oral health, early dental visit at age one, improved dietary and nursing habits, oral hygiene habits to be inculcated in early childhood and the appropriate use of fluoride. Early identification of ECC was encouraged using the 'lift the lip' examination of maxillary anterior teeth and further referrals encouraged. Since this is a recently launched program, the full outcome is unlikely to have taken full effect at the time of this study.

The results of this study show that knowledge is not necessarily translated into good practices, indicating lack of motivation among parents (Berkowitz, 2003), as seen in other studies (Amin & Harrison, 2009; Rajab et al., 2002; Syahrial et al., 1995) . Cultural practices specific to the region can be one of the obstacles to improvement in attitudes and oral health practices among the public (Amin & Harrison, 2009; Ismail, 2003). Different cultural backgrounds should be evaluated in separate cultural contexts (Skaret et al., 2008). Certain practices exist over many generations and remain persistent, many times overriding information obtained through books, media pamphlets, brochures and advertisements. In one study, prolonged breast feeding was practiced in Pohnpean women for purposes of birth control (Riedy et al., 2001). Weaning from the bottle was at 2-3 years, since it was child-centered and not based on knowledge gained through other sources (Riedy et al., 2001). In one study, professional advice regarding dietary practices was considered unrealistic and too complicated and believed that sugars had an important place in the life of the child (Amin & Harrison, 2009). In our study, it was noted that parents had the habit of biting hard food into smaller pieces before giving it to the child. A similar practice of mothers feeding their children rice that was pre-chewed by them for 20 seconds has been reported in a previous study and is probably a cultural practice of the south-east Asian region. In the above mentioned Myanmar community, ECC was considered inevitable and parents were not aware of the etiology (van Palenstein Helderman et al., 2006). Hence culturally appropriate and targeted strategies aimed at these modifiable practices need to be wisely promoted so that the oral health burden carried by these children can be reduced (Amin & Harrison, 2009; Schluter et al., 2007).

Other reasons for poor attitude and practice may be varied viz, inadequate time to deal with children, in cases of working parents, single mothers or large families and other social problems. This is in line with other studies which found that social problems can be a causative factor for caries and the family dynamics is an important aspect to be considered with regard to ECC (Amin & Harrison, 2009; Mattila et al., 2000). This is one aspect of ECC that needs to be further explored. One of the problems faced by parents of the 21st century is the free access of sweets to young children, either through close family and friends or through pocket money obtained by the children at an early age (Roberts et al., 2003). Hence a considerable majority of the parents have less control when it comes to the intake of sweets of their children. However, this may not apply to ECC, where the child is too young to exert his/her own independence. Furthermore, with modern day media exposure, commercials can distort or convey contradicting messages to the public, leaving them perplexed, which may explain why 52% of parents thought that effective cleaning of teeth can be achieved by the child himself/herself. On the other hand, we can assume that the public is not informed about details of prevention, for example: implicating that sweetened food causes caries but not being aware that feeding milk at night (which has hidden sugar) can also cause caries. These facts point to the need for further and continued dental awareness programs, highlighting more accurate and detailed information on preventive measures.

The limitation of this study was the small number of subjects. Further studies with larger samples can help clarify and motivate necessary policy changes. In addition, as stated by Hawley and Holloway (Hawley & Holloway, 1994), this approach to assess knowledge, attitude and practice can be notoriously inaccurate, for when approached face to face by a professional person; subjects will attempt to say what they knew, rather than what is in fact practiced.

5. Conclusion

We concluded that parents showed relatively good knowledge, but poor attitude and practice towards the oral health of their children. It is possible that parents are not informed about the details of oral disease and how it is caused. As previously suggested, in-depth education about caries etiology is more likely to bring about behavior change in parents (Hoeft et al., 2010). Consequently, more effort is required to improve knowledge, attitude and practice of oral health among parents and caretakers. However, some aspects of knowledge were better than other countries, especially knowledge about dietary factors causing caries. Health education should focus on parental responsibilities for oral health and mothers should be encouraged to give practical and emotional support to their children with regard to oral hygiene habits. Cultural practices of this region were evident in the practices of this population. Focus on modifying these behaviours will require considerable effort on the part of health educationists. Further studies should assess social concerns and study family dynamics.

6. References

Abiola Adeniyi, A., Eyitope Ogunbodede, O., Sonny Jeboda, O., & Morenike Folayan, O. (2009). Do Maternal Factors Influence the Dental Health Status of Nigerian Pre-

School Children? *Int J Paediatr Dent*, Vol.19, No.6, (Nov 2009), pp. 448-54, ISSN 1365-263X

Alexander, K., & Mazza, D.(2010) How to Perform a 'Healthy Kids Check'. *Aust Fam Physician*, Vol.39, No.10, (Oct 2010), pp. 761-5, ISSN 0300-8495

Almeida, A. G., Roseman, M. M., Sheff, M., Huntington, N., & Hughes, C. V. (2000). Future Caries Susceptibility in Children with Early Childhood Caries Following Treatment under General Anesthesia. *Pediatr Dent*, Vol.22, No.4, (Jul-Aug 2000), pp. 302-6, ISSN 0164-1263

Amin, M. S., & Harrison, R. L. (2009). Understanding Parents' Oral Health Behaviors for Their Young Children. *Qual Health Res*, Vol.19, No.1, (Jan 2009), pp. 116-27, ISSN 1049-7323

Berg, J. H., & Slayton, R. L. (ed(s).). (2009).*Early Childhood Oral Health,* Wiley-Blackwell, ISBN 978-0-8138-2416-1, Singapore

Berkowitz, R. J. (2003). Causes, Treatment and Prevention of Early Childhood Caries: A Microbiologic Perspective. *J Can Dent Assoc*, Vol.69, No.5, (May 2003), pp. 304-7, ISSN 1488-2159

Blinkhorn, A. S., Wainwright-Stringer, Y. M., & Holloway, P. J. (2001). Dental Health Knowledge and Attitudes of Regularly Attending Mothers of High-Risk, Pre-School Children. *Int Dent J*, Vol.51, No.6, (Dec 2001), pp. 435-8, ISSN 0020-6539

Casamassimo, P. S., Thikkurissy, S., Edelstein, B. L., & Maiorini, E. (2009). Beyond the Dmft: The Human and Economic Cost of Early Childhood Caries. *J Am Dent Assoc*, Vol.140, No.6, (Jun 2009), pp. 650-7, ISSN 1943-4723

Chan, S. C., Tsai, J. S., & King, N. M. (2002). Feeding and Oral Hygiene Habits of Preschool Children in Hong Kong and Their Caregivers' Dental Knowledge and Attitudes. *Int J Paediatr Dent*, Vol.12, No.5, (Sep 2002), pp. 322-31, ISSN 0960-7439

Clarke, P., Fraser-Lee, N. J., & Shimono, T. (2001). Identifying Risk Factors for Predicting Caries in School-Aged Children Using Dental Health Information Collected at Preschool Age. *ASDC J Dent Child*, Vol.68, No.5-6, (Sep-Dec2001), pp. 373-8.

Da Silva, K. (2007). A Role for the Family in Children's Oral Health. *N Y State Dent J*, Vol.73, No.5, (Aug-Sep 2007), pp. 55-7.

Douglass, J. M., Douglass, A. B., & Silk, H. J. (2004). A Practical Guide to Infant Oral Health. *Am Fam Physician*, Vol.70, No.11, (Dec 1 2004), pp. 2113-20.

Douglass, J. M., Montero, M. J., Thibodeau, E. A., & Mathieu, G. M. (2002). Dental Caries Experience in a Connecticut Head Start Program in 1991 and 1999. *Pediatr Dent*, Vol.24, No.4, (Jul-Aug 2002), pp. 309-14, ISSN 0164-1263

Drury, T. F., Horowitz, A. M., Ismail, A. I., Maertens, M. P., Rozier, R. G., & Selwitz, R. H. (1999). Diagnosing and Reporting Early Childhood Caries for Research Purposes. A Report of a Workshop Sponsored by the National Institute of Dental and Craniofacial Research, the Health Resources and Services Administration, and the Health Care Financing Administration. *J Public Health Dent*, Vol.59, No.3, (Summer 1999), pp. 192-7, ISSN 0022-4006

Dykes, J., Watt, R. G., & Nazroo, J. (2002). Socio-Economic and Ethnic Influences on Infant Feeding Practices Related to Oral Health. *Community Dent Health*, Vol.19, No.3, (Sep 2002), pp. 137-43, ISSN

Edelstein, B., Vargas, C. M., Candelaria, D., & Vemuri, M. (2006). Experience and Policy Implications of Children Presenting with Dental Emergencies to Us Pediatric Dentistry Training Programs. *Pediatr Dent*, Vol.28, No.5, (Sep-Oct 2006), pp. 431-7, ISSN 0164-1263

Finlayson, T. L., Siefert, K., Ismail, A. I., Delva, J., & Sohn, W. (2005). Reliability and Validity of Brief Measures of Oral Health-Related Knowledge, Fatalism, and Self-Efficacy in Mothers of African American Children. *Pediatr Dent*, Vol.27, No.5, (Sep-Oct 2005), pp. 422-8, ISSN 0164-1263

Finlayson, T. L., Siefert, K., Ismail, A. I., & Sohn, W. (2007). Maternal Self-Efficacy and 1-5-Year-Old Children's Brushing Habits. *Community Dent Oral Epidemiol*, Vol.35, No.4, (Aug 2007), pp. 272-81, ISS N 1600-0528

Gussy, M. G., Waters, E. B., Riggs, E. M., Lo, S. K., & Kilpatrick, N. M. (2008). Parental Knowledge, Beliefs and Behaviours for Oral Health of Toddlers Residing in Rural Victoria. *Aust Dent J*, Vol.53, No.1, (Mar 2008), pp. 52-60, ISSN 0045-0421

Hallett, K. B. (2000). Early Childhood Caries--a New Name for an Old Problem. *Ann R Australas Coll Dent Surg*, Vol.15(Oct 2000), pp. 268-75, ISS N

Hallett, K. B., & O'Rourke, P. K. (2003). Social and Behavioural Determinants of Early Childhood Caries. *Aust Dent J*, Vol.48, No.1, (Mar 2003), pp. 27-33, ISSN 0045-0421

Hawley, G., & Holloway, P. (1994). Measuring Health Behaviours--Which Tools Should We Use? *Community Dent Health*, Vol.11, No.3, (Sep 1994), pp. 129-30, ISSN 0265-539X

Hoeft, K. S., Barker, J. C., & Masterson, E. E. (2010). Urban Mexican-American Mothers' Beliefs About Caries Etiology in Children. *Community Dent Oral Epidemiol*, Vol.38, No.3, (Feb 10 2010), pp. 244-55, ISS N 1600-0528

Hood, C. A., Hunter, M. L., & Kingdon, A. (1998). Demographic Characteristics, Oral Health Knowledge and Practices of Mothers of Children Aged 5 Years and under Referred for Extraction of Teeth under General Anaesthesia. *Int J Paediatr Dent*, Vol.8, No.2, (Jun 1998), pp. 131-6, ISSN 0960-7439

Horton, S., & Barker, J. C. (2008). Rural Latino Immigrant Caregivers' Conceptions of Their Children's Oral Disease. *J Public Health Dent*, Vol.68, No.1, (Winter 2008), pp. 22-9, ISSN 0022-4006

Ismail, A. I. (2003). Determinants of Health in Children and the Problem of Early Childhood Caries. *Pediatr Dent*, Vol.25, No.4, (Jul-Aug 2003), pp. 328-33, ISSN 0164-1263

Jackson, R. (2006). Parental Health Literacy and Children's Dental Health: Implications for the Future. *Pediatr Dent*, Vol.28, No.1, (Jan-Feb 2006), pp. 72-5, ISSN 0164-1263

Jin, B. H., Ma, D. S., Moon, H. S., Paik, D. I., Hahn, S. H., & Horowitz, A. M. (2003). Early Childhood Caries: Prevalence and Risk Factors in Seoul, Korea. *J Public Health Dent*, Vol.63, No.3, (Summer 2003), pp. 183-8, ISSN 0022-4006

Kanellis, M. J., Damiano, P. C., & Momany, E. T. (2000). Medicaid Costs Associated with the Hospitalization of Young Children for Restorative Dental Treatment under General Anesthesia. *J Public Health Dent*, Vol.60, No.1, (Winter 2000), pp. 28-32, ISSN 0022-4006

Mattila, M. L., Rautava, P., Sillanpaa, M., & Paunio, P. (2000). Caries in Five-Year-Old Children and Associations with Family-Related Factors. *J Dent Res*, Vol.79, No.3, (Mar 2000), pp. 875-81, ISSN 0022-0345

Meyer, K., Geurtsen, W., & Gunay, H. (2010). An Early Oral Health Care Program Starting During Pregnancy: Results of a Prospective Clinical Long-Term Study. *Clin Oral Investig*, Vol.14, No.3, (Jun 2010) , pp. 257-64, ISSN 1436-3771

Mohebbi, S. Z., Virtanen, J. I., Murtomaa, H., Vahid-Golpayegani, M., & Vehkalahti, M. M. (2008). Mothers as Facilitators of Oral Hygiene in Early Childhood. *Int J Paediatr Dent*, Vol.18, No.1, (Jan 2008), pp. 48-55, ISSN 0960-7439

Oral Health Division, Ministry of Health Malaysia.(2003). *Guidelines on Oral Healthcare for Pre-School Children*, Government printers, Kuala Lumpur

Oral Health Division, Ministry of Health Malaysia.(2004). *Oral Healthcare for Antenatal Mothers*, Government Printers, Kuala Lumpur

Oral Health Division, Ministry of Health Malaysia.(2007). *The National Oral Health Survey of Preschool Children 2005 (NOHPS 2005)*, Government printers, Kuala Lumpur

Oral Health Division, Ministry of Health Malaysia.(2008). *Guidelines Early Chilhood Oral Healthcare*, Government printers, Kuala Lumpur

Oral Health Division, Ministry of Health Malaysia.(2009). *National Oral Health Survey of School Children 2007 (NOHSS 2007)*, Government printers, Kuala Lumpur

Orenuga, O. O., & Sofola, O. O. (2005). A Survey of the Knowledge, Attitude and Practices of Antenatal Mothers in Lagos, Nigeria About the Primary Teeth. *Afr J Med Med Sci*, Vol.34, No.3, (Sep 2005), pp. 285-91.

Pahel, B. T., Rozier, R. G., & Slade, G. D. (2007). Parental Perceptions of Children's Oral Health: The Early Childhood Oral Health Impact Scale (ECOHIS). *Health Qual Life Outcomes*, Vol.5 (2007), pp. 6, ISSN 1477-7525

Petersen, P. E., Danila, I., & Samoila, A. (1995). Oral Health Behavior, Knowledge, and Attitudes of Children, Mothers, and Schoolteachers in Romania in 1993. *Acta Odontol Scand*, Vol.53, No.6, (Dec 1995), pp. 363-8, ISSN 0001-6357

Petersen, P. E., & Esheng, Z. (1998). Dental Caries and Oral Health Behaviour Situation of Children, Mothers and Schoolteachers in Wuhan, People's Republic of China. *Int Dent J*, Vol.48, No.3, (Jun 1998), pp. 210-6, ISSN 0020-6539

Plutzer, K., & Spencer, A. J. (2008). Efficacy of an Oral Health Promotion Intervention in the Prevention of Early Childhood Caries. *Community Dent Oral Epidemiol*, Vol.36, No.4, (Aug 2008), pp. 335-46, ISSN 0301-5661

Rajab, L. D., Petersen, P. E., Bakaeen, G., & Hamdan, M. A. (2002). Oral Health Behaviour of Schoolchildren and Parents in Jordan. *Int J Paediatr Dent*, Vol.12, No.3, (May 2002), pp. 168-76, ISSN 0960-7439

Riedy, C. A., Weinstein, P., Milgrom, P., & Bruss, M. (2001). An Ethnographic Study for Understanding Children's Oral Health in a Multicultural Community. *Int Dent J*, Vol.51, No.4, (Aug 2001), pp. 305-12, ISSN 0020-6539

Roberts, B. P., Blinkhorn, A. S., & Duxbury, J. T. (2003). The Power of Children over Adults When Obtaining Sweet Snacks. *Int J Paediatr Dent*, Vol.13, No.2, (Mar 2003), pp. 76-84, ISSN 0960-7439

Savage, M. F., Lee, J. Y., Kotch, J. B., & Vann, W. F., Jr. (2004). Early Preventive Dental Visits: Effects on Subsequent Utilization and Costs. *Pediatrics*, Vol.114, No.4, (Oct 2004), pp. e418-23, ISSN 1098-4275

Schluter, P. J., Durward, C., Cartwright, S., & Paterson, J. (2007). Maternal Self-Report of Oral Health in 4-Year-Old Pacific Children from South Auckland, New Zealand:

Findings from the Pacific Islands Families Study. *J Public Health Dent*, Vol.67, No.2, (Spring 2007), pp. 69-77, ISSN 0020-4006

Schroth, R. J., Brothwell, D. J., & Moffatt, M. E. (2007). Caregiver Knowledge and Attitudes of Preschool Oral Health and Early Childhood Caries (Ecc). *Int J Circumpolar Health*, Vol.66, No.2, (Apr 2007), pp. 153-67.

Silver, D. H. (1992). A Comparison of 3-Year-Olds' Caries Experience in 1973, 1981 and 1989 in a Hertfordshire Town, Related to Family Behaviour and Social Class. *Br Dent J*, Vol.172, No.5, (Mar 7 1992), pp. 191-7, ISSN 0007-0610

Singh, P., & King, T. (2003). Infant and Child Feeding Practices and Dental Caries in 6 to 36 Months Old Children in Fiji. *Pac Health Dialog*, Vol.10, No.1, (Mar 2003), pp. 12-16.

Skaret, E., Espelid, I., Skeie, M. S., & Haugejorden, O. (2008). Parental Beliefs and Attitudes Towards Child Caries Prevention: Assessing Consistency and Validity in a Longitudinal Design. *BMC Oral Health*, Vol.8 (2008), pp. 1, ISSN 1472-6831

Southward, L. H., Robertson, A., Wells-Parker, E., Eklund, N. P., Silberman, S. L., Crall, J. J., Edelstein, B. L., Baggett, D. H., Parrish, D. R., & Hanna, H. (2006). Oral Health Status of Mississippi Delta 3- to 5-Year-Olds in Child Care: An Exploratory Study of Dental Health Status and Risk Factors for Dental Disease and Treatment Needs. *J Public Health Dent*, Vol.66, No.2, (Spring 2006), pp. 131-7, ISSN 0020-4006

Syahrial, D., Abdul-Kadir, R., Yassin, Z., & Jali, N. M. (1995). Knowledge and Attitudes of Parents of Children with Nusing Bottle Syndrome in Serdang, Malaysia. *J Nihon Univ Sch Dent*, Vol.37, No.3, (1995), pp. 146-51.

Szatko, F., Wierzbicka, M., Dybizbanska, E., Struzycka, I., & Iwanicka-Frankowska, E. (2004). Oral Health of Polish Three-Year-Olds and Mothers' Oral Health-Related Knowledge. *Community Dent Health*, Vol.21, No.2, (Jun 2004), pp. 175-80, ISSN 0265-539X

Talib, N. A. (2010) "National Oral Health Plan (Nohp) for Malaysia 2011-2020." 5.9.2011, Available from http://ohd.moh.gov.my/v2/images/pdf/1nohpa.pdf.

Tate, A. R., Ng, M. W., Needleman, H. L., & Acs, G. (2002). Failure Rates of Restorative Procedures Following Dental Rehabilitation under General Anesthesia. *Pediatr Dent*, Vol.24, No.1, (Jan-Feb 2002), pp. 69-71, ISSN 0164-1263

Tickle, M., Milsom, K. M., Humphris, G. M., & Blinkhorn, A. S. (2003). Parental Attitudes to the Care of the Carious Primary Dentition. *Br Dent J*, Vol.195, No.8, (Oct 25 2003), pp. 451-55, ISSN 0007-0610

Tsai, A. I., Chen, C. Y., Li, L. A., Hsiang, C. L., & Hsu, K. H. (2006). Risk Indicators for Early Childhood Caries in Taiwan. *Community Dent Oral Epidemiol*, Vol.34, No.6, (Dec 2006), pp. 437-45, ISSN 0301-5661

van Palenstein Helderman, W. H., Soe, W., & van 't Hof, M. A. (2006). Risk Factors of Early Childhood Caries in a Southeast Asian Population. *J Dent Res*, Vol.85, No.1, (Jan 2006), pp. 85-88.

Vargas, C. M., & Ronzio, C. R. (2006). Disparities in Early Childhood Caries. *BMC Oral Health*, Vol.6 No.Suppl 1, (August 2006), pp. S3, ISSN 1472-6831

Wigen, T. I., Espelid, I., Skaare, A. B., & Wang, N. J. (2011). Family Characteristics and Caries Experience in Preschool Children. A Longitudinal Study from Pregnancy to 5 Years of Age. *Community Dent Oral Epidemiol*, Vol.39, No.4, (Aug 2011), pp. 311-17, ISSN 1600-0528

Williams, N. J., Whittle, J. G., & Gatrell, A. C. (2002). The Relationship between Socio-Demographic Characteristics and Dental Health Knowledge and Attitudes of Parents with Young Children. *Br Dent J*, Vol.193, No.11, (Dec 7 2002), pp. 651-4, ISSN 0007-0610

Yin, H. S., Johnson, M., Mendelsohn, A. L., Abrams, M. A., Sanders, L. M., & Dreyer, B. P. (2009). The Health Literacy of Parents in the United States: A Nationally Representative Study. *Pediatrics*, Vol.124 Suppl 3(Nov 2009), pp. S289-98, ISSN 1098-4275

Zeedyk, M. S., Longbottom, C., & Pitts, N. B. (2005). Tooth-Brushing Practices of Parents and Toddlers: A Study of Home-Based Videotaped Sessions. *Caries Res*, Vol.39, No.1, (Jan-Feb 2005), pp. 27-33, ISSN 0008-6568

Gingivitis in Children and Adolescents

Folakemi Oredugba and Patricia Ayanbadejo
Faculty of Dental Sciences, College of Medicine, University of Lagos
Nigeria

1. Introduction

Gingivitis or inflammation of the gingiva, is the commonest oral disease in children and adolescents. It is characterized by the presence of gingival inflammation without detectable bone loss or clinical attachment loss. The causes and risks are as varied in children as in adults and range from local to systemic causes. The most important local predisposing factor in children is poor oral hygiene which stems from children's dependence on adults for assistance with routine oral hygiene. It also stems from age limitation in perception of the need for regular and efficient tooth brushing.

When plaque and food debris accumulate in poor oral hygiene, micro-organisms also accumulate and the process of inflammation starts. This leads to gingivitis, which, if not taken care of can progress to gradual destruction of supporting soft and hard tissues of the teeth. This is evident in the very young and those with disabilities, where manual dexterity is not well developed.

Gingivitis in children is also commonly seen during eruption and exfoliation of both primary and permanent teeth and exfoliation of primary teeth. This process, although physiological, if not managed carefully, may contribute to discomfort during tooth brushing, mastication and also cause restlessness in the affected children. During puberty, it may be a response to hormonal changes in the developing adolescent, though more pronounced when there is plaque accumulation.

In children with compromised immunity, chronic malnutrition, exanthematous fevers such as malaria, measles or chicken pox, the gingivitis may be acute and necrotic. The systemic effect and local destruction of soft and hard tissues may contribute to increased morbidity and poor aesthetics in affected children.

Habitually leaving the mouth open, either spontaneously or due to pathology in the oropharynx, may also contribute to gingivitis. During childhood and adolescence, appliances, either habit breakers or removable and fixed appliances may be required. Most children at this age present with gingivitis. This is a result of non compliance with routine tooth brushing which is further made difficult by orthodontic wires and elastics. One of the pre-conditions for appliance therapy is a commitment to efficient routine tooth brushing because the use of an appliance in the presence of plaque and debris accumulations is deleterious to the periodontal structures.

Gingivitis may also be a complication of chronic use of certain medications whose side effects include dryness of the mouth. It predisposes to gingival inflammation which is due to a low output of saliva. This type of gingivitis is frequently encountered in children and adolescents on antidepressants and other medications, which if used on long term basis and in the presence of plaque and debris, predispose to gingivitis.

Several studies on the oral health of the young population in developing countries show that poor gingival health is rampant, especially in those residing in the rural and remote areas and in those of the lower socioeconomic strata. This condition is even more significant in those who are institutionalized, those with intellectual disabilities, for example, Down syndrome, Autism Spectrum Disorders; those with multiple disabilities and generally those who have musculo-skeletal disorders who may not be able to carry out effective tooth brushing. The main problem with these individuals is neglect on the part of parents and care givers who are supposed to be responsible for their daily hygiene. When compared with children and adolescents without disabilities, their oral health has been found to be poorer.

The situation can however be controlled with regular dental visits, which is still alien to the population at large, where oral health education will be re-inforced. The school health programme has also been recommended as an important means by which oral health education can be provided and established for children and adolescents. The programme is being supported by Faculty and corporate bodies across the globe and it is believed that this will gradually expose the population to good oral health practices and improve gingival health. This Chapter aims to discuss the various forms of gingivitis encountered in children and adolescents including those with special health care needs and provide a summary of recommendations given from the different studies carried out.

2. Plaque induced gingivitis

Gingivitis is also regarded as the most common periodontal disease in children, with the primary aetiology as plaque (Oh et al, 2002). In poor oral hygiene, food debris, plaque and micro-organisms also accumulate and the process of inflammation starts. This leads to gingivitis, which, if not taken care of can progress to gradual destruction of supporting soft and hard tissues of the teeth (Fig 1).

2.1 Histopathology

Inflammation represents the body's protective response to injury and tissue destruction. This response consists of a spectrum of highly coordinated events that occur at cellular and tissue level. Its purpose is to destroy, dilute or sequestrate the injurious agent and the injured tissue in order to permit healing.

Inflammation is a defensive mechanism intended to protect the host, but can also be potentially harmful. Clinical signs of inflammation are redness (due to open blood vessels), heat (due to warmth of blood), swelling (due to oedema), pain (due to stimulation of pain receptors) and loss of function due to oedema (Ramzi et al, 2002).

Gingival inflammation is the result of plaque or bacterial biofilm. This biofilm develops and matures over a period of several weeks, initially developing supragingivally with mainly aerobic bacteria (Serio et al, 2009). Over time, the flora changes from predominantly gram positive to gram negative, from facultative aerobes to strictly anaerobic species, with more motile forms present. Mature subgingival biofilm takes up to twelve weeks to develop (Lovegrove et al, 2004) and contains gram negative bacteria such as *P. gingivalis, B. forsythus, and P. intermedia*, among many others (Fleming, 1999).

These bacteria possess complex carbohydrate and proteins on their cell walls called endotoxins or lipopolysaccharides (LPS). When these molecules are detected by the host, a protective response ensues, resulting in inflammation, recruitment of white blood cells (WBCs) and release of cytokines and chemical mediators.

As the biofilm accumulates, gingivitis develops over a period of several days in the presence of periodontal bacteria (Loe et al, 1965). Gingivitis may be a non-specific bacterial infection dependent on the level of plaque present (Goodson et al, 2004).

Nevertheless, the prevalence and severity of inflammation of the oral tissues (gingivitis and periodontitis) is low in healthy young children and gradually increases with increasing age (Matsson, 1993; Papaioannou et al, 2009). With increasing age, the proportions of periodontal pathogens also increase (Papaioannou, 2009; Kimura et al, 2002).

Page and Shroeder (1976), reported the sequence of changes during the development of gingivitis and peridontitis under four stages, according to prominent histopathological signs. They termed the stages, Initial, Early, Established and Advanced lesions.

In health, hallmark features of gingival connective tissue are an even collagen density throughout the gingiva and absence of clusters of inflammatory cells.

In the initial lesion, which occours within 2 to 4 days after allowing plaque to accumulate, an increased volume of junctional epithelium (JE) is occupied by polymorphonuclear leucocytes (PMNL). Blood vessels subjacent to the JE become dilated and exhibit increased permeability. A small cellular infiltrate of PMNL and mononuclear cells forms and collagen content in the infiltrated areas markedly decreases.

In the Early stage, which is about 4 to 7 days of plaque accumulation, gingivitis in humans evolves at this stage, the differentiating sign being accumulation of large numbers of lymphocytes as an enlarged infiltrate in the connective tissue. There are altered fibroblasts and earlier changes are quantitatively increased.

In the Established stage, which is about 2 to 3 weeks of plaque accumulation, there is preponderance of plasma cells in an expanded inflammatory lesion with continuance of earlier changes. The Established lesion may persist for a long time before becoming 'aggressive' and progressing to the advanced lesion.

In the Advanced lesion, the infiltrate is dominated by plasma cells. Collagen destruction continues with loss of alveolar bone and apical migration of JE, with "pocket" formation now being apparent. Throughout the sequence, viable bacteria remain outside the gingiva, on the surface of the tooth and in the periodontal pocket against, but not invading the soft tissue.

However, a notable finding by Longhurst (1980) is that the histopathology of chronic gingivitis in children corresponds to the plasma cell-dominated established lesion of the adult, but has an inflammatory infiltration with a great majority of lymphocytes. This is analogous to the Early lesion as described by Page and Shroeder (1976) for the adult. Other reports on the nature of cellular infiltrates in various stages of periodontal disease had indicated that in mild gingivitis, the predominant lymphocyte was the T-cell while in more severe gingivitis and peridontitis the B-cell line predominates. This implies that gingivitis in children is T-cell dominated, although the degree of delineation is not quite established. It also indicates an age-related difference in immunologic response (Koch & Poulsen, 2009).

In a study assessing the prevalence of three microorganisms, *Porphyromonas gingivalis*, *Actinobacillus actinomycetemcomitans* and *Tannerella forsythensis*, in the bacterial plaque of children with and without gingivitis, it was found that the organisms causing gingivitis were endogenous in healthy mouths. They start to cause disease when their numbers increase significantly (Gafan et al, 2004)

In Nigeria, gingivitis has been reported to be more prevalent in children from lower socioeconomic background (Oredugba, 2006). This was attributed to low educational level which causes low perception of need for adequate oral hygiene. In a recent study among Finnish school children, those whose mothers had a college or university education had a smaller chance of presenting with visible plaque accumulation than those from mothers with a lower educational level (Leroy et al, 2011). The study also found an association between bacterial plaque accumulation and the presence of gingivitis.

Poor oral hygiene and gingivitis have been reported to be more prevalent in children with cognitive and developmental disabilities. The Oral Hygiene Index (OHI) scores have been found to be higher in children and adolescents with disabilities than in control groups in studies carried out in some developing countries (Oredugba, 2006; Oredugba & Akindayomi, 2008; Nahar et al, 2010). In the study carried out in Bangladesh, as many as 64% of those with disabilities had gingivitis compared with 27.5% of controls. The prevalence of gingivitis has also been found to be influenced by other demographic factors such as place of residence, age and severity of disability and cognition.

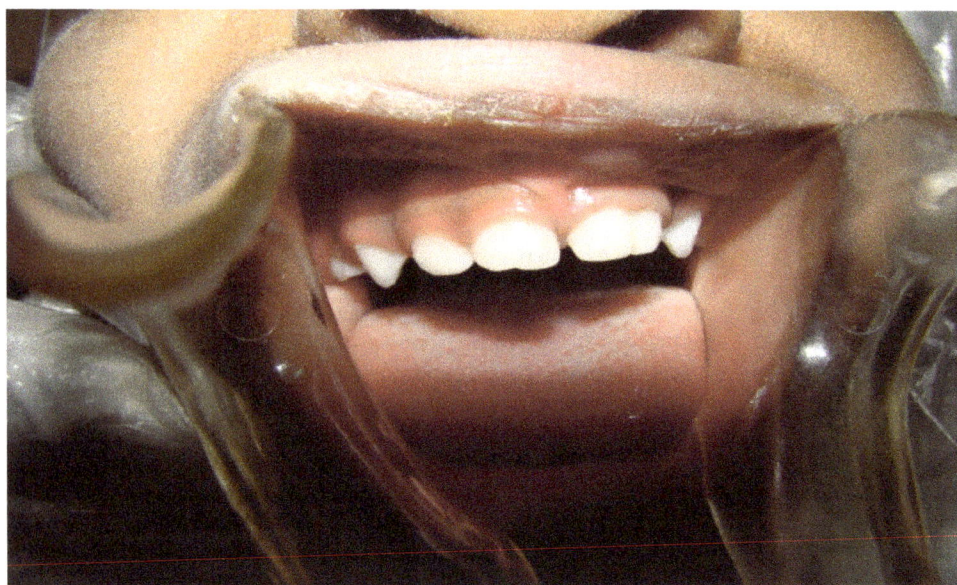

Fig. 1. Gingivitis of the anterior maxillary teeth in a four year old boy

Since most of the affected children do not brush their teeth, or brush only once a day or occasionally, mouth washes containing chemical anti-plaque agents which reduce bacterial plaque accumulation and therefore the incidence of gingival and periodontal diseases are important in such individuals. Chlorhexidine is currently the most effective chemical anti-plaque agent used in dentistry (Twetman, 2004). It causes an immediate reduction in the number of salivary bacteria and possesses a broad spectrum against gram positive and negative bacteria, fungi and lipophylic viruses (Jones, 2000). Its effect is both bactericidal and bacteriostatic and clinical efficacy results from its interaction with bacterial cell membrane causing cell lysis and prevention of adhesion of new bacteria in the oral cavity. These findings point to the need for motivation of parents and caregivers to commence and encourage effective tooth brushing which will lay a foundation for good oral health in their children and wards (Meyer et al, 2010). This is especially so in those with intellectual disabilities and the very young children.

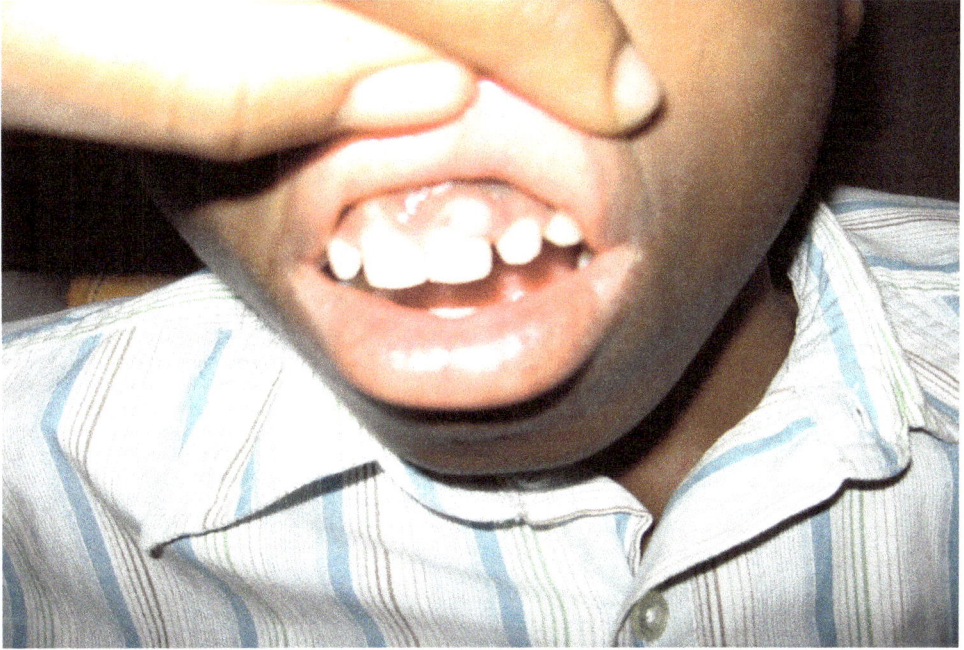

Fig. 2. Gingivitis in a nine year old boy due to mouth breathing

Gingivitis in the maxillary anterior region is also a common finding in mouth breathers (Fig 2). This habit is common among young children and it predisposes to dryness of the gingiva when the lubricating effect of saliva is absent. This habit can be corrected with the use of a removable appliance. Children who use orthodontic appliances for correction of malocclusion are predisposed to gingivitis. However effective tooth brushing and use of chlorhexidine mouthwash will reduce plaque accumulation and gingivitis.

3. Eruption gingivitis

This is gingival inflammation occouring around an erupting permanent tooth. The child may be experiencing discomfort which will therefore make tooth brushing difficult. Sometimes, the child refuses tooth brushing completely. This will lead to plaque accumulation and inflammation. Also during the eruptive phase, the epithelium displays degenerative changes at the site of fusion between dental and oral epithelia. These areas are vulnerable to plaque accumulation and sets up a bacterial reaction (Koch & Poulsen, 2009).

4. Infective gingivitis

These are of viral or bacterial origin and caused by viruses or bacteria which are normal commensals of the oral cavity becoming virulent when present in high proportions.

4.1 Herpetic gingivo-stomatitis

Also known as acute herpetic gingivo-stomatitis and affects both the gingivae and other parts of the oral mucus membrane. It is commonly seen in children less than three years of age. It is caused by the herpes simplex virus type 1. Infection usually follows bouts of childhood fevers such as malaria, measles and chicken pox and it may assume epidemic proportions among children attending same pre-school or crèche centres. The onset of generalized gingivitis is preceded by a prodromal period with symptoms such as irritability, malaise, vomiting and fever and the appearance of small vesicles which rupture to reveal small yellowish painful ulcers with erythematous margins. The condition is associated with drooling of saliva, inability to chew and swallow and the child may become increasingly uncooperative during tooth brushing (Fig 3).

The condition is self limiting and the management is to encourage bed rest, plenty of fluid and maintenance of good oral hygiene through gentle debridement. Analgesics are prescribed to relieve the pain and antibiotics are useful in preventing superimposed bacterial infection. The application of a mild topical anaesthetic gel has been found useful in young children and reduces irritability.

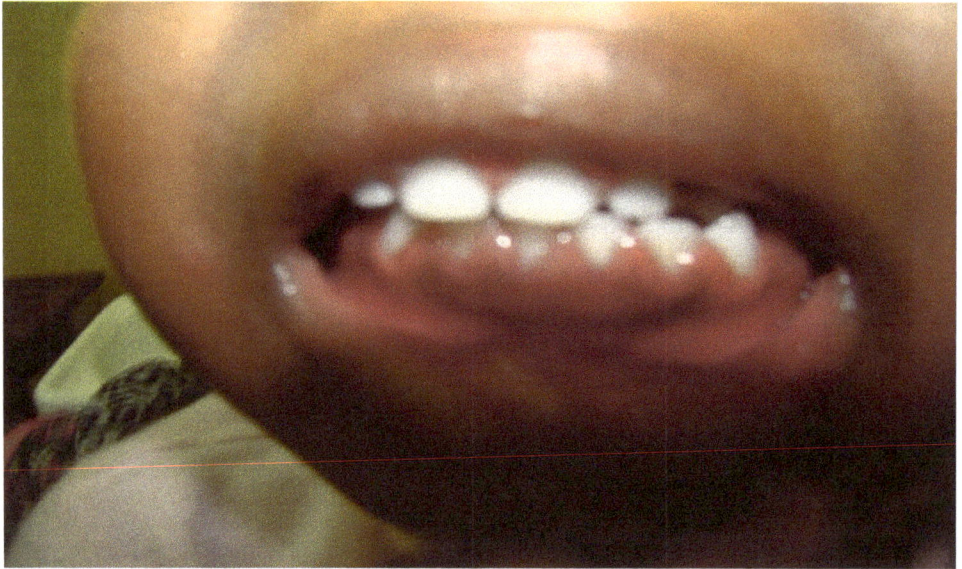

Fig. 3. Acute herpetic gingivostomatitis in a 2 1/2 year old girl

4.2 HIV-associated gingivitis

Oral manifestations of human immunodeficiency virus (HIV) disease are an important part of the natural history of HIV disease (Lamster et al, 1998). Many studies have reported that hairy leukoplakia, pseudomembranous candidiasis, Kaposi sarcoma, non-Hodgkin's lymphoma, linear gingival erythema, necrotizing ulcerative gingivitis and periodontitis were common lesions seen in patients with HIV infection and AIDS. It was also reported that the higher prevalence and incidence rates of these conditions correlated with the falling CD4 counts and higher viral load of the patients (Han & Liu, 2010). However the use of highly active antiretroviral therapy (HAART) was associated with decreases in the prevalence of oral diseases.

In a study comparing the oral microbiology of HIV-positive children with that of controls, the prevalence of gingivitis was significantly higher in the HIV-positive group (89.4%) than in the healthy group (40.5%) (Portela et al, 2004). It was also found that the frequency of yeast isolation correlated positively with the severity of the gingival condition in the HIV-infected group, because 95% of infants who presented with Candida had inflammation of the gingivae. In the study, multiple candida species were isolated from the subgingival crevices of children with positive HIV infection. These include C. *albicans, C. dubliniensis, C. globrata and C. tropicalis.* Apart from yeast infection, fusobacterial and spirochaetal infections have been found in HIV positive children, with a high proportion of those who manifested the AIDS disease having necrotizing gingivitis. These findings confirm the multiple microbial colonization of the gingival lesions in HIV infection.

4.3 Acute necrotizing ulcerative gingivitis (ANUG)

This is an acute multiple bacterial infection of the gingivae. The lesion starts at the interdental papilae, spreading along the gingival margins and if untreated, starts to destroy the underlying connective tissue and bone. There is a characteristic necrotic odour associated with this condition and the mouth becomes progressively painful with sloughing off of the necrotic ulcers on the gingivae. The ulcers become erythematous and bleed following minimal trauma, especially tooth brushing. Systemic upset may not be associated, but the regional lymph nodes are enlarged and tender. If untreated, destruction of the soft tissues of the mouth and cheek and facial bones result, a condition referred to as Cancrum oris or Noma (Figs 4-6).

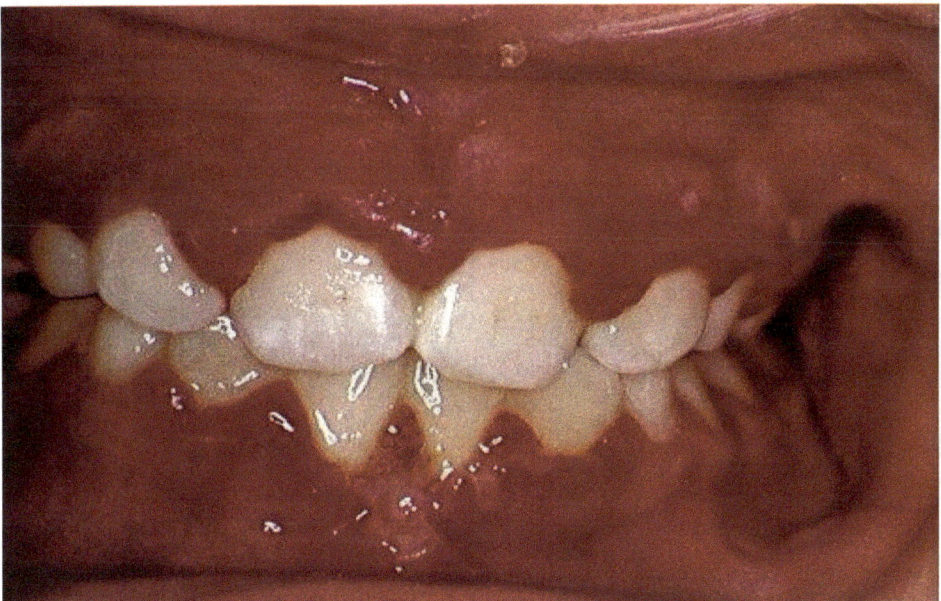

Fig. 4. Early stage of acute necrotizing ulcerative gingivitis (ANUG)

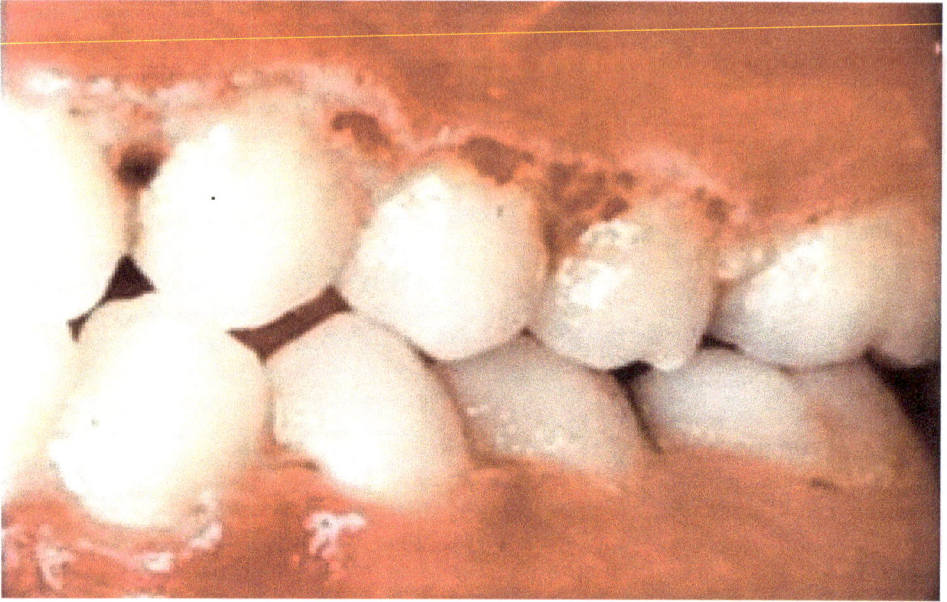

Fig. 5. Advanced stage of acute necrotizing ulcerative gingivitis

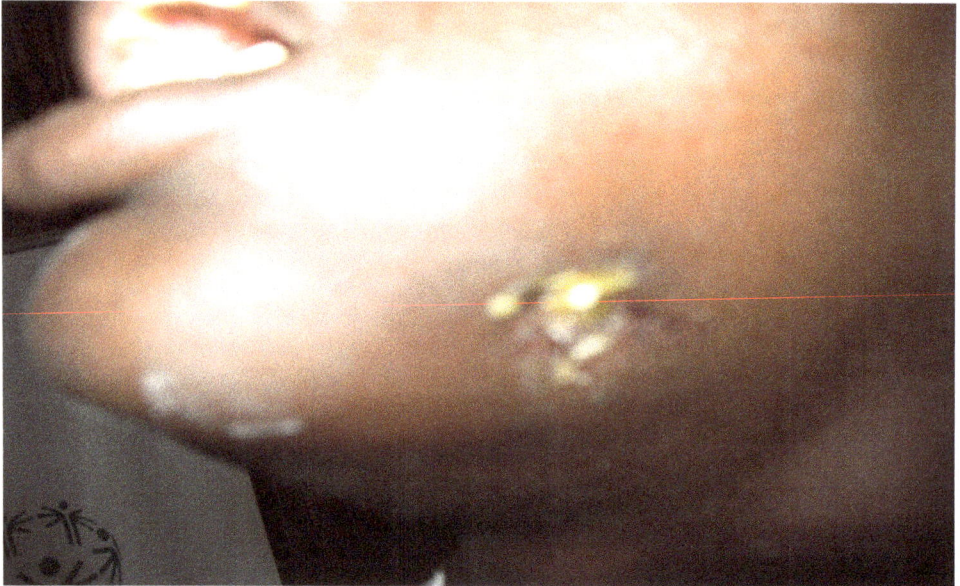

Fig. 6. Cancrum oris in a 14 year old boy

It occours with low frequency (<1%) in children in developed countries but still seen in higher proportions (2-5%) in children and adolescents in developing countries in Africa, Asia and South America. It is also frequently seen in children and adolescents with intellectual disabilities and some other medically compromising conditions who may not be able to comply with routine oral hygiene practices.

Predisposing factors include poor oral hygiene, malnutrition, depressed immunity and long term hospitalization. It used to be known as "trench mouth" because it was seen frequently in soldiers occupying trenches during the World War I. It was also called "Vincent's angina", after the French physician Henri Vincent (1862- 1950). Later, it was seen in children from low socio-economic families who were malnourished and with poor oral hygiene.

The bacteria implicated earlier were *Fusobacteria fusiformis and Borrelia vincentii*. However, modern electron microscope studies have shown the lesion to be colonized by various species of gram negative anaerobes and spirochaetes such as *Treponema species, Bacteroides, Veilonella, Fusobacteria and Actinomyces.*

The treatment of choice is regular gentle debridement of the gingivae and irrigation with an oxidising antiseptic such as hydrogen peroxide, until the infection clears. Diet and oral hygiene counseling is also useful and this should be followed up to ensure speedy healing. Metronidazole is used because it is effective against obligate anaerobes which are found in large numbers in the lesion. To prevent secondary infection, penicillin is prescribed.

5. Malnutrition-induced gingivitis

Adolescence is a time of rapid growth, independent food choices and food fads. (Bello & Al-Hammad, 2006). It is also a period of heightened caries activity as a result of increased intake of cariogenic substances and inattentiveness to oral hygiene procedures (Majewski, 2001).

Biological antioxidants form an important part of our diet and together with intracellular antioxidants and antioxidant enzyme systems may prevent various pathological diseases (O'Brien, 1994; Battino et al, 2002). Saliva, which bathes the oral tissues, contains pure salivary secretions, crevicular fluid, proteins, carbohydrates, enzymes, ions, antioxidants and microorganism, and is usually a reflection of plasma. One of the most important functions of salivary enzymes such as peroxidase is the control of oral bacteria that form dental plaque and imbalance in oral ecology which lead to dental caries and chronic inflammatory periodontal diseases (Tulunoglu et al, 2006).

There is evidence that different foods, such as dietary proteins and carbohydrates can affect the buffering capacity of saliva (Mundorff-Shrestha et al, 1994) and protein deficiency influences markedly the composition of whole saliva in man (Johansson et al, 1984; Agarwal et al, 1984). Chronic deficiencies of iron, the B group vitamins and folic acid also predispose to glossitis and gingivitis, especially in young children.

6. Gingivitis associated with hormonal changes

Hormones have been found to have strong effects on mucosal, connective tissue and bones. For an individual, birth is a borderline between the sterile intrauterine life and the extra-uterine existence with a continous exposure to microorganisms (Kononen, 1999). The microbial community is further shaped by diet, personal oral hygiene (Crielaard et al, 2011) and other parameters such as hormones and various systemic conditions. The microbiome analysis by Crielaard et al (2011) showed that the salivary microbiome of children is already complex by the age of three years matures with increasing age, but at the age of puberty, still differs from the adult microbiome. A higher amount of plaque has also been found in the primary dentition compared with the mixed and permanent dentitions, but the prevalence and severity of inflammation of the oral tissues (gingivitis and periodontitis) is low in healthy young children and gradually increases with increasing age (Papaioannou et al, 2009).

Pubertal gingivitis has been seen with increasing frequency in young teenagers and has been ascribed to the "rush" of sex hormones which also affects the reaction of tissues to corticosteroids. The same pattern has been described in pregnant women who are more predisposed to gingivitis during pregnancy. The condition ranges from localized inflammation of one or two papillary gingivae, also called 'pregnancy epulis', to generalized marginal gingivitis. This condition is not severe if plaque is well controlled. Most cases resolve as soon as debridement is commenced.

7. Drug-induced gingivitis

Drug-induced gingival enlargement (DIGE) and gingivitis are side effects and unwanted outcomes of antiepileptic therapy with phenytoin, or immunosuppressive therapy with systemic cyclosporine. Patients on these medications develop varying degrees of gingival overgrowth (Trackman & Kantaki, 2004; Cury et al, 2009). Gingival enlargement is the most significant oral finding (Robbins, 2009) and can occour in up to 50% of patients taking Phenytoin (Thomason et al, 1992). Valproic acid and Carbamazepine have also been demonstrated to cause gingival enlargement, especially on the labial surfaces of the anterior maxillary and mandibular teeth (Figs 7a & 7b). It is strongly correlated to poor plaque control. Where the oral hygiene is good and food debris and plaque are not allowed to accumulate, this side effect of anticonvulsive therapy is not observed or not so significant. Treatment includes meticulous oral hygiene and in severe cases where the enlarged tissue interferes with function and aesthetics, surgical resection is advised. (Robbins, 2009). A more frequent recall and oral hygiene interval has also been suggested for such patients on antiepileptic drug therapy to reduce the risk of gingival hyperplasia.

7.1 Plasma Cell Gingivitis (PCG)

Plasma cell gingivitis is characterized by diffuse and massive infiltration of plasma cells into the subepitheial gingival tissue (Macleod & Ellis, 1989). It is a rare benign inflammatory condition with no clear aetiology, but an exaggerated response to bacterial plaque, immunological reaction to allergens in food such as strong spices, chilli pepper, medications, toothpaste or herbs such as khat has been reported (Halbach, 1972; Kalix, 1988; Macleod & Ellis, 1989; Serio et al, 1991; Marker & Krogdahl, 2001). The diagnosis requires haematological screening in addition to clinical and histopathological examination in order to exclude leukemia. Further, serological examination is needed to exclude connective tissue disease – first and foremost lupus erythematosus (Al-Meshal, 1988; Neville et al, 1995). In affected children, standard professional oral hygiene procedures and non- surgical periodontal therapy including antimicrobials are associated with marked improvement of clinical and patient related outcomes (Arduino et al, 2011).

8. Gingivitis as a manifestation of systemic disease

Subjects with developmental disabilities, mental retardation, cerebral palsy and autism have been shown to require special care for maintaining oral hygiene and receiving dental treatment (Surabian, 2001 A & B; Oredugba & Akindayomi, 2008). A considerably higher frequency of inflamed gingival surfaces and pathological gingival pockets are present in children with severe mental retardation as compared with healthy children, in spite of similar frequencies of dental care (Forsberg, 1985). This has been attributed to their lack of cooperation during tooth brushing at home and during treatment. A lot of patience is required by parents and care givers in order to provide effective home oral hygiene care for this group of individuals. Oral health education is also desirable to create awareness of need for good oral health for all individuals, irrespective of age and mental status.

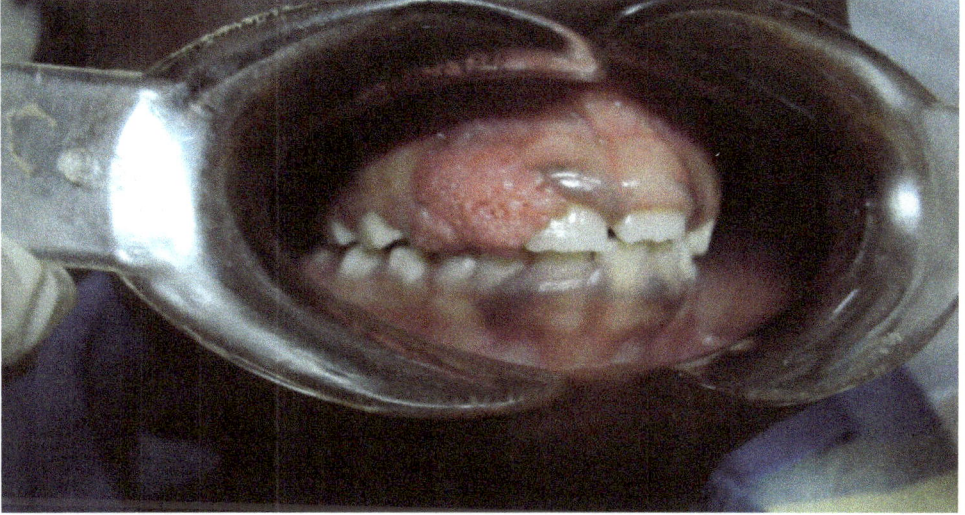

Fig. 7a. Hyperplasic gingivae and generalized gingivitis in a 7 year old boy on carbamazepine for epilepsy

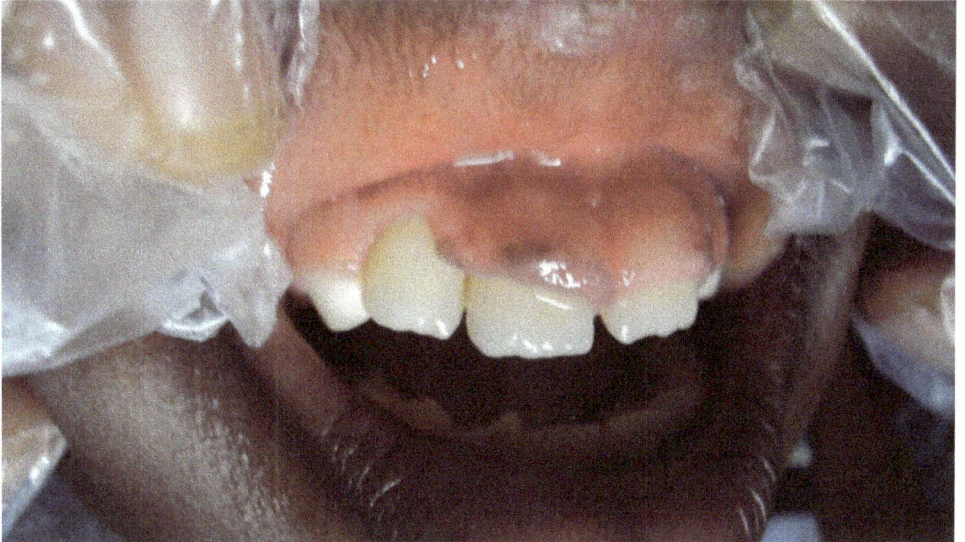

Fig. 7b. Post-operative appearance after excision of hyperplastic mass and removal of plaque

8.1 Gingivitis and orofacial clefts

Children with clefts have been found to show an increase in gingival inflammation when compared with control subjects (Lucas et al, 2000; Perdikogianni et al, 2009)). The cleft deformity, the soft tissue folds, the shallow vestibule, the dental arch irregularities, the long term orthodontic treatment and scar tissue observed in the region, after surgical closure of the cleft defect hinder optimal oral hygiene control (Stec et al, 2007). Parents and care givers should be educated on the method of plaque control as early as possible after presentation in the dental clinic to control plaque, thereby reducing inflammatory gingival and periodontal diseases. For the very young patients, chlorhexidine wipe after careful toothbrushing will reduce bacterial load and recurrent respiratory tract infections which follow aspiration of oral contents.

8.2 Gingivitis and neuromuscular disorders

Reduced muscle strength and motor function characterize conditions such as cerebral palsy (CP), poliomyelitis, myotonic dystrophy and Duchenne muscular dystrophy. Individuals affected by these conditions also have oral motor dysfunction, impairment of lip and tongue motility, lip force and chewing capacity which contribute to poor oral self cleansing ability and plaque and calculus accumulation. Several studies have shown poor oral hygiene and a higher prevalence of gingivitis and periodontal disease in these groups of individuals (Balasubramaniam et al, 2008; Symons et al, 2002; Engvall et al, 2009). According to findings from a recent study of a group of Nigerian individuals with CP and controls, gingivitis was more prevalent among those with CP (Oredugba, 2011). Mouth breathing and food pouching contribute to gingivitis especially in the anterior region in individuals with CP (Scully & Cawson, 2005). Gingival and periodontal diseases have been reported to be common, especially in older children with CP due to poor oral hygiene and complications of oral habits, physical disabilities, malocclusion and gingival hyperplasia caused by medications (National Institute of Dental and Craniofacial Research, 2004). Mouth breathing worsens the periodontal state and papillary hyperplastic gingivitis may be seen even in the absence of phenytoin (Scully & Cawson, 2005). Early routine oral care and close supervision will prevent the untoward consequence of periodontal disease.

8.3 Gingivitis and metabolic conditions

Diabetes mellitus (DM) is one of the most common chronic metabolic diseases of glucose metabolism which affects almost all the organs of the body. The Type 1 DM is the juvenile onset type which affects young people. Diabetes-related abnormalities include impaired hepatic glucose uptake, alterations in immune function, early cellular senescence and premature apoptosis (Crofford, 1995; Acikgoz et al, 2004). The oral environment is characterized by the presence of moisture, warmth and a constant reservoir of micro organisms and so, individuals with diabetes are at increased risk for oral diseases such as gingivitis and periodontal disease. Good and sustained glycaemic control will however reduce this risk considerably.

8.4 Gingivitis and haematological conditions

Gingivitis may be seen in patients affected by haematological conditions such as haemophilia, aplastic anaemia and leukaemia. Oral hygiene maintenance may be impaired because of their reluctance to brush their teeth for fear of increased gingival bleeding (Oyaizu et al, 2005). In very young children, the gingival bleeding may be experienced for the first time during exfoliation of primary teeth and eruption of the first set of permanent teeth **(Figs 8a & 8b)**.

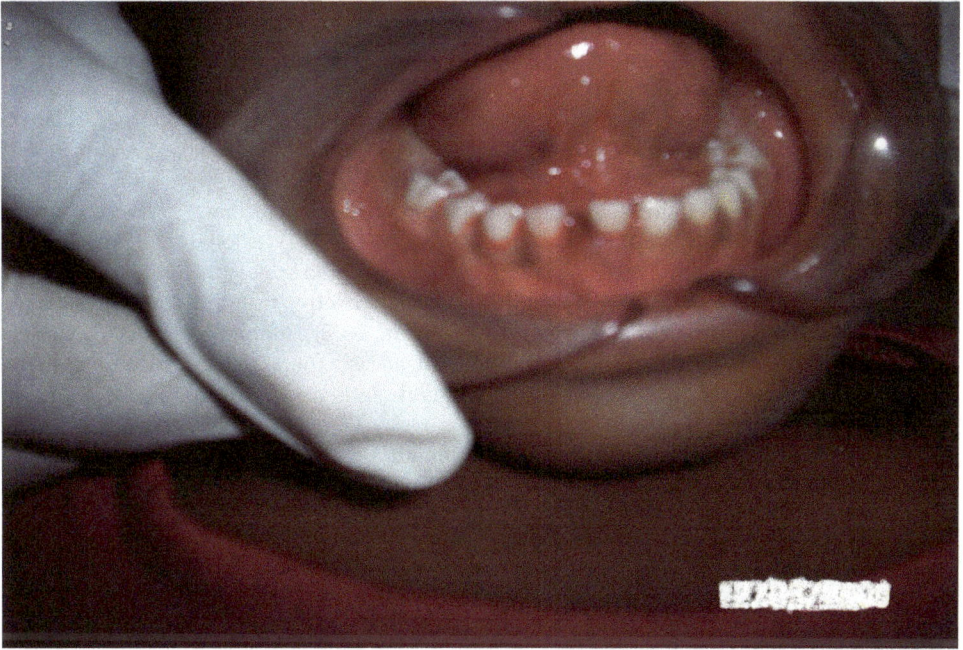

Fig. 8a. Gingival bleeding and gingivitis associated with plaque accumulation in a 3 year old haemophiliac *(Reproduced with permission from Nigerian Dental Journal, 2010,Vol.18,1)*

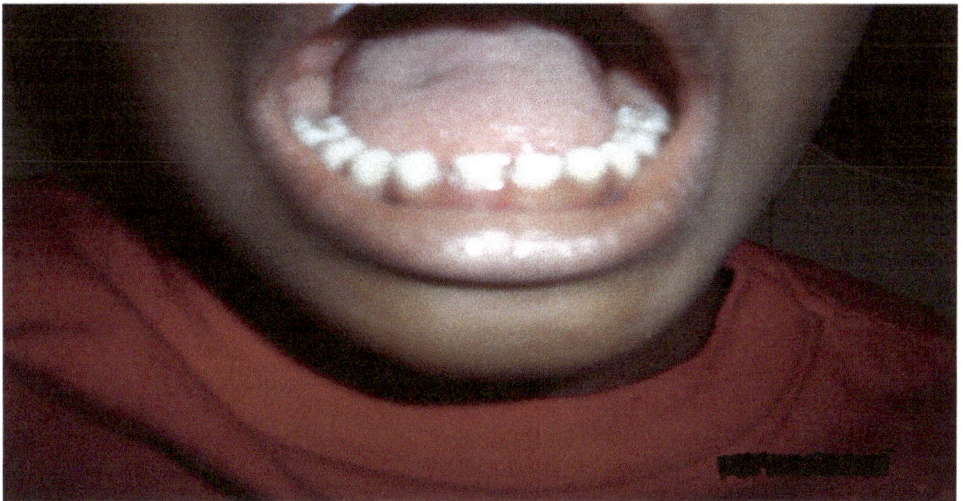

Fig. 8b. Clinical appearance after administration of Factor VIII and removal of plaque *(Reproduced with permission from Nigerian Dental Journal, 2010,Vol.18,1)*

Patients with aplastic anaemia have a weak immune response due to the concurrent immuno suppressive therapy and neutropenia (Agnihotri et al, 2009). Opportunistic infections from normal oral bacteria, periodontal pathogens or mixed odontogenic pathogens may also develop.

Oral findings in aplastic anaemia include gingival haemorrhage, mucosal petechiae, purpura and ecchymoses due to thrombocytopaenia (Neville et al, 2004). Ulcerative lesions with erythematous margins, especially of the gingiva, may develop in association with secondary infection (Oyaizu et al, 2005). Gingival hyperplasia, swelling and submucosal haemorrhage may also be present (Luker et al, 1991; Brennan et al, 2001). Patients with leukaemia present with bleeding diathesis, petechiae, oral ecchymosis, gingival haemorrhage and progressive gingival enlargement (Weckx et al, 1990; Genc et al, 1998). The change in gingival morphology and its cyanotic appearance may result from reactive hyperplasia, dense leukaemic infiltration of connective tissue and compression of local vasculature, causing ischaemia (Abdullah et al, 2002; Cooper et al, 2000). Caries, calculus and poor oral hygiene, place the patient at risk for oral pain, bleeding, super infection and tissue necrosis, exacerbating gingival signs and symptoms (Cooper et al, 2000).

Severe persistent gingival inflammation and stomatitis are some of the features of severe congenital neutropenia heightened by susceptibility to bacterial infections due to impaired bone marrow myelopoiesis and an absolute neutrophil count (ANC) in the peripheral blood of $< 0.2 \times 10\ ^9/L$ (Okada et al, 2001; Zeidler et al, 2009). Periodontal manifestations may range from marginal gingivitis to rapidly progressive periodontal disease with advancing bone loss, which may affect both primary and permanent dentitions, but primarily the permanent dentition (Zeidler et al, 2000). Although an individual's susceptibility to gingivitis and periodontal disease is influenced by many factors such as systemic diseases and genetics, evidence indicates that prevention of gingival inflammation by dental plaque control reduces the severity of disease in this group of individuals (Antonio et al, 2010). Such individuals should be motivated to maintain good oral hygiene. In most haematologic conditions, the most important part of patient management is making the patients and their relatives aware of the importance of preventive measures and the need for medical as well as dental appointments at appropriate intervals (Ranjith et al,2008).

While it is difficult to determine the relative importance of each aetiologic or facilitating factor for gingival and periodontal diseases, there is increasing data that indicates that environmental, dietary, behavioural and systemic factors, (including the genetic complement of the host) have an important role in gingival and periodontal disease initiation, progression and response to treatment (Hart, 2001; Shenkein, 2001)

9. Conclusion

Several factors such as genetics, systemic conditions, medications, diet and individual host response to infection have been identified in the aetiology of gingivitis in children. However, the most significant facilitating factor is dental plaque which could be controlled by mechanical means and use of topical chemical agents. Parents, relatives and care givers should be educated on the need for effective plaque control to prevent the condition.

10. References

Abdullah, BH; Yahyah, HI; Kumoona, RK; Hilmi, FA. & Mirza, KB. (2002). Gingival fine needle aspiration cytology in acute leukaemia. *Journal of Oral Pathology and Medicine*, Vol.31, pp. 55-58

Acikgoz, G; Devrim, I. & Ozdamar, S. (2004). Comparison of keratinocyte proliferation in diabetic and non- diabetic inflamed gingiva. *Journal of Periodontology*, Vol. 75, pp. 989-994

Agarwal, PK; Agarwal, KN. & Agarwal, DK. (1984). Biochemical changes in saliva of malnourished children. *American Journal of Clinical Nutrition*, Vol. 39, pp. 181-184

Agnihotri, R; Bhat, KM; Bhat, GS. & Pandurang, P. (2009). Periodontal management of a patient with severe aplastic anaemia: a case report. *Special Care Dentistry*, Vol. 29, pp. 141-144

Al-Meshal, IA. (1988). Effect of (alpha) chationone, an active principle of Catha edulis Forssk (khat) on plasma amino acid levels and other biochemical parameters in male wistar rats. *Phytotherapy Research*, Vol. 2, pp. 63–66

Antonio, AC; Alcantara, PC; Ramos, MEB. & de Souza, PR. (2010). The importance of dental care for a child with severe congenital neutropaenia: a case report. *Special Care Dentistry*, Vol. 30, pp. 261-265

Arduino, PG; D'Aiuto, F; Cavallito, C; Carcieri, P; Carbone, M; Conrotto, D; Defabianis, P. & Broccoletti, R. (2011). Professional oral hygiene as a therapeutic option for pediatric patients with plasma cell gingivitis: preliminary results of a prospective case series. *Journal of Periodontology*, May 12, (doi:10.1902/jop.2011.100663

Balasubramaniam, R; Sollecito, TP. & Stoopler, ET. (2008). Oral health considerations in muscular dystrophies. *Special Care Dentistry*, Vol. 28, pp. 243-253

Battino, M; Ferreiro, MS; Garllado, I; Newman, HN. & Bullon, P. (2002). The antioxidant capacity of saliva. *Journal of Clinical Periodontology*, Vol. 29, pp. 189-194

Bello, LL. & Al-Hammad, N. (2006). Pattern of fluid consumption in a sample of Saudi Arabian adolescents aged 12-13 years. *International Journal of Paediatric Dentistry*, Vol. 16, pp. 168-173

Brennan, MT; Sankar, V. & Baccaglini, L. (2001). Oral manifestations in patients with aplastic anaemia. *Oral Surgery Oral Medicine Oral Pathology Oral Radiology and Endodontics*, Vol. 92, pp. 503-508

Cooper, CL; Loewen, R. & Shore, T. (2000). Gingival hyperplasia complicating acute myelomonocytic leukaemia. *Journal of Canadian Dental Association*, Vol. 66, pp. 78-79

Crielaard, W; Zaura, E; Schuller, AA; Huse, SM; Montijn, RC. & Keijser, BJF. (2011). Exploring the oral microbiota of children at various developmental stages of their dentition in relation to their oral health. *BioMedCentral Medical Genomics* Vol. 4, 22

Crofford, OB. (1995). Diabetic control and complications. *Annual Review of Medicine*, Vol. 46, pp. 267-279

Cury, PR; Arsati, F; de Magalhaes, MH; de Araujo, VC; de Araujo, NS. & Barbuto, JA. (2009). Antigen-presenting cells in human immuno-suppressive drug-induced gingival enlargement. *Special Care Dentistry*, Vol. 29, pp. 80-84

Fleming, T. (1999). Periodontitis. *Annals of Periodontology. International Workshop for Classification of Periodontal Diseases and Conditions*, Vol. 4, pp. 32-35

Forsberg, H; Quick-Nilsson, I; Gustavson, KH. & Jagell, S. (1985). Dental health and dental care in severely mentally retarded children. *Swedish Dental Journal*, Vol. 9, pp. 15-28

Gafan, GP; Lucas, VF; Roberts, GJ; Petrie, A; Wilson, M. & Spratt, DA. (2004). Prevalence of periodontal pathogens in dental plaque of children. *Journal of Clinical Microbiology*, Vol. 42, pp. 4141-4146

Genc, A; Atalay, T; Gedikoglu, G; Zulfikar, B. & Kullu, S. (1998). Leukemic children: clinical and histopathological gingival lesions. *Journal of Clinical Pediatric Dentistry*, Vol. 22, pp. 253-256

Goodson, JM; Palys, MD; Carpino, E et al (2004). Microbiological changes associated with dental prophylaxis. *Journal of American Dental Association*, Vol. 35, pp. 1559-1564

Halbach, H. (1972). Medical aspects of the chewing of khat leaves. *Bullettin of the World Health Organization* Vol. 47, pp. 21–29

Han, Y. & Liu, HW. (2010). Progress on study on oral lesions in patients with AIDS. *Beijing Da Xue Xue Bao*, Vol. 42, pp. 117-121

Hart, TC. (2001). Genetic aspects of periodontal diseases. In: Bimstein, E; Needleman, HL; Karinbux, N. & Van Dyke, TE. *Periodontal and Gingival Health and Diseases. Children, Adolescents and Young Adults*. London, England:Martin Dunitz Ltd, pp. 189-204

Johansson, I; Ericsson, T. & Steen, L. (1984). Studies of the effect of diet on saliva secretion and caries development: the effect of fasting on saliva composition of female subjects. *Journal of Nutrition*, Vol. 114, pp. 2010-2020

Jones, CG. (2000). Chlorhexidine: is it still the good standard? *Periodontology*, Vol 15, pp. 55-62

Kalix, P. (1988). Khat: A plant with amphetamine effects. *Journal of Substance Abuse and Treatment*, Vol. 5, pp. 163–169

Kimura, S; Ooshima, T; Takiguchi, M; Sasaki, Y; Amano, A; Morisaki, I. & Hamada, S. (2002). Periodontopathic bacterial infection in childhood. *Journal of Periodontology*, Vol. 73, pp. 20-26

Kononen, E. (1999). Oral colonization by anaerobic bacteria during childhood: role in health and disease. *Oral Diseases*, Vol. 5, pp. 278-285

Lamster, IB; Grbic, JT; Mitchell-Lewis, DA; Begg, MD. & Mitchell, A. (1998). New concepts regarding the pathogenesis of periodontal disease in HIV infection. *Annals of Periodontology*, Vol. 3, pp. 62-75

Leroy, R; Jara, A; Martens, L. & Declerck, D. (2011). Oral hygiene and gingival health in Flemish pre-school children. *Community Dental Health,*Vol. 28, pp. 75-81

Loe, H; Theilade, E. & Jensen, SB. (1965). Experimental gingivitis in man. *Journal of Periodontology*, Vol. 36, pp. 177-187

Lovegrove, JM. (2004). Dental plaque revisited: bacteria associated with periodontal disease. *Journal of New Zealand Society of Periodontology*, Vol. 87, pp. 7-21

Lucas, VS; Gupta, R; Ololade, O; Gelbier, M. & Roberts, GJ. (2000). Dental health indices and caries associated microflora in children with unilateral cleft lip and palate. *Cleft Palate and Craniofacial Journal*, Vol. 37, pp. 447-452

Luker, J; Scully, C. & Oakhill, A. (1991). Gingival swelling as a manifestation of aplastic anaemia. *Oral Surgery Oral Medicine Oral Pathology*, Vol. 71, pp. 55-56

Macleod, RI. & Ellis, JE. (1989). Plasma cell gingivitis related to the use of herbal tooth-paste. *British Dental Journal*, Vol. 166, pp. 375–376

Majewsky, R. (2001). Dental caries in adolescents associated with caffeinated carbonated beverages. *Pediatric Dentistry* Vol. 23, pp. 198-203

Marker, P. & Krogdahl, A. (2002). Plasma cell gingivitis apparently related to the use of khat: report of a case. *British Dental Journal*, Vol. 192, pp. 311-313

Matsson, L. (1993).Factors influencing the susceptibility to gingivitis during childhood – a review. *International Journal of Paediatric Dentistry*, Vol. 3, pp. 119-127

Meyer, AC; Tera T; da Rocha, AC. & Jardini MAN. (2010). Clinical and microbiological evaluation of the use of toothpaste containing 1% chlorhexidine and the influence of motivation on oral hygiene in patients with motor deficiency. *Special Care Dentistry*, Vol. 30, pp. 140-145

Mundorff-Shrestha, SA; Featherstone, JDB. & Eisenberg, AD. et al (1994). Cariogenic potential of foods. *Caries Research*, Vol. 28, pp. 106-115

Nahar, SG; Hossain, MA; Howlader, MB. & Ahmed, A. (2010). Oral health status of disabled children. *Bangladesh Medical Research Council Bulletin*, Vol. 36, pp. 61-63

National Institute of Dental and Craniofacial Research. (2004). Practical oral care for people with cerebral palsy. *National Oral Health Information Clearinghouse, Bethesda, MD.*

Nejat, R; Nejat, D. & Nejat, M. (2007). Periodontal inflammation: the oral-body connection. *The Academy of Dental Therapeutics and Stomatology*. September, PennWell Publications

Neville, BW; Damm, DD; Allen, CM. & Bouquot, JE. (1995). *Oral and Maxillofacial Pathology*. Philadelphia: WB Saunders Company, pp. 126–127

Neville, BW; Damm, DD; Allen, CM. & Bouquot, JE. (2004). Hematological disorders. In: Neville BW, Damm DD, Allen CM, Bouquot JE (eds). *Oral and Maxillofacial Pathology*. Philadelphia, PA. WB Saunders Company, pp. 497-531

O'Brien, PJ. (1994). Antioxidants and cancer: molecular mechanisms. In: Amstrong D (ed). *Free Radicals in Diagnostic Medicine*. 2nd edition, New York. Plenum Press. Pp. 215-232

Oh, TJ; Eber, R. & Wang, HL. (2002). Periodontal disease in the child and adolescent. *Journal of Clinical Periodontology*, Vol. 29, pp. 400-410

Okada, M; Kobayashi, M; Hino, T; Kurihara, H. & Miura, K. (2001). Clinical periodontal findings and microflora profiles in children with chronic neutropenia under supervised oral hygiene. *Journal of Periodontology*, Vol. pp. 72, 945-952

Oredugba, FA. & Akindayomi, Y. (2008). Oral health status and treatment needs of children and young adults attending a day centre for individuals with special needs. *BioMedCentral Oral Health*, Vol. 8, 30

Oredugba, FA. (2006). Use of oral health care services and oral findings in children with special needs in Lagos, Nigeria. *Special Care Dentistry*, Vol. 26, pp. 59-65

Oredugba, FA. (2011), Comparative oral health of children and adolescents with cerebral palsy and controls. *Journal of Disability and Oral Health*, Vol. 12, pp. 81-87

Page, RC. & Shroeder, HE. (1976). Pathogenesis of inflammatory periodontal disease. *Laboratory Investigations*, Vol. 33, pp. 235-249

Papaioannou, W; Gizani, S; Haffajee, AD; Quirynen, M; Mama-Homata, E. & Papagiannoulis, L. (2009). The microbiota on different oral surfaces in healthy children. *Oral Microbiology and Immunology*, Vol. 24, pp. 183-189

Perdikogianni, H; Papaioannou, W; Nakou, M; Oulis, C. & Papagianoulis, L. (2009). Periodontal and microbiological parameters in children and adolescents with cleft lip and/palate. *International Journal of Paediatric Dentistry*, Vol. 19, pp. 455-467

Portela, MB; Souza, IPR; Costa, EMMB; Hagler, AN; Soares, RMA. & Santos, ALS. (2004). Differential recovery of Candida species from subgingival sites in human immunodeficiency virus-positive and healthy children from Rio de Janeiro, Brazil. *Journal of Clinical Microbiology*, Vol. 42, pp. 5925-5927

Ramzi, S; Contran, SL; Robins, V; Kumar, V; Robbins J. & Perkins A. (2002) *Basic Pathology,* 7th Edition. Harcourt Publishers Limited.

Ranjith, A; Nandakumar, K. & Glanzmann, A. (2008). Thrombasthenia; a rare hematological disorder with oral manifestations: a case report. *Journal of Contemporary Dental Practice,* Vol. 9, pp. 107-113

Robbins, MR. (2009). Dental management of special needs patients who have epilepsy. *Dental Clinics of North America,* Vol. 53, pp.295-309

Schenkein, HA. (2001). Pathogenesis of aggressive periodontitis. In: Bimstein, E; Needleman, HL; Karinbux, N. & Van Dyke, TE. *Periodontal and Gingival Health and Diseases. Children, Adolescents and Young Adults.* London, England: Martin Dunitz Ltd, pp. 147-197

Scully, C. & Cawson, RA. (2005). Neurological disorders I: Epilepsy, stroke and craniofacial neuropathies. In: Medical Problems in Dentistry. 5th Edition, Elsevier, Churchill Livingstone, pp. 297-298

Serio, FG. & Duncan, TB. (2009). The pathogenesis and treatment of periodontal disease. *Academy of Dental Therapeutics and Stomatology.* PennWell Publications, pp. 1-12

Serio, FG; Siegel, MA. & Slade, BF. (1991). Plasma cell gingivitis of unusual origin. *Journal of Periodontology,* Vol. 62, pp. 390–393

Stec, M; Szczepanska, J; Pypec, J. & Hirschfelder, U. (2007). Periodontal status and oral hygiene in two populations of cleft patients. *Cleft Palate and Craniofacial Journal,* Vol. 44, pp. 73-78

Surabian, SR. (2001). Developmental disabilities and understanding the needs of patients with mental retardation and Down syndrome. *Journal of Californian Dental Association,* Vol. 29, pp. 415-423

Surabian, SR. (2001). Developmental disabilities: epilepsy, cerebral palsy and autism. *Journal of Californian Dental Association,* Vol. 29, pp. 424-432

Symons, AI; Townsend, GC. & Hughes, TE. (2002). Dental characteristics of children with Duchenne muscular dystrophy. *Journal of Dentistry for Children,* Vol. 69, pp. 277-283, 234

Thomason, JM; Seymour, RA. & Rawlins, MD. (1992). Incidence and severity of phenytoin-induced gingival overgrowth in epileptic patients in general medical practice. *Community Dentistry and Oral Epidemiology,* Vol. 20, pp. 288-291

Trackman, PC. & Kantaki, A. (2004). Connective tissue metabolism and gingival overgrowth. *Critical Review of Oral Biology and Medicine* Vol. 15, pp. 165-175

Tulunoglu, O; Demirtas, S. & Tulunoglu, I. (2006). Total antioxidant levels of saliva in children related to caries, age and gender. *International Journal of Paediatric Dentistry* Vol. 16, pp. 186-191

Twetman, S. (2004). Antimicrobials in future caries control? A review with special reference to chlorhexidine treatment. *Caries Research,* Vol. 38, pp. 223-229

Weckx, LL; Hidal, LB. & Marcucci, G. (1990). Oral manifestations of leukaemia. *Ear Nose and Throat Journal,* Vol. 69, pp. 341-342, 345-346

Zeidler, C; Boxer, L; Dale, DC; Freedman, MH; Kinsey, S. & Welte, K. (2000). Management of Kostmann syndrome in the G-CSF era. *British Journal of Haematology,* Vol. 109, pp. 490-495

Zeidler, C; Germeshausen, M; Klein, C.& Welte, K. (2009). Clinical implications of ELA 2-, HAX 1-, and G-CSF receptor (CSF3R) mutations in severe congenital neutropenia. *British Journal of Haematology,* Vol. 144, pp. 459-467

The Principles Prevention in Dentistry

Jalaleddin Hamissi

Department of Periodontics & Preventive Dentistry, Faculty of Dentistry,
Qazvin University of Medical Sciences, Qazvin
Iran

1. Introduction

1.1 What is health promotion?

Health promotion is the science and art of helping people and society change their lifestyles to achieve optimal health. It places an emphasis on improving quantity and quality of life for all and enables the improvement of health. Therefore, health promotion includes the use of any preventive, educational, administrative policy, program, or law to achieve this outcome. (1, 2, 3) Health promotion practice and policy is currently undergoing a process of fundamental change. The focus of many health education interventions has been on defined diseases, targeted at changing the behaviors of high-risk individuals. Health professionals have dominated this approach in terms of programme development, implementation, and evaluations. This health education model has been very popular with the dental profession as it fits the clinical approach to care and treatment of individual patients. Recent effectiveness reviews of the oral health education and promotion literature have however, recognized the limitations of many educational interventions to produce sustained improvements in oral healths. Another one of the common finding of the reviews was the lack of theory underpinning many interventions (4-8).

2. Oral health promotion

2.1 What is oral health promotion?

Oral health is a vital part of general health and hence affects the total well-being of individuals; thus, special attention must be given to this subject. Health education is part of the wider aspect of oral health promotion which involves local, national and even international cooperation. Oral health promotion attempts to make the healthier choices (9).

Oral health promotion has developed and progressed a great deal in the last 20 years. In line with developments in public health, oral health promotion has changed focus to encompass a broader approach. It is important to highlight these developments as they are very relevant to the way in which oral health promotion interventions are evaluated (10, 11, 12).

Oral health promotion is aimed at four preventable oral diseases: dental caries, disease of supporting structures, oral pharyngeal cancers, and craniofacial injuries. The poor, minorities, and the elderly share a disproportionate amount of preventable oral disease. Since prevention is vital to health promotion, the goal of any oral health program should be to empower people to attain equity in health and to reduce the incidence and prevalence of oral diseases through education and interventions (1).

Many oral health professionals may feel very uncertain and anxious about how they can become involved in this health practice, which seems so far removed from prevention and clinical dentistry.

The behavior of oral health providers and their attitudes towards their own oral health reflect their understanding of the importance of preventive dental procedures and improving the oral health of their patients (13, 14).

Oral health related behaviors are not just simple actions, but are enmeshed in more complex socio-environmental conditions (15), which include educational programs, such as tobacco prevention and cessation programmes, and public school oral hygiene instruction.

It is about making wider changes, which will enable people to make healthier choices. Oral health professionals must take an active role in changing the perceptions related to oral healths by being involved in local initiatives that promotes health so that oral health becomes an integrated part of general health.

2.2 The Ottawa Charter

In 1986, WHO produced a document called *The Ottawa Charter* (16), which set out strategies for effective health promotion, including:

- Building healthy public policy.
- Local authority healthy eating policies.
- Creating supported environments.
- Developing individual knowledge and skill in those who deal with the public, including doctors, dental personnel, pharmacists, caterers, teachers and nursery staff.
- Supporting community action by working with voluntary groups in communities to care for the health in their particular community.
- Re-orientating health services towards prevention and ensuring that all health professionals give the same message.

2.3 Describing people's needs

If oral health promotion is to be effective, the Ottawa Charter needs to be in affect (for authorities, organizations, groups and individuals), continually revised, and delivered to the public in acceptable ways. In order to do this, it is necessary to define the needs of the people rather than their 'wants'. Epidemiological surveys show that people in poorer, deprived areas suffer far greater dental disease than those in wealthier areas and needs expressed by people in poorer areas are more likely to be free treatment, rather than water fluoridation. This is known as '*felt need*'.

The overall aim of oral health promotion is to influence the social norms of a community towards change and improvement (e.g. water fluoridation, smoking cessation, etc.).

The need for a dental health programme to target this specific segment of the population should be through systematic public and school oral health promotion programmes. Parents could also benefit from oral health education and should be advised regarding the necessity of regular dental follow-ups with dietary instructions to maintain good oral hygiene (17).

3. Oral public health

Nowadays, oral health is recognized as equally important in relation to general health (12). A recent document has set out new oral health objectives for the year 2020 (18).These includes paying special attention to high-risk groups. The current unequal distribution of caries in developed countries, where the highest percentage is reported, demonstrates the need to identify such risk groups (19).

In terms of prevention of oral diseases, the relationship between periodontal and caries status of professionals is significant. The oral health concern of an individual is dependent on the attitude of a person. These attitudes naturally reflect their own experiences, cultural perceptions, familial beliefs, and other life situations and strongly influence the oral health behavior (20). In numerous developing countries, the prevention of oral health programs does not benefit the general population. This is due in part to the incidence of dental caries that is expected to increase in the near future in many countries as a result of increased sugar consumption and insufficient exposure to fluoride. In addition, with the increased use of tobacco in developing countries, the risk of periodontal disease, tooth loss, and oral cancer is also on the rise. Periodontal disease and tooth loss are also linked to chronic diseases such as diabetes mellitus and in several countries research has shown that the growing incidence of diabetes has a negative impact on the oral health of people.

3.1 Oral health education
3.1.1 What is health education?
Health education is the profession of educating people about health (21). Areas within this profession include environmental health, physical health, social health, emotional health, intellectual health, and spiritual health (22). Health education also provides the decision-making basics needed for achieving and maintain health. It is a process of communicating information about evidence-based methods of disease prevention and encouraging responsibility for self-care (23).

3.2 Oral health
The major challenges for oral health in the near future will be to turn knowledge and experience of disease prevention into action. Oral health advances and knowledge have yet to be achieved in developing countries. Clear differences have widened the gap between the poor and wealthy countries. In the year 2007, the WHO General Assembly declared that a mechanism to provide essential oral health care coverage for the population so to promote the availability of oral health services should be directed towards disease prevention and health promotion for poor and disadvantage countries. It further stated that for these countries, particularly for schoolchildren, the development and implementation of preventive programmes as a part of activities in schools for promoting health, with aiming to introduce healthy lifestyle and self-care practices in children need to be considered (24, 25).

In the twenty-first century in the USA, a healthy smile is necessary for social mobility and acceptance, interpersonal relations, employability, and a good self-image. Poor oral health may lead to pain and infection, absence from school or work, poor nutrition, poor general health, an inability to speak or eat properly, and even early death. Studies done in the late 1990s showed that poor oral health may also lead to low birth-weight babies, heart disease, and stroke. Up until the late 1990s, when the new HIV medications became available, over 90 percent of persons with AIDS had HIV-related oral diseases; therefore, it is clear that oral diseases play a significant role in compromising the overall health potential of individuals.

Oral health promotion as an emerging discipline needs to be based upon an appropriate, rigorous, high quality theory if it is to develop and mature. Within public health, discussions and debates are focusing on the value of new theories and concepts. It is important that oral health promoters engage in an informed debate over the theoretical nature of their work. As Hochbaum and colleagues have stated 'Any profession that is not based on sound and continuously evolving theories that yield new understanding of its problems and yields new methods, is bound to stagnate and fall behind in the face of changing challenges.(26).

3.3 Oral health prevention programs

Oral disease, affects children, adults and families across the world every day, although they are nearly 100% preventable. While oral diseases are significant, their relationship to overall general health is often overlooked. It is the role of the dental public health to prevent and control dental diseases and promote dental health through organized community efforts.

This type of Oral Disease Prevention Program should be part of the Center for Health Promotion at all Departments of Health in the Ministry of Health and Medical Education. Moreover, this public health program should work to build the substructure and capacity of oral health within the community.

For those that have the Oral Disease Prevention Program (ODPP) in place, it works with partners throughout to reduce the prevalence and impact of oral disease. It also works to improve oral health care access and addresses oral health disparities in many countries.

Priority is given to diseases linked by common, preventable and lifestyle related risk factors (e.g. unhealthy diet, tobacco use, etc.), including oral health. Key socio-environmental factors involved in the promotion of oral health are also identified.

High relative risk of oral disease relates to socio-cultural determinants such as poor living conditions, low education, and lack of traditions, beliefs and culture in support of oral health. Communities and countries with inappropriate exposure to fluorides imply higher risk of dental caries and settings with poor access to safe water. Furthermore, control of oral disease depends on availability and accessibility of oral health systems but reduction of risks to disease are only possible if services are oriented towards primary health care and prevention.

Clinical and public health research has shown a number of individual, professional and community preventive measures are effective in preventing most oral diseases. This, together with insufficient emphasis on primary prevention of oral diseases, poses a considerable challenge for many countries, particularly the developing countries and countries with economies and health systems in transition.

Most of the evidence relates to dental caries prevention and control of periodontal diseases. Gingivitis can be prevented by good personal oral hygiene practices, including brushing and flossing which are important also for the control of advanced periodontal lesions. Community water fluoridation is effective in preventing dental caries in both children and adults. Water fluoridation benefits all residents served by community water supplies regardless of their social or economic status. Salt and milk fluoridation schemes are shown to have similar effects when used in community preventive programmes. Professional and individual measures, including the use of fluoride mouth rinses, gels, toothpastes and the application of dental sealants are additional means of preventing dental caries. In a number of developing countries the introduction of affordable fluoridated toothpaste has been shown to be a valuable strategy, ensuring that people are exposed appropriately to fluorides.

Individuals can take actions for themselves and for persons under their care, to prevent disease and maintain health. With appropriate diet and nutrition, primary prevention of many oral, dental and craniofacial diseases can be achieved. Lifestyle behavior that affects general health such as tobacco use, excessive alcohol consumption and poor dietary choices affect oral and craniofacial health as well. These individual behaviors are associated with increased risk of craniofacial birth defects, oral and pharyngeal cancers, periodontal disease, dental caries, oral candidiasis and other oral conditions.

Opportunities exist to expand oral disease prevention and health promotion knowledge and practices among the public through community programmes and in health care settings. Oral health care providers can also play a role in promoting healthy lifestyles by incorporating tobacco cessation programmes and nutritional counseling into their practices.

However, there are profound oral health disparities across regions, countries and within countries. These may relate to socioeconomic status, race or ethnicity, age, gender or general health status. Although common dental diseases are preventable, not all community members are informed of or are able to benefit from appropriate oral health-promoting measures. Under-served population groups are found in both developed and developing countries. In many countries, moreover, oral health care is not fully integrated into national or community health programmes.

The major challenges of the future will be to translate knowledge and experiences about disease prevention into action programmes. Social, economic and cultural factors and changing population demographics impact the delivery of oral health services in countries and communities and how people care for themselves. Reducing disparities requires far-reaching wide-ranging approaches that target populations at highest risk of specific oral diseases and involves improving access to existing care. Meanwhile, in several developing countries the most important challenge is to offer essential oral health care within the context of primary health programmes. Such programmes should meet the basic health needs of the population, strengthen active outreach to the community, organize primary care, and ensure effective patient referral.

To implement oral disease prevention programmes globally, existing partnerships must be strengthened, notably with national and international nongovernmental organizations and WHO Collaborating Centers on Oral Health. The WHO Regional Offices play an important roles in the implementation process. WHO coordinates, in collaboration with the international oral health community, global alliances with a view to sharing responsibilities for implementation of a global strategy. One major responsibility for WHO is map the changing patterns of oral diseases and to analyze their determinants, with particular reference to poor or disadvantaged populations. WHO's work for oral health also focuses on devising tools for intersectorial collaboration, community participation, supportive policy decisions, oral health care reform, and development of community-based strategies for oral disease control.

4. Major oral diseases

Oral disease is one of the most prevalent diseases in the world, causing considerable morbidity, particularly for disadvantaged populations and it has many risks common to other diseases affected by lifestyles. There are many different types of oral diseases, but they are generally differentiated as being of hard / soft tissue in origin. Hard-tissue oral diseases are those of the teeth, supporting bone and jaw; whereas soft tissue diseases affect the tissues in and around the mouth, including the tongue, lips, cheek, gums, salivary glands, and roof and floor of the mouth. Some oral diseases may result in both hard and soft tissue disorders and conditions such as cleft palate or oral-facial injuries. The major oral diseases and conditions are:

- Dental caries (tooth decay, cavities)
- Periodontal disease (gum disease)

- Malocclusion (crooked teeth)
- Edentulism (complete tooth loss)
- Oral cancer
- Craniofacial birth defects such as cleft lip and cleft palate
- Soft tissue lesions
- Oral-facial injuries
- Temporomandibular dysfunction (TMD)

4.1 What is caries?
Caries is the progressive destruction of enamel, dentine and cementum, initiated by microbial activity at a susceptible tooth surface. *Caries* is a Latin word meaning *decay*.

5. Dental caries & tooth loss

5.1 Overview
Dental caries is commonly known as tooth decay. In the minds of the lay person, and surprisingly even within dentistry, dental caries is often thought of as holes in the teeth rather than an entire disease process. Although dental caries is the most commonly investigated oral disease, most studies have only focused on children and thus studies on caries among adolescents and young adults are scarce. It is still one of the most common chronic diseases affecting children and adolescents in the world today (27, 28). Dental caries is a disease which afflicts humans of all ages, in all regions of the world. Subsequently, several studies have been carried out around the world to assess dental caries prevalence among children. In particular, there has been some discussion of early sociobiological factors affecting dental caries later in life.

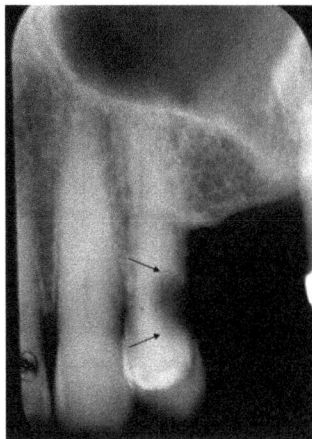

Fig. 1. Radiograph illustrating a large carious lesion on the distal root surface of a maxillary first bicuspid tooth (arrows)

The current unequal distribution of caries in developed countries, where the highest percentages has been reported demonstrates the need to identify such risk groups. With the enlarged use of fluoride, the detection of caries is not as simple as before. Yet, in 2009 many of us are still diagnosing caries the same way as in the early 1900s. The goal now is to be minimally invasive — to catch caries at its earliest stages and attempt to remineralize incipient caries in teeth through the use of ozone and MI paste. Decay is difficult to detect in radiographs unless they are larger than 2 to 3 mm deep into dentin, or one-third of the buccolingual distance. A sharp explorer has a high specificity, but a low sensitivity for caries. Therefore, a lot of incipient caries can be missed if we rely on an explorer and radiographs alone. However, it has been known for over 100 years that dental decay is caused by multifactorial, transmissible diseases that involve dissolution of mineralized tooth structure by acids produced by dental plaque bacteria (29).Two groups of bacteria are responsible for initiating caries: *Streptococcus mutans* and *Lactobacillus*. If left untreated, the disease can lead to pain, tooth loss and infection (30).

A substrate (fermentable carbohydrate) and a susceptible host. The results of bacterial metabolism of carbohydrates include lactic acid and uric acid, which can lead to demineralization of the enamel and dentin. When the tooth root is exposed, the cementum covering the root surface is also affected. Dental caries can occur as coronal caries, root caries (Fig 1) and recurrent caries (caries associated with existing dental restorations).

5.2 Types of caries
There are three main types of caries as follows:
1. *Smooth surface caries* (Fig .2).
2. *Pit and fissure caries*-common in newly erupted teeth (Fig .3).
3. *Root caries*-Common in elderly, when root surfaces are exposed (Fig .4).
    Gross caries (Fig.5).

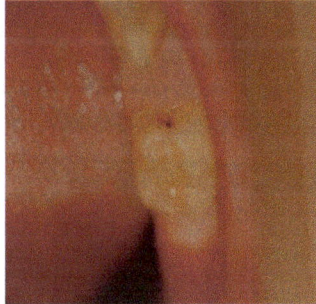

Fig. 2. Smooth surface caries on lower molar

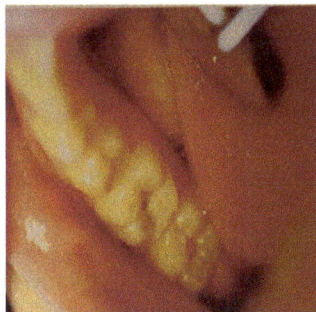

Fig. 3. Pit and fissure caries in lower molar

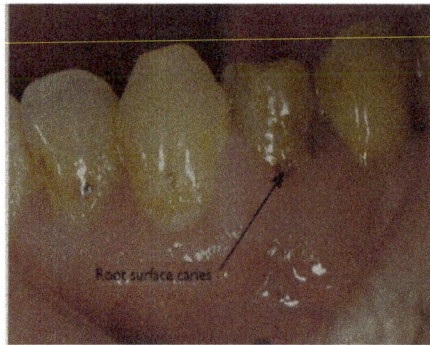

Fig. 4. Root Caries

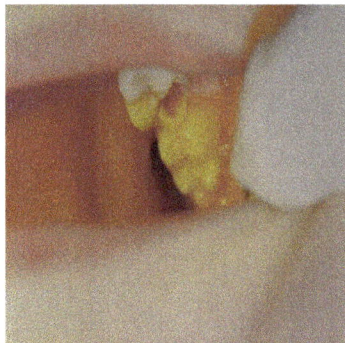

Fig. 5. Gross caries with collapse of overlying tooth cusp

5.3 Development of caries

There are four factors to develop dental caries:

- Susceptible tooth
- Bacterial plaque
- Bacterial substrate (fermentable carbohydrate, which feeds plaque bacteria).
- Time.

Susceptible tooth + bacterial plaque + substrate + time = Caries

The most common sites where caries can occurs are:

1. Occlusal surfaces of newly erupted pre-molars and molars
2. Contact areas between adjacent teeth
3. Exposed root surfaces

The least common sites for caries to occur are smooth surfaces

Improved ways for the detection of caries include the use of devices that detect caries through fluorescence and a low power laser to scan for tooth decay. New methods will soon appear to improve the ability of dentists to detect caries earlier than before. With this enhanced knowledge, dentists will be able to establish better protocols for caries intervention and treatment.

5.4 Epidemiology of caries

Epidemiology is the study of the incidence and severity of diseases within population groups. A number of studies have contributed to existing knowledge of the cause and development of dental caries.

Dental caries remain a major problem in many developing countries. Although decaling in most western countries over the past decades, caries continue to be the principal reason for dental treatment and tooth loss.

The application of specific agents for caries prevention in children and adolescents has been on the increase in the dental profession. These techniques include professional or at-home applications of fluorides, dental sealants, antimicrobials such as chlorhexidine, and xylitol chewing gum with studies supporting their use. For caries prevention, in order for these regimens to be as effective as possible, this evidence must transfer into increased use in the practice of clinical dentistry.

6. What is Gingivitis?

Gingivitis (*inflammation of the gingival* tissue) is a term used to describe non-destructive periodontal disease (31). The most common form of gingivitis is in response to bacterial biofilms (also called plaque) adherent to tooth surfaces, termed *plaque-induced gingivitis*, and is the most common form of periodontal disease. In the absence of treatment, gingivitis may progress to periodontitis, which is a destructive form of periodontal disease (32). While in some sites or individuals, gingivitis never progresses to periodontitis (33), data indicates that periodontitis is always preceded by gingivitis (34). According to the World Workshop in Clinical Periodontics in year 1999; there are two primary groups of gingival diseases, each with numerous subgroups (35):

6.1 Dental plaque-induced gingival diseases
- Gingivitis associated with plaque only
- Gingival diseases modified by systemic factors
- Gingival diseases modified by medications
- Gingival diseases modified by malnutrition

6.2 Non-plaque-induced gingival lesions
1. Gingival diseases of specific bacterial origin
2. Gingival diseases of viral origin
3. Gingival diseases of fungal origin
4. Gingival diseases of genetic origin
5. Gingival manifestations of systemic conditions
6. Traumatic lesions
7. Foreign body reactions
8. Not otherwise specified

6.3 Symptoms
- Bleeding
- Bright red or red-purple appearance (Healthy gums are pink and firm in appearance)
- Tender when touched, sometimes painless

- Mouth sores
- Swollen gingiva
- Shiny appearance

6.4 Treatment

The objectives of treatment are to reduce inflammation. The teeth are cleaned with scaling or root planning thoroughly by the dentist or dental hygienist. Careful oral hygiene is necessary after scaling and polishing. It is recommended that professional tooth cleaning be done twice per year or more frequently for severe cases in addition to brushing and flossing, antibacterial mouth rinses or other aids that may be suggested.

Orthodontic appliances may be advised for the treatment of malpositioned teeth or replacement of dental and other related illnesses.

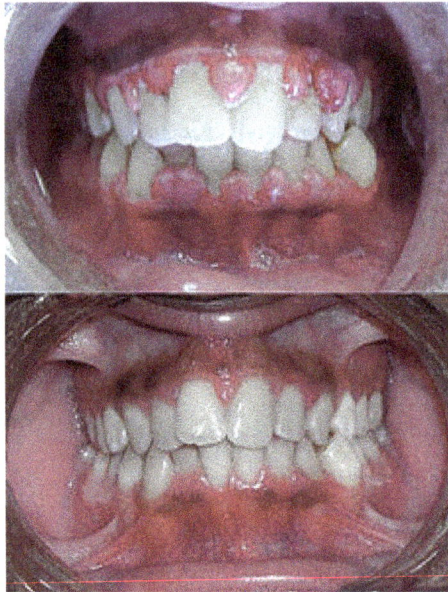

Fig. 6. Severe gingivitis before (**top**) and after (**bottom**) a thorough mechanical debridement of the teeth and adjacent gum tissues.

6.5 Complications

- Recurrence of gingivitis
- Periodontitis
- Infection or abscess of the gingiva or the jaw bones

6.6 Prevention

Good oral hygiene is the best prevention against gingivitis because it removes the dental plaques that causes the disorder. The teeth should be brushed at least twice daily and flossed at least once per day. For people who are prone to gingivitis, brushing and flossing may be recommended after every meal. Regular scaling and polishing professionally is important to removes plaque that may develop even with careful brushing and flossing. Many dentists recommend having the teeth professionally cleaned at least every 6 months.

7. What is periodontal disease?

Periodontal disease is a type of disease that affects one or more of the periodontal apparatus tissues:
*   alveolar bone
*   periodontal ligament
*   cementum
*   gingiva

While many different diseases affect the tooth-supporting structures, plaque-induced inflammatory lesions make up the vast majority of periodontal diseases (34) and have traditionally been divided into two categories (36):
1. Gingivitis
2. Periodontitis.

Although in some sites or individuals, gingivitis never progresses to periodontitis (33), data indicates that gingivitis almost always precedes periodontitis.

7.1 Epidemiology of periodontal disease

As recently as the mid-1960s, the main model for the epidemiology of periodontal diseases included these principles:
1. All individuals were considered more or less equally susceptible to severe periodontitis;
2. Gingivitis usually progressed to periodontitis with consequent loss of bony support and eventually loss of teeth;
3. Susceptibility to periodontitis increased with age and was the main cause of tooth loss after age 35 (37-40).

Data on the prevalence of periodontitis are dependent on how the disease is defined and the age group from which they were taken. Some 5% to 20% of any population suffers from severe, generalized periodontitis, although mild to moderate periodontitis affects a majority of adults. For those who are most susceptible, periodontitis becomes evident in teenage and early adult years rather than the later years. There are some risk factors for periodontitis include smoking, genetic predisposition, probably psychosocial stress, diabetes, and several uncommon systemic diseases. Improved molecular biology techniques for measuring bacteria and inflammatory cytokines have aided recent research in both epidemiology and clinical studies, and in the future are likely to permit more accurate diagnosis in the clinic (41).

7.2 Periodontal disease and associated factors

Plaque is the primary cause of gingival disease. There are factors that can contribute to periodontal disease which includes:
*   **Hormonal changes**, such as those occurring during pregnancy, puberty, menopause, and monthly menstruation, make gingiva more sensitive, which makes it easier for gingivitis to develop.
*   **Illnesses** may affect the condition of gingiva gums. This includes diseases such as cancer or HIV that interfere with the immune system. Since diabetes affects the body's ability to use blood sugar, patients with this disease are at higher risk of developing infections, including periodontal disease.

- **Medications** could affect oral health because some drugs could lessen the flow of saliva, which has a protective effect on teeth and gums. Some drugs, such as the anticonvulsant medication *Dilantin* and the anti-angina drug *Procardia* and *Adalat* can cause gingival hyperplasia.
- **Bad habits** such as smoking make it harder for gum tissue to healing itself.
- **Poor oral hygiene habits** such as not brushing or flossing on a daily basis make it easier for gingivitis to progress.
- **Family history of dental disease** can be a contributing factor for the development of gingivitis and periodontitis.

8. Malocclusion

Malocclusion is the misalignment of the upper and lower teeth when biting or chewing. A malocclusion is a misalignment of teeth and/or incorrect relation between the teeth of the two dental arches. The term was coined by Edward Angle, the "father of modern orthodontics" (42).

Alternative Names

Crowded teeth; Misaligned teeth; Crossbite; Overbite; Underbite; Open bite

How to identify Malocclusion?

- Pain arising from pressure to the jaw
- Problems in speech and ability to eat
- Breathing through the mouth
- Difficulty in keeping the lips closed

8.1 Cause

Causes and symptoms

Malocclusions are most often inherited, but may be acquired. Inherited conditions include too many or too few teeth, too much or too little space between teeth, irregular mouth and jaw size and shape, and atypical formations of the jaws and face, such as a cleft palate. Malocclusions may be acquired from habits like finger or thumb sucking, tongue thrusting, premature losses of teeth from an accident or dental disease, and possibly from medical conditions such as enlarged tonsils and adenoids that lead to mouth breathing.

Malocclusions may cause no symptoms, or they may produce pain from the increased stress on oral structures. Teeth may show abnormal signs of wear on the chewing surfaces or decay in areas of tight overlap and chewing may be difficult. Crowding of teeth is recognized as an affliction that stems in part from a modern western lifestyle. It is unknown whether it is due to the consistency of western diets, a result of mouth breathing; or the result of an early loss of deciduous teeth due to decay.

Other theories state that the malocclusion could be due to trauma during development that affects the permanent tooth bud, ectopic eruption of teeth, supernumerary teeth, and early loss of the primary tooth.

Causes of malocclusion include:

- Childhood habits such as thumb sucking, tongue thrusting, pacifier use beyond age 3, and prolonged use of a bottle

- Extra teeth, lost teeth, impacted teeth, or abnormally shaped teeth
- Ill-fitting dental fillings, crowns, appliances, retainers, or braces
- Misalignment of jaw fractures after a severe injury
- Tumors of the mouth and jaw

During active skeletal growth (43) mouth breathing, finger sucking, thumb sucking, pacifier sucking, onychophagia (nail biting), dermatophagia, pen biting, pencil biting, abnormal posture, deglutition disorders and other habits greatly influence the development of the face and dental arches (44).

Pacifier sucking habits are also correlated with otitis media. Dental caries, periapical inflammation and tooth loss in the deciduous teeth alter the correct permanent teeth eruptions.

Complications

- Tooth decay
- Discomfort during treatment
- Irritation of mouth and gums (gingivitis) caused by appliances
- Chewing or speaking difficulty during treatment

8.2 Treatment of malocclusion

Crowding of the teeth are treated with orthodontics, often with tooth extraction and dental braces, followed by growth modification in children or jaw surgery (orthognathic surgery) in adults. This could be as follows:

- **Use of brackets**

  Malocclusion is commonly treated by using dental brackets. The constant and gently pressure provided by braces will enable teeth straightening and help push teeth back to their correct position. Braces consist of brackets that are fixed to the teeth, and wires that connect the brackets. Since the braces cannot be removed, extra attention should be paid in keeping the teeth clean and getting rid of food particles that are likely to get stuck in the braces.

- **Removal of teeth**

  This will help in instances of overcrowding, where it would make room for the other teeth to move into the correct position.

- **Reshaping, and bonding or capping teeth**

  This will treat rough or irregular teeth removing resistance in forming a proper bite.

- **Surgery**

  Requirement of surgery is rare. Surgery can be used to reshape the jaw or to stabilize the jaw bone through wires, plates or screws where required.

  Malocclusion can be treated in the majority of cases. Consulting a dentist early when malocclusion is suspected can ensure proper and effective treatment which will help in maintaining proper dental health.

8.3 Prevention

Many types of malocclusion are not preventable. Control of habits such as thumb sucking may be necessary in some cases. However, early detection and treatment may optimize the time and method of treatment needed.

9. Edentulism

Edentulism or tooth losses is considered as a major health problem that has serious emotional, social, and psychological consequences affecting a person's self-confidence, self-esteem, and overall health. Edentulism is a condition when one or more teeth are missing, have fallen out, or need removing due to injury or some dental disease. It can be full or partials, depending on the severity of the condition.

Edentulism is the condition of being toothless to at least some degree; it is the result of tooth losses. Loss of some teeth results in *partial edentulous,* while loss of all teeth results in *complete edentulism*. Organisms that never possessed teeth can also be described as *edentulous*.

Tooth loss among elderly people is usually attributed to plaque accumulation, gum recessions, and dry mouth.

9.1 Cause

The etiology, or cause of edentulism, can be multifaceted. While the extraction of non-restorable or non-strategic teeth by a dentist does contribute to edentulism, the predominant cause of tooth loss in developed countries is periodontal disease. While the teeth may remain completely decay-free, the bone surrounding and providing support to the teeth may reabsorb and disappear, giving rise to tooth mobility and eventual tooth loss. In the photo at right, tooth #21 (the lower left first premolar, to the right of #22, the lower left canine) exhibits 50% bone loss, presenting with a distal horizontal defect and a mesial vertical defect. Tooth #22 exhibits roughly 30% bone loss (45).

9.2 Other causes of edentulism

Other causes of edentulism include the following:

- **Poor oral hygiene habits:** Not brushing or flossing daily can cause the development and progression of tooth decay and gingival disease, increasing the risk of tooth loss.
- **Poor diet:** Foods and drinks high in sugar, carbohydrates and acid may cause irreversible tooth and gum damage, resulting in tooth loss.
- **Bad habits:** Smoking, chewing tobacco and/or drug use can damage teeth to the point of tooth loss.
- **Lack of education about tooth loss:** A lack of education about the causes and consequences of tooth loss prevents people from taking the proper preventative lifestyle and oral health care measures, or from getting periodic dental maintenance or necessary restorative treatment.
- **Fear and embarrassment:** Many people suffer from dental phobia, or anxiety/fear of going to the dentist, and do not seek dental treatment, even do they know they have a problem or pain. Others are embarrassed or ashamed to seek dental treatment because they feel they will be blamed for the condition of their teeth. Ignoring tooth decay or other serious dental problems can prolong and aggravate the condition and eventually lead to tooth loss.
- **Finances:** Some people have to postpone or forgo dental visits and treatments, including regular check-ups and cleanings, due to high dental care costs and/or lack of insurance coverage. Unfortunately, prolonging or eliminating dental care increases the chances of developing serious problems and, subsequently, greater expense for treatments.

- **Trauma:** Babies and young children are most susceptible to losing teeth prematurely due to trauma, because their tooth roots and gums are still developing. If parents do not take the proper and often immediate steps to deal with dental trauma, their children's oral health can be permanently affected. Adults, particularly those who participate in sports or suffer accidents affecting the face, also are at risk for tooth loss.
- **Systemic conditions:** Such as heart disease, respiratory disease, diabetes, HIV infection, malnutrition and immunosuppression are all associated with forms of periodontitis that often result in tooth loss.
- **Medical treatments:** Certain treatments, such as chemotherapy, head radiation therapy and immunosuppressive medications, weaken the immune system. These treatments may increase the risk of tooth infections and, therefore, the need for tooth extraction.

9.3 Treatments for tooth loss

- Patients and their dentists should develop a treatment plan that emphasizes prevention and early detection of oral diseases in order to keep the remaining teeth, especially in cases of partial edentulism. Prevention and detection strategies include patient education about edentulism causes, consequences and treatments, and following preventive oral health practices (e.g., daily oral health care), as well as preventative and therapeutic treatment.
- However, if tooth loss is unavoidable, there are several options for restoring your teeth and your smile.
- **Dental implants** are artificial tooth roots surgically attached to the jaw to secure a replacement tooth, bridge or denture. Permanent and stable, implant-supported restorations look, feel and function like natural teeth. Dental implants also can be used with a denture for better stabilization. Some implants take two to six months for the bone and implant to bond together (osseointegrate). During this time, a removable temporary tooth replacement can be worn over the implant site. Research also has advanced to where an implant can be placed immediately following tooth extraction in certain cases.
- **Dentures** are removable replacements for missing teeth and adjoining tissues. Partial dentures fill in the spaces created by missing teeth, keep remaining teeth from shifting and are an option if you have some natural teeth remaining. If you have lost most or all of your teeth, complete or full dentures are recommended. "Immediate" dentures are inserted immediately after removal of the natural teeth; "conventional" dentures are placed in the mouth about three to six months after tooth removal.
- A **dental bridge** is a false tooth that is fused between two porcelain crowns to fill in or bridge the space left by a missing tooth. The two crowns holding the dental bridge in place are cemented to your teeth on each side of the space; the bridge is secured into place and is irremovable. Some bridges also may contain two or more false teeth between the crown components, depending on the case.

9.4 Edentulism affects several areas of life

- **Low self-esteem**: Edentulism prevents people from feeling confident about their appearances. Many adults hesitate to venture into the public without teeth. They feel embarrassed to talk, smile and lack the confidence to meet people.
- **Impaired speech**: Edentulism affects speech; a lot of sounds and words we utter, depend on our front teeth. Using dentures too affects speech, especially if the dentures

are not well fitted. The individual usually tenses the facial muscles to hold the dentures in place, or constantly uses the tongue to rearrange it; resulting in slurred speech and clicking noises.

- **Increased health risk**: Edentulous individuals are at an increased risk for cardiovascular diseases.
- **Changed appearance**: Edentulous individuals have to deal with altered appearance, loss of teeth, and changes in their facial structure such as recessed cheeks, unsupported lips, collapsed jawline, which makes the chin and nose to be appear closer. There is a huge change in a person's looks because the teeth, which support the facial muscles, are no longer present.
- **Facial ageing**: Total tooth loss accelerates facial ageing because the bone reduces in height and thickness; jawbone begins to shrink making the face look older.

10. Oral cancer

Cancer is one of the most common worldwide causes of morbidity and mortality today, with more than 10 million new cases and more than 6 million deaths each year (45). More than 20 million people around the world live with a diagnosis of cancer, and more than half all cancer cases happen in the developing countries; about 20% of all deaths in high-income countries and 10% in low-income countries. By the year 2020, there will be every year 15 million new cancer cases and 10 million cancer deaths. The cancer epidemic in high-income countries, and increasingly in low/middle-income countries, is also due to high or increasing levels of prevalence of cancer risk factors (46). It is estimated that around 43% of cancer deaths are due to *tobacco use, unhealthy diets, alcohol consumption, inactive lifestyles* and *infection* (47). And the world's most avoidable cause of cancer is tobacco user. In addition to lung cancer, tobacco consumption causes cancer of the oral cavity, pharynx, larynx, esophagus, stomach, pancreas, liver, kidney, ureter, urinary bladder, uterine cervix and bone marrow (myeloid leukemia). Exposure to environmental tobacco smoke (passive smoking) increases risk of lung cancer. Tobacco user and alcohol consumption act synergistically to cause cancer of the oral cavity, pharynx, larynx and esophagus. Cancer incidence and survival rates are clearly linked to socioeconomic factors. Infectious agents are responsible for almost 25% of cancer deaths in the developing and 6% in industrialized countries (47, 48).

The worldwide occurrence of oral cancer is high particularly among men; it is the eighth most common cancer (49, 50, 51). Cancer is one of the major threats to public health and increasingly in the developing world. Cancer is a silent epidemic that has not yet attracted major attention among health policy-makers and public health administrators.

10.1 Treatment and prevention

Treatment aims and therapy of disease prolong life and improve the quality of life. The most efficient treatment care is early detection programmes and following evidence-based standards. Treatment guidelines and praxis guides improve treatment outcome by setting standards for patient management. The formulation of guidelines and their adaptation to various resource settings help to assure quality including equitable and sustainable access to treatment resources.

To ensure that prevention of oral cancer is an integral part of national cancer control programmes, and to involve oral health professionals or primary health care personnel with relevant training in oral health in detection, early diagnosis and treatment, the WHO Global Oral Health Programme. intends to work for the integration of oral cancer prevention into cancer prevention.

10.2 Craniofacial birth defects such as cleft lip and cleft palate

Craniofacial defects such as cleft lip and cleft palate are among the most common of all birth defects. They can be isolated or one component of an inherited disease or syndrome. Both genetic and environmental factors contribute to oral clefts. Although clefts can be repaired to varying degrees with surgery, researchers are working to understand the developmental processes that lead to clefting and how to prevent the condition or more effectively treat it.

Cleft lip and cleft palate are birth defects that occur when a baby's lip or mouth do not form properly. Together, these birth defects commonly are called "orofacial clefts". These birth defects happen early during pregnancy. A baby can have a cleft lip, a cleft palate, or both.

Children with a cleft lip with or without a cleft palate or a cleft palate alone often have problems with feeding and talking. They also might have ear infections, hearing loss, and problems with their teeth.

The Centers for Disease Control and Prevention (CDC) recently estimated that each year 2,651 babies in the United States are born with a cleft palate and 4,437 babies are born with a cleft lip with or without a cleft palate (53). Cleft lip is more common than cleft palate. Isolated orofacial clefts, or clefts that occur with no other birth defects, are one of the most common birth defects in the United States. About 70% of all orofacial clefts are isolated clefts.

10.2.1 Cleft lip

The lip forms between the fourth and seventh weeks of pregnancy. A cleft lip happens if the tissues that make up the lip do not join completely before birth. This results in an opening in the upper lip. The opening in the lip can be a small slit or it can be a large opening that goes through the lip into the nose. A cleft lip can be on one or both sides of the lip or in the middle of the lip, which occurs very rarely. Children with a cleft lip also can have a cleft palate.

10.2.2 Cleft palate

The roof of the mouth is called the "palate." It is formed between the sixth and ninth weeks of pregnancy. A cleft palate happens if the tissue that makes up the roof of the mouth does not join correctly. Among some babies, both the front and back parts of the palate are open. Among other babies, only part of the palate is open.

10.2.3 Causes and risk factors

Just like the many families affected by birth defects, CDC wants to find out what causes them. Understanding the risk factors that can increase the chance of having a baby with a birth defect will help us learn more about the causes. CDC currently is working on one of the largest studies in the United States—the National Birth Defects Prevention Study—to understand the causes of and risk factors for birth defects. This study is looking at many possible risk factors for birth defects, such as orofacial clefts.

The causes of orofacial clefts among most infants are unknown. Some children have a cleft lip or cleft palate because of changes in their genes. Cleft lip and cleft palate are thought to be caused by a combination of genes and other factors, such as exposures in the environment, maternal diet, and medication use (54).

Recently, CDC reported on important findings about some factors that increase the risk of orofacial clefts:

- Smoking—Women who smoke during pregnancy are more likely to have a baby with an orofacial cleft than women who do not smoke (55).
- Diabetes—Women with diabetes diagnosed before pregnancy have been shown to be an increased risk of having a child with a cleft lip with or without cleft palate (56).

CDC continues to study birth defects, such as orofacial clefts and how to prevent them.

10.2.4 Causes of cleft lip and cleft palate

The specific causes or risk factors for developing cleft lip or palate are not well understood. Potential causes/risk factors include:

- **Genetics** - Sometimes cleft lips/palates run in families.
- **Syndromes** - A cleft lip and/or palate may occur with other birth defects as part of a genetic syndrome.
- **Environment** - Some studies suggest a link between maternal drug use (such as antiseizure medication), alcohol abuse, or smoking, maternal illness or infection, or deficiency of folic acid may be related to the development of a cleft lip or palate.
- **Spontaneous** - Most cleft lip/palate anomalies occur randomly and without any clear cause or fault.

10.2.5 Diagnosis

Orofacial clefts sometimes can be diagnosed during pregnancy, usually by a routine ultrasound. Most often, orofacial clefts are diagnosed after the baby is born. However, sometimes minor clefts (e.g., submucous cleft palate and bifid uvula) might not be diagnosed until later in life.

10.2.6 Treatments

Services and treatment for children with orofacial clefts can vary depending on the severity of the cleft; the presence of associated syndromes or other birth defects, or both; and the child's age and needs. Surgery to repair a cleft lip usually occurs in the first few months of life and is recommended within the first 12 months of life. Surgery to repair a cleft palate is recommended within the first 18 months of life (57). Many children will need additional surgeries as they get older. Although surgical repair can improve the look and appearance of a child's face, it also may improve breathing, hearing, speech, and language. Children born with orofacial clefts also might need different types of treatments and services, such as special dental or orthodontic care or speech therapy (58).

Because children and individuals with orofacial clefts often require a variety of services that need to be provided in a coordinated manner, services and treatment by cleft teams is recommended. Cleft teams provide a coordinated, interdisciplinary team approach to care for children with orofacial clefts. These teams usually consist of experienced and qualified physicians and health care providers from different specialties. Cleft teams and centers are located throughout the United States and other countries. Resources are available to help in choosing a cleft team. With treatment, most children with orofacial clefts do well and lead a healthy life.

10.3 Soft tissue lesions

Oral malignancies are the sixth most common cancer around the globe (59). Oral mucosal lesions could be due to infection (bacterial, viral, fungal), local trauma and or irritation (traumatic keratosis, irrigational fibroma, burns), systemic disease (metabolic or immunological), or related to lifestyle factors such as the usage of tobacco, areca nut, betel quid, or alcohol (60).

10.3.1 History of the procedure

Benign soft tissue tumors are fairly common and are treated with surgery alone. Prior to the 1970s, surgery was the primary therapy for malignant soft tissue tumors, and most patients with high-grade tumors had a poor prognosis and a significant mortality rate. Since the mid-1970s, radiation therapy, chemotherapy, and advanced surgical techniques have helped increase long-term survival and decrease the need for ablative surgery (61). Future advances in molecular oncology may further improve diagnostic, prognostic, and treatment protocols for patients with soft tissue sarcomas (62, 63).

10.3.2 Epidemiology

Overall, age-adjusted annual incidence of soft tissue sarcomas range from 15-35 per 1 million population. The rate increases steadily with age and is slightly higher in men than in women. Moreover, malignant soft tissue tumors occur twice as often as primary bone sarcomas.

Approximately 45% of sarcomas occur in the lower extremities, 15% in the upper extremities, 10% in the head-and-neck region, 15% in the retro peritoneum, and the remaining 15% in the abdominal and chest wall. Visceral sarcomas, arising from the connective tissue stroma in parenchymal organs, are not common.

The different types of soft tissue tumors have distinct age distributions.

- Rhabdomyosarcoma is seen more frequently in children and young adults.
- Synovial sarcoma arises in young adults.
- Malignant fibrous histiocytoma and liposarcoma generally occur in older adults.

Benign deep masses in adults usually are due to intramuscular lipoma.

In general, the prognosis in older patients with a diagnosis of high-grade sarcoma is poor. and the incidence of soft tissue tumors is slightly higher in males than in females (64, 65, 66).

11. Oral-facial injuries

11.1 Oral Injury prevention and emergency care

Oral and facial trauma surgery involves procedures that repair injuries to the face or mouth. The extent and types of surgery depend on the degree and forms of injury. In all traumatic injuries, it is important to recognize whether other structures may have been damaged such as the face, jaws or teeth.

11.2 Temporomandibular dysfunction

Temporomandibular joint disorder (TMJD or TMD), or TMJ syndrome, is a term covering acute or chronic inflammation of the temporomandibular joint, which connects the mandible to the skull. The disorder and subsequent dysfunction can result in major pain and damage. Since the disorder exceeds the boundaries between several health-care areas in particular, dentistry and neurology, there are different treatments.

The temporomandibular joint is predisposed to many conditions that affect other joints in the body, including ankylosis, trauma, arthritis, dislocations, developmental anomalies, and neoplasia. An older name in 1934 was characterized by James B Costen as Costen's syndrome (67, 68).

Symptoms

The symptoms associated with TMJ disorders may be:
1. Biting or chewing difficulty and discomfort
2. Clicking, popping, or grating sound when opening / closing the mouth
3. Earache (particularly in the morning)
4. Headache (particularly in the morning)
5. Hearing loss
6. Migraine (particularly in the morning)
7. Reduced ability to open and close the mouth
8. Tinnitus
9. Neck and shoulder pain
10. Dizziness
11. Jaw pain or tenderness of the jaw
12. Dull, aching pain in the face

Causes

There are many external factors that place excessive strain on the TMJ. These are not limited to the following:
Bruxism has been exposed to be a contributory factor in the majority of TMD cases (69). Over-opening the jaw beyond its range for the individual or unusually aggressive or repetitive sliding of the jaw sideways (laterally) or forward (protrusive). These movements may also be due to parafunctional habits or a malalignment of the jaw or dentition. This may be due to:

- Bruxism (repetitive unconscious clenching or grinding of teeth, often at night).
- Trauma
- Malalignment of the occlusal surfaces of the teeth due to defective crowns or other restorative procedures.
- Jaw thrusting (causing unusual speech and chewing habits).
- Excessive gum chewing or nail biting.
- Size of food bites eaten.
- Degenerative joint disease, such as osteoarthritis or organic degeneration of the articular surfaces, recurrent fibrous and/or bony ankylosis, developmental abnormality, or pathologic lesions within the TMJ
- Myofascial pain dysfunction syndrome
- Lack of overbite

Patients with TMD often experience pain such as migraines or headaches. There is evidence that some people who use a biofeedback headband to reduce night time clenching experience a reduction of TMD (70). The dentist must ensure a correct diagnosis and not mistake trigeminal neuralgia as a temporomandibular disorder (71, 72).

Treatment

If the occlusal surfaces of the teeth or supporting structures have been changed due to inappropriate dental treatment, periodontal disease, or trauma, the proper occlusion may need to be restored. Patients with bridges, crowns, or onlays should be checked for bite differences. These discrepancies, if present, may cause a person to make contact with posterior teeth during sideways chewing motions. These unsuitable contacts are called interferences, and if present, they can cause a patient to subconsciously avoid those motions, as they will have a painful response. The result may cause spasms of the chewing muscles. Treatment could be including of adjusting the restorations or replacing them.

12. References

[1] Duhl Guide to community preventive services (2002): A commentary. Am J Prev Med.23 (1):10-11.

[2] World Health Organization (1998). WHO /HPR/HEP/98.1 Health Promotion Glossary.

[3] Green LW, Kreuter MW (2002).Commentary on the emerging guide to community preventive services from a health promotion perspective. Am J Prev Med. (23) 1:7-9.

[4] Brown L (1994). Research in dental health education and health promotion: a review of the literature. Health Educ Queraterly.21:83–102.

[5] Schou L, Locker D (1994). Oral Health: a Review of the Effectiveness of Health Education and Health Promotion. Amsterdam: Dutch Centre for Health Promotion and Health Education.

[6] Kay L, Locker D (1996). Is dental health education effective? A systematic review of current evidence. Community Dent Oral Epidemiol. 24:231–5.

[7] Sprod A, Anderson R, Treasure E (1996). Effective oral health promotion. Literature Review. Cardiff: Health Promotion Wales, UK.

[8] Kay L, Locker D (1998). A Systematic Review of the Effectiveness of Health Promotion Aimed at Promoting Oral Health. London: Health Education Authority.

[9] Bilinkhorn, A.S (2001) Notes on Oral Health, 5th edn.Eden Bianchi Press, Manchester, UK.

[10] Springett, J (2001).Appropriate approaches to the evaluation of health promotion. Critical Public Health, 11:139-152.

[11] World Health Organization (2001).Evaluation in health promotion. Principles and perspectives. Copenhagen: World Health Organization.

[12] Peterson PE. The world Oral Health Report 2003. Oral Health Programme, Noncommunicable Disease Prevention and Health Promotion. Geneva, Switzerland: World Health Organization, 2003; 1-45. Available at:http://www.who.int

[13] Nusair KB, Alomari Q, Said K (2006). Dental health attitudes and behaviour among dental students in Jordan. Community Dent Health. 23:147-151.

[14] Al-Wahadni AM, Al-Omiri MK, Kawamura M (2004). Differences in self-reported oral health behavior between dental students and dental technology/dental hygiene students in Jordan. J Oral Sci .46:191-197.

[15] Sheiham, A (2000). Improving oral health for all: focusing on determinants and conditions. Health Education Journal, 59: 351-363.

[16] Ottawa Charter for Health Promotion (hpr). First International Conference of Health Promotion. Ottawa, Canada, 21 Nov; 1986, Available at:http//www.who.int/hpr/archive/does/Ottawa.html.Acessed February 2004.

[17] Hamissi J, Ramezani GH, Ghodousi A (2008). Prevalence of dental caries among high school attendees in Qazvin, Iran. J Indian Soc Pedod Prevent Dent: 26; 6: 53-55.

[18] Hobdell M, Petersen PE, Clarkson J, et al (2003). Global goals for oral health 2020. Int Dent J.53:285-8.

[19] Tickle M (2002). The 80:20 phenomenons: Help or hindrance to planning caries prevention programs. Community Dent Health. 19:39-42

[20] Chen MS (1986). Children's preventive dental behavior in relation to their mother's socioeconomic status, health beliefs, and dental behaviors. ASDC J Dent Child, 53(2): 105-109.

[21] McKenzie, J., Neiger, B., Thackeray, R. (2009). Health Education and Health Promotion. Planning, Implementing, & Evaluating Health Promotion Programs. (pp. 3-4). 5th edition. San Francisco, CA: Pearson Education, Inc.

[22] Donatelle, R. (2009). Promoting Healthy Behavior Change. Health: The basics. (pp. 4). 8th edition. San Francisco, CA: Pearson Education, Inc.

[23] De Biase CB. Dental hygiene in Review. Baltimore, MD: Lippincott Williams &Wilkins, 2001.

[24] Petersen, P.E (2008). Promotion of oral health and integrated disease prevention in the 21th century the WHO approach, Developing Dentistry, vol. 9, no. 1, pp. 3–5.

[25] Petersen, P.E (2009). Global policy for improvement of oral health in the 21st century – implications to oral health research of World Health Assembly 2007, World Health Organization, Community Dentistry and Oral Epidemiology, vol. 37, no. 1, pp. 1–8.

[26] Hochbaum G, Sorenson S, James R, et al (1992). Theory in health education practice. Health Education Quarterly. 19:295–313.

[27] Featherstone JDB (1999). Prevention and reversal of dental caries: role of low level fluoride. Community Dent Oral Epidemiol ; 27:31–40.

[28] Featherstone JDB (2000). The science and practice of caries prevention. J Am Dent Assoc. 131:887–899.

[29] Tinanoff N, Reisine S (2009). Update on early childhood caries since the Surgeon General's Report. Acad Pediatr. 9:396–403.

[30] Cavities/tooth decay (2008), hosted on the Mayo Clinic website. Page accessed May 25, 2008.

[31] The American Academy of Periodontology (1989). Proceedings of the World Workshop in Clinical Periodontics. Chicago: The American Academy of Periodontology. I/23-I/24.

[32] Parameter on Plaque-Induced Gingivitis (2000). Journal of Periodontology. 71 (5 Suppl): 851–2.

[33] Ammons, WF; Schectman, LR; Page, RC (1972). Host tissue response in chronic periodontal disease. 1. The normal periodontium and clinical manifestations of dental and periodontal disease in the marmoset. Journal of periodontal research 7 (2): 131–43.

[34] Page, RC; Schroeder, HE (1976). Pathogenesis of inflammatory periodontal disease. A summary of current work". Laboratory investigation; a journal of technical methods and pathology 34 (3): 235–49.

[35] Armitage, Gary C. (1999). Development of a Classification System for Periodontal Diseases and Conditions. Annals of Periodontology 4 (1): 1–6.

[36] Armitage GC (2004). Periodontal diagnoses and classification of periodontal diseases. Periodontol.2000 34: 9–21.

[37] Belting CM (1957). A review of the epidemiology of periodontal diseases. J Periodontol. 28:37-46.

[38] Kreshover SJ, Russell AL (1958). Periodontal disease. J Am Dent Assoc .56:625-629.

[39] Russell AL (1967). Epidemiology of periodontal disease. Int Dent J.17:282-296.

[40] Waerhaug J (1966). Epidemiology of periodontal disease: Review of literature. In: Ramfjord SP, Kerr DA, Ash MM, eds. World Workshop in Periodontics. Ann Arbor, MI: University of Michigan. 181-211.

[41] Position Paper (2005). Epidemiology of Periodontal Diseases J Periodontol 76:1406-1419.

[42] Gruenbaum, Tamar (2010). Famous Figures in Dentistry Mouth – JASDA. 30 (1):18

[43] Aznar T., Galán A. F., Marín I, et al (2006). Dental Arch Diameters and Relationships to Oral Habits. Angle Orthod. 76 (3): 441–445.

[44] Yamaguchi H., Sueishi K., H; Sueishi, K (2003). Malocclusion associated with abnormal posture. Bull Tokyo Dent Coll. 44 (2): 43–54.

[45] Abrams, H (1987). Incidence of anterior ridge deformities in partially edentulous patients. J Prosthet Dent. 57:191-194.

[46] World Health Organization (2004). The world health report 2004: changing history. Geneva.

[47] Stewart BW, Kleihues P, (2003). World cancer report. Lyon: WHO International Agency for Research on Cancer.

[48] Lopez AD, Mathers CD, Ezzati M, et al (2006). Global burden of disease and risk factors. Washington: The Word Bank/Oxford University Press.

[49] Jamison DT, Breman JG, Measham AR, et al (2006). Disease control priorities in developing countries. 2nd ed. Washington: The World Bank/Oxford University Press.

[50] Stewart BW, Kleihues P (2003). World cancer report. Lyon: WHO International Agency for Research on Cancer.

[51] Petersen PE (2003). The world oral health report 2003: continuous improvement of oral health in the 21st century – the approach of the WHO global oral health programme. Community Dent Oral Epidemiol.31 (Supp. 1): 3-24.

[52] Petersen PE, Bourgeois D, Bratthall D, et al (2005). Oral health information systems – towards measuring progress in oral health promotion and disease prevention. Bull World Health Organ. 83:686–93.

[53] World Health Organization (2002). National cancer control programmes: policies and managerial guidelines: executive summary. Geneva.

[54] Parker SE, Mai CT, Canfield MA, et al (2010).For the National Birth Defects Prevention Network. Updated national birth prevalence estimates for selected birth defects in the United States, 2004-2006. Birth Defects Res A Clin Mol Teratol. 2010 Sept 28. (Pub ahead of print).

[55] Little J, Cardy A, Munger RG (2004). Tobacco smoking and oral clefts: a meta-analysis. Bull World Health Organ. 82(3):213-8.

[56] Honein MA, Rasmussen SA, Reefhuis J, et al (2007). Maternal smoking, environmental tobacco smoke, and the risk of oral clefts. Epidemiology.18 (2):226–33.

[57] Correa A, Gilboa SM, Besser LM, et al (2008). Diabetes mellitus and birth defects. Am J Obstet Gynecol.199 (3): 237.1-9.

[58] American Cleft Palate-Craniofacial Association (2009). Parameters for evaluation and treatment of patients with cleft lip/palate or other craniofacial anomalies. Revised edition. Chapel Hill, NC. P. 1-34.

[59] Yazdy MM, Autry AR, Honein MA, et al (2008). Use of special education services by children with orofacial clefts. Birth Defects Res A Clin Mol Teratol. 82:147-54.

[60] Parkin DM, Bray F, Ferlay J, et al (2005): Global cancer statistics, 2002. CA: Cancer Journal for Clinicians. 55:74-108.

[61] Mehrotra R, Pandya S, Chaudhary AK, et al (2008): Prevalence of oral pre-malignant and malignant lesions at a tertiary level hospital in Allahabad, India. Asian Pac J Cancer Prev. 9(2):263-5.

[62] Conrad EU, Bradford L, Chansky HA (1996). Pediatric soft-tissue sarcomas. Orthop Clin North Am. 27 (3):655-64.

[63] Ludwig JA (2008). Personalized therapy of sarcomas: integration of biomarkers for improved diagnosis, prognosis, and therapy selection. Curr Oncol Rep.10 (4):329-37.

[64] Ordóñez JL, Martins AS, Osuna D, et al (2008). Targeting sarcomas: therapeutic targets and their rational. Semin Diagn Pathol. 25 (4):304-16.

[65] Enneking WF (1984). Staging of musculoskeletal neoplasms. In: Uhthoff HK, ed. Current Concepts of Diagnosis and Treatment of Bone and Soft Tissue Tumors. Heidelberg: Springer-Verlag.

[66] Potter DA, Glenn J, Kinsella T (1985). Patterns of recurrence in patients with high-grade soft-tissue sarcomas. J Clin Oncol. 3(3):353-66.

[67] Gustafson P (1994). Soft tissue sarcoma. Epidemiology and prognosis in 508 patients. Acta Orthop Scand Suppl. 259:1-31.

[68] Costen JB (1997). A syndrome of ear and sinus symptoms dependent upon disturbed function of the temporomandibular joint. Ann Otol Rhinol Laryngol 106 (10 Pt 1): 805–19.

[69] Michael LA (1997). Jaws revisited: Costen's syndrome. Ann Otol Rhinol Laryngol 106 (10 Pt 1): 820–2.

[70] van der Meulen MJ, Ohrbach R, Aartman IH, et al (2010). Temporomandibular disorder patients' illness beliefs and self-efficacy related to bruxism. J Orofac Pain 24 (4): 367–372.

[71] Crider A, Glaros AG, Gevirtz RN (2005). Efficacy of biofeedback-based treatments for temporomandibular disorders. Appl Psychophysiol Biofeedback 30 (4): 333-45.

[72] Drangsholt, M; Truelove, EL (2001). Trigeminal neuralgia mistaken as temporomandibular disorder. J Evid Base Dent Pract.1 (1): 41–50.

[73] Vickers ER, Cousins MJ (2000). Neuropathic orofacial pain. Part 2-Diagnostic procedures, treatment guidelines and case reports. Aust Endod J 26 (2): 53–63.

Part 2

Research in Oral Health

Antidepressants: Side Effects in the Mouth

Patrícia Del Vigna de Ameida, Aline Cristina Batista Rodrigues Johann,
Luciana Reis de Azevedo Alanis, Antônio Adilson Soares de Lima
and Ana Maria Trindade Grégio
Pontifícia Universidade Católica do Paraná & Universidade Federal do Paraná
Brazil

1. Introduction

Oral reactions to medications are common and affect patients' quality of life. Almost all classes of drugs, particularly those used continuously, such as antidepressants, anti-hypertensives, anxiolytics, hypnotics, diuretics, antipsychotics among others, including vitamins, minerals and phyto-pharmaceuticals, may cause oral alterations. If not suitably treated, these may aggravate the patient's general state of health and affect his/her oral health (Lamy, 1984; Smith & Burtner, 1994; Rees, 1998; Ciancio, 2004; American Dental Association [ADA], 2005; Scelza et al., 2010).

Prescribed and over-the-counter medications are frequently used in large quantities and by many adults, particularly by those over the age of 65 years. The abusive use of drugs, mainly by elderly patients, may generate oral side effects (Lamy, 1984; Ciancio, 2004; ADA, 2005).

The number of prescriptions in the USA is mainly due to the therapeutic advances in the treatment of various medical conditions and the increase in the geriatric population. Josephe et al. (2003) observed that 21% of the 1,800 patient dental records reviewed showed antidepressant use. It is suspected that the prevalence of oral lesions increases in direct relation to the increase in the use of necessary drugs, mainly to control chronic diseases. Over 200 drugs are involved in adverse reactions and side effects on oral tissues. Smith & Burtner (1994) founded as oral side-effects of the most frequently prescribed drugs: dry mouth (80.5%), dysgeusia (47.5%) and stomatitis (33.9%).

Xerostomia, a subjective dry mouth sensation, is a side effect of around 400 medications. Moreover, it is one of the major problems in the USA at present, affecting millions of persons. Diminishment or absence of saliva may affect the emotional well being, cause significant morbidity and a reduction in the patient's quality of life (Ciancio, 2004; Fox et al., 1985; Sreebny & Schwartz, 1986; Sreebny & Valdini, 1987; Butt, 1991; Guggenheimer & Moore, 2003). Thus, a dental and medical record of the patient is necessary, with regular updating of the prescribed medications, because of the potential side effects of drugs and interactions among them. It is also important for dentists to know about the problems related to medication and the impact of this on diagnosis and the treatment plan (Keene et al., 2003).

2. Antidepressant

Psychotropic drugs are those that act on the central nervous system (SNC) producing alterations in behaviour, mood and cognition, and that may lead to dependence.

The use of psychotropic has increased over the last few decades in several countries. This growth has been attributed to the increased frequency of psychiatric disturbance diagnoses in the population, the introduction of new psycho pharmaceuticals on the pharmaceutical market and the new therapeutic indications of existent psychotropics (Rodrigues, 2006).

Patients that take psychotropic medications for long periods may experience behaviours that have a negative impact on oral health. These medications may cause lethargy, fatigue and lack of motor control and memory that may impair the individual's ability to practice a good oral hygiene technique (McClain et al., 1991). Furthermore, a large number of medications used for the treatment of psychiatric diseases, have the side effects of dry mouth, diminished salivary flow speed and/or alteration in saliva composition (Sreebny & Schwartz, 1997; Loesche et al., 1995; Bardow et al., 2001). Zaclikevis et al. (2009) observed that psychotropic drugs caused hyposalivation in rats and acinar hypertrophy in their parotid glands. De Almeida et al. (2009) observed that psychotropic users presented a significant decrease in the stimulated salivary flow rate compared with the control group.

Antidepressants are medications prescribed to patients of all ages (Von Knorring & Wahlin, 1986; Meskin & Berg, 2000), for the treatment of a variety of psychiatric diseases (depression, affective disease, insomnia, anxiety, the panic syndrome and bipolar disorder). In addition, they are also prescribed for the treatment of some medical conditions, such as rheumatoid arthritis, dietary disorders, fibromyalgia, migraine, trigeminal neuralgia, pre-menstrual tension (Keene et al., 2003).

Antidepressant drugs were discovered in the early 1950s, with the development of the monoamine-oxidase inhibitors (MAOIs). MAO is the enzyme responsible for the degradation of various neurotransmitters, including adrenalin, serotonin, noradrenalin and dopamine. It is believed that MAO inhibition alleviates depression, allowing serotonin and noradrenalin to accumulate at the synaptic junction, in the storage locations, in the SNC and the independent sympathetic system (Perry et al., 1997). The following are examples of this class of antidepressants: tranylcypromine, moclobemide and selegiline.

In addition to the MAOIs, there are tricyclic antidepressants (TCAs) that are relatively non selective, acting not only on the serotonergic and noradrenergic systems, but also on the muscarinic, histaminergic and α- adrenergic systems (Messer et al., 1997). Their efficiency appears to be related to the increase in serotonin and noradrenalin, and to a lesser extent, of dopamine, at the synaptic gap (Stahl, 1992). Amitriptyline, imipramine, clomipramine and nortriptyline are some examples of tricyclic antidepressants.

The selective serotonin recapture inhibitors (SSRIs), such as: citalopram, fluoxetine, fluvoxamine, paroxetine and sertraline, represent another class of antidepressants that increase the availability of serotonin at the post-synaptic terminals by means of blocking recapture at the pre-synaptic terminal (Coccaro & Siever, 1985; Friedlander et al., 2002; Preskorn et al., 2004). The SSRIs appear to have fewer side effects than the TCAs, which present significant anticolinergic and cardiovascular effects (Keene et al., 2003).

The serotonin-noradrenalin recapture inhibitors are a new class of antidepressants, of which the venlafaxine, mirtazapine, trazodone and nefazodone form part (Feighner, 1999). Venlafaxine, especially, is a potent pre-synaptic inhibitor of serotonin and noradrenalin recapture, and a moderate inhibitor of dopamine recapture (Feighner, 1999; Barman Balfour & Jarvis, 2000; Wellington K, Perry, 2001).

Bupropion, an atypical antidepressant, exercises its effect by preventing the reuptake of noradrenalin and dopamine at the synaptic gap, thus facilitating neural transmission

(Goodnick PJ, Dominguez, 1998). The antidepressant effect of lithium, a mood stabilizing agent used to treat the depressive phase of bipolar disorder, may derive from its ability to increase the serotonin levels in the SNC (Schou, 1999).

The majority of antidepressant medications prescribed is associated with a number of significant oral reactions (Friedlander & Mahler, 2001). These complications, including xerostomia, sialoadenitis, gingivitis, dysgeusia, glossitis, tongue edema and discoloration and stomatitis, almost always appear due to dysfunction of the salivary gland induced by the medication. But in patients that make use of mirtazapine, the development of stomatitis may represent the initial signs of bone marrow suppression induced by the medication, such as: agranulocytosis, leukopenia or granulocytosis, a potentially fatal event (Friedlander & Norman, 2002). Bertini et al. (2009) reports a case of ulceration of the oral mucosa induced by antidepressant medication.

Rindal et al. (2005) suggest that antidepressant drugs do not generate a raise in the overall restoration risk level when compared with a group on non-xerogenic drug. Instead, that antidepressant medication raises the quantity of disease for persons already at risk. The non-xerogenic group had a superior restoration rate than the no medication group but not as high as the antidepressant group rate.

Studies that assessed the oral health of patients that use antidepressants observed extensive tooth losses. This may occur because of various factors: lack of interest in oral hygiene, preference for carbohydrates (probably because of the reduction of serotonin in the SNC), preference for sweetened foods because of alterations in the sense of taste (dysgeusia), by the diminishment of saliva release and by the high lactobacillus counts (Rundegren et al., 1985; Christensen & Somers, 1996; Anttila et al., 1999).

Persons with depression are also at high risk of developing periodontal disease, because neglected oral hygiene, increased smoking and altered immune response, associated with xerostomia facilitate increased colonization by pathologic bacteria in the mouth, leading to collapse of the periodontium (Moss et al., 1996; Elter et al., 1999). Patients that receive SSRIs or atypical antidepressants may sometimes develop movement disorders that include bruxism or tooth-grinding, which may aggravate the patient's periodontal status (Brow & Hong, 1999). These drugs raise the extrapyramidal serotonin levels, thus inhibiting the dopaminergic pathways that control the movements (Bostwick & Jaffee, 1999).

There is consensus among various authors that xerostomia is the main and the commonest side effect of antidepressant drugs (Smith & Burtner, 1994; Pajukoski et al., 2001; Ciancio, 2004; Scully, 2003; Josephe et al., 2003; Thomson et al., 2006; Uher et al., 2009), in addition to this, patients that receive antidepressant therapy frequently complain about diminished salivation and changes in salivary viscosity (Astor et al., 1999).

2.1 Role of saliva in oral health

Saliva is a true mirror of the body that contains a large number of organic and inorganic compounds, and can be seen as a very important health indicator. Salivary secretion is controlled by the autonomic nervous system through receptors present in the salivary gland. Many studies show that medicine and diseases can affect the function of salivary glands as regards the quality and quantity of saliva secreted (Greabu et al. 2009; Gregio et al., 2006).

Salivary secretion is complex and occurs subsequent to neurotransmitter stimuli. The principal control of secretion is derived from sympathetic and parasymphatetic innervation which regulates the secretory function on the acinar cell level and controls the reabsorption process in the striated ducts of salivary glands. Parasympathetic stimulation increases the volume of secreted saliva, whereas sympathetic stimulation mainly affects protein content and composition. The salivary gland may serve as a model to determine the peripheral effects of different antidepressants on the monoaminergic and the cholinergic systems. Salivary gland function depends on the integrity of both parasympathetic and sympathetic innervation. Normal salivation is an essential demand for oral health, due to its important contributions to the oral defense mechanisms. Diminished salivary secretion could lead to serious disease and deterioration of the mucosa (Von Knorring & Mornstad, 1986; Hunter& Wilson, 1995) The saliva has several important functions in the mouth, including protection of the oral mucosa, chemical buffering, digestion, taste, antimicrobial action, and maintaining the integrity of the teeth. Due to its glycoprotein contents saliva has a viscous aspect that protects the oral mucosa by the formation of a barrier against noxious stimuli, microbial toxins, and minor trauma. Its fluid nature facilitates the removal of cell debris and non-adherent bacteria (Edgar, 1992).

2.2 Antidepressant and xerostomia

Xerostomia means a subjective dry mouth sensation and represents a symptom related by the patient. It may occur in the presence of systemic diseases or conditions, such as displayed on Table 1, or as consequence of use of drugs (Table 2) (Lamy, 1984; Sreebny & Schwartz, 1997; Stack & Papas, 2001; Scully, 2003; Guggenheimer & Moore, 2003). Between the drugs stands out the antidepressants (Table 3). Patients with xerostomia displayed various degrees of discomfort related to the quality of life according to the aetiology of their conditions (Cho et al., 2010). Around 1 in 5 people complain of dry mouth, and a rising occurrence in the elderly, it is essential to have a complete understanding of this subject (Hopcraft & Tan, 2010).

Of the conditions mentioned above, salivary hypofunction secondary to the use of medications is the commonest (Nederfors, 1996; Fox, 1998). They inhibit the cholinergic signals in the salivary tissues and thus diminish the excretion of fluids by the glands, and interferences in central pathways (serotoninergics and dopaminergics) may also alter salivary composition (Atkinson & Baum, 2001). The normal stimulated salivary flow rate is between 0.7 to 1 mL/min, whereas hyposalivation is considered when the salivar production is under 0.7 mL/min (Tenovuo & Lagerlöf, 1994).

Aging has a minimum impact on salivary flow, but the advance of age and the appearance of chronic diseases lead to the use of drugs that may diminish the salivary flow by up to 40% (Sreebny & Schwartz, 1997; Ben-Aryeh et al., 2001). Complaints of xerostomia may increase three-fold in elderly patients that receive xerogenic medication (Osterberg et al., 1984).

In a study comparing the use of escitalopram and nortriptyline, Uher et al. (2009) observed that dry mouth was the most commonly reported adverse effect, and that it was more common during treatment with either nortriptyline or escitalopram than in the medication-free state. The authors also demonstrated a positive correlation with the dose of both antidepressants.

There is evidence that the prevalence of dry mouth is correlated to polymedication (Locker, 1995; Nederfors et al., 1997). But, Persson et al. (1991) verified that the use of up to 4 different xerogenic medications did not result in significantly additional reduction in the salivary flow speed in his patients.

Diseases/Conditions
Salivary aplasia
Dehydration
Sarcoidosis
Cystic fibrosis
Psycogenic
Sjögren´s syndrome
Primary biliary cirrhosis
Infections (HIV, HTLV-1, Hepatitis C)
Radiation therapy
Renal dialysis
Vasculits
Bone marrow transplantation
Anxiety
Depression
Graft vs host disease
Diabetes type 1 or 2
Diabetes insipidus
Haemorrhage
Chemotherapy
Tabagism
Oral respiration

Table 1. Systemic diseases or conditions related with xerostomia

The subjective dry mouth sensation may occur even in the presence of a normal salivary flow that is, not necessarily being associated with a diminution in the amount of saliva (Fox et al., 1985; Närhi, 1994). According to Mandel & Wotman (1994) the quality of salivary secretion (especially the mucin content) is more important than the quantity in the dry mouth sensation. The type of saliva (rest or stimulated), procedures and time of collection, composition and source (larger or smaller salivary glands) are factors that can contribute to the patient's report of dry mouth and it relationship with hyposalivation (Mandel & Wotman, 1994; Von Knorring & Mörnstad, 1981). According to Nagler (2004), in up to one third of cases, xerostomia does not reflect a real reduction in salivary flow speed.

As regards dry mouth, it is due to the reduction in saliva secretion or when its composition is altered, and it may cause various clinical problems (Table 4) (Nagler, 2004; Ursache et al., 2006; Tuner et al., 2007).

Drugs
Skeletal muscle relaxants
Antihypertensive agents
Anti-Parkison agents
Antihistamines
Antipsychotics
Diuretics
Antispasmodics - Scopolamine
Atropine
Muscarinic receptor antagonists for treatment of overactive bladder
Barbiturates
Clonidine
Lithium carbonate
Phenylbutazone
Psychotropics
Tri-iodothyronine
Anticonvulsivants
Antidysrhythimic
Anti-incontinence agent
Ophtalmic formulation
Smoking cessation agent
Appetite suppressants
Antimigraine agents
Antidepressants
Descongestionants
Bronchodilators
Alfa receptor antagonist for treatment of urinary retention
Benzodiazepines- Lorazepam
Opioids- morphine
Hypnotics
Retinoids
Cytokines
Anti-HIV drugs
H2 antagonists and proton pump inhibitors
Cytotoxic agents
Drugs of abuse
Anxiolytics

Table 2. Drugs related with xerostomia

Antidepressant
Serotonin agonists
Noradrenalin re-uptake blockers
Serotonin re-uptake inhibitors
Noradrenalin and Serotonin re-uptake blockers
Atipical antidepressants
Tricyclic antidepressants
Heterocyclic antidepressants
Monoamine oxidase inhibitors
Venlafaxine
Buspirone
Alprazolan

Table 3. Antidepressant related with xerostomia

Dental caries
Dry lips (Fig.1)
Colourless oral mucosa
Dry mouth (Fig.2)
Dysgeusia
Partially no papilla tongue
Atrophied papilla and deep fissures (Fig.3)
Dysphagia
Gingivitis
Halitosis
Mastication problems
Burning sensation in the mouth
Mucositis
Candidiasis
Poorly fitting prostheses
Sleeping difficulty
Difficulty with speech
Traumatic oral lesions
Halitosis
Ulceration
Periodontal disease
Saliva composition changes

Table 4. Oral effects of hipossalivation

A variety of technique have used to evaluate xerostomia: questionnaire; visual analogue-scale; clinical inspection if a tongue blade adheres to the buccal mucosa or if a patient can chew and swallow dried food without water; by quantifying the volume of residual saliva on mucosal surfaces using filter paper and micro-moisture meter and calculating thickness; and mucosal wetness devices (Osailan et al., 2011). Also, sialometry (salivary flow rate measurement) is indicated as part of the diagnostic procedures for hyposalivation (Tenovuo & Lagerlöf, 1994), and the composition of saliva can be verified by means of biochemical salivary exams.

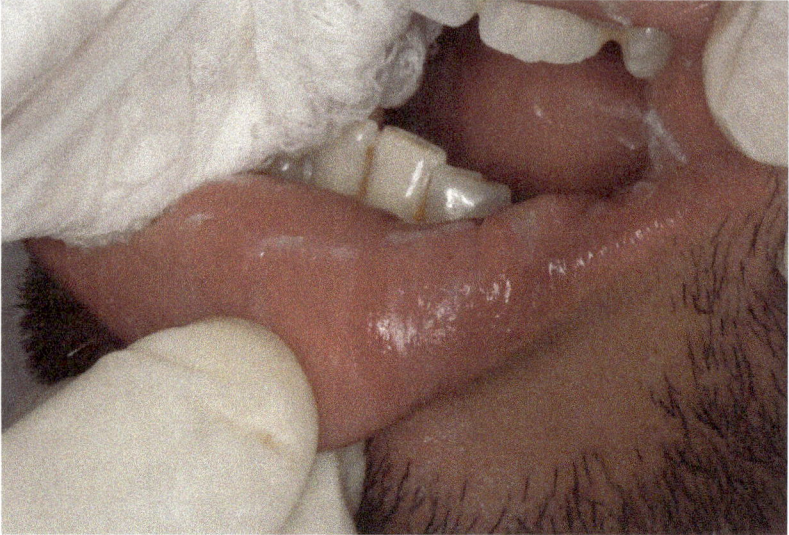

Fig. 1. Clinical presentation: A patient in a coma state showing intense dry lip mucosa

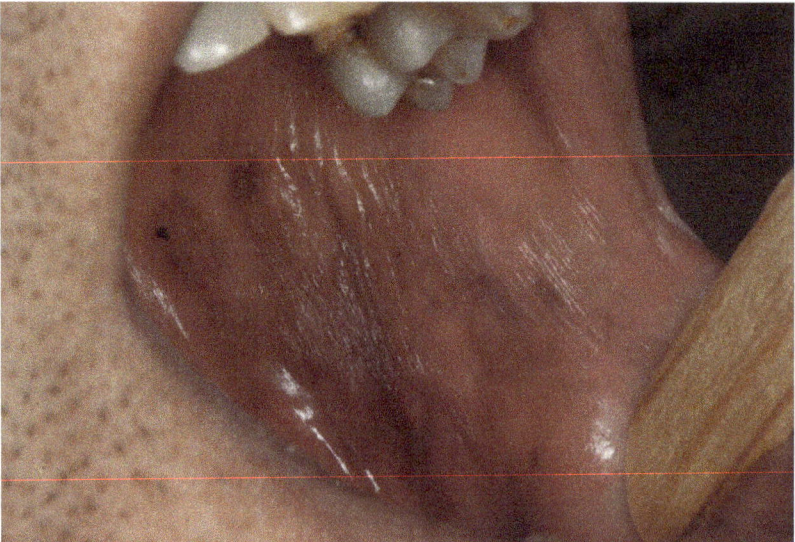

Fig. 2. Clinical presentation: A patient showing dry mucosae after use of medications

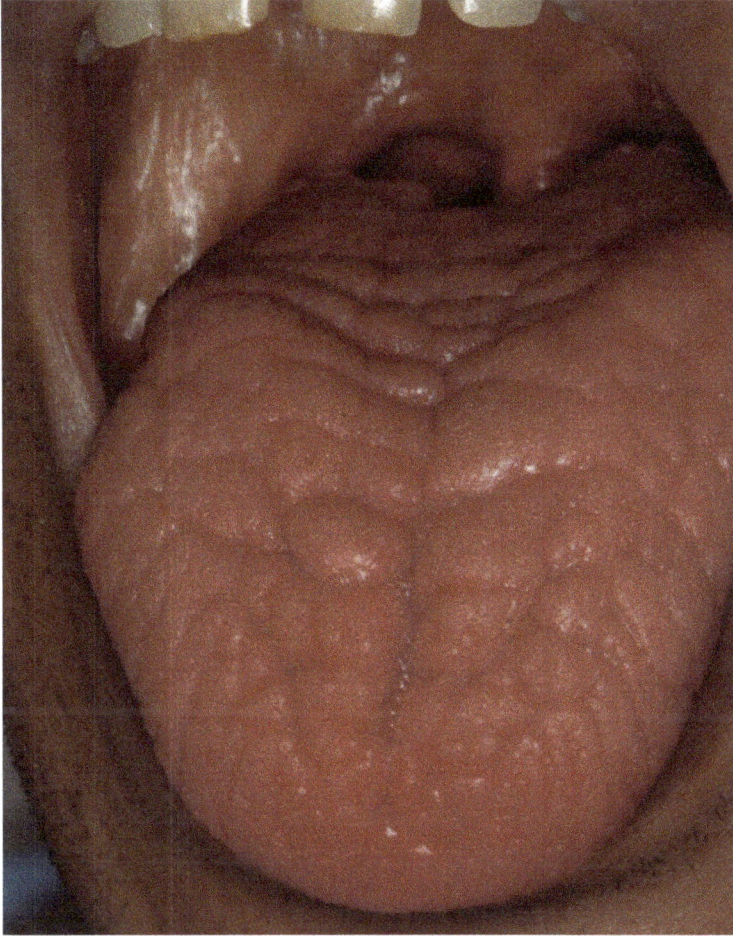

Fig. 3. Clinical presentation: A patient treated with medication showing tongue with atrophied papilla and deep fissures

Antidepressants have anticolinergic or antimuscarinic action, which acts to block the actions of the parasympathetic system by inhibiting the effects of acetylcholine on the salivary gland receptors. This results in a dry mouth sensation, probably because the sympathetic portion of the independent nervous system predominates over the "blocked" parasympathetic system (Wynn et al., 2001). According to Schubert & Izutsu (1987), the drugs may affect the salivary flow and its composition by interferences in the acinary and duct functions, and by means of alterations in the blood flow of the salivary glands. According to Douglas (2002) diminishment of the salivary flow is due to the reduction in the blood flow of the gland, produced by adrenergic sympathetic vasoconstriction. Therefore, when there is sympathetic hyperactivity the mouth presents dry.

It is important to emphasize that the dry mouth sensation and alteration in salivary composition may occur during periods of stress and/or acute anxiety, frequently present in depressive disorders, due to predominant stimulation of the sympathetic system, irrespective of the use of anxiolytic and/or antidepressant medication (Guggenheimer & Moore, 2003). Isolated depression is related to diminishment of salivary secretion and to xerostomia, due an anticolinergic action (Stack & Papas, 2001; Brown, 1970). Therefore, it may be difficult to determine whether these side effects and their intensity arise from the medical condition that led to the treatment, or from the medication prescribed for it (Smith & Burtner, 1994), it probably is as a result of both.

2.3 Treatment of hyposalivation

Various treatments are proposed for enhanced salivary secretion, among them, the use of a salivary flow stimulating drug pilocarpine chloride which acts by stimulating the parasympathetic ANS (Vivino et al., 1999). This drug has been used because it stimulates the cholinergic receptors, among them the muscarinicM3 receptor present in the salivary glands, resulting in the expulsion of the stored salivary contents (Ferguson, 1993), thus an increase in saliva production and release was observed with the use of cholinergic drugs.

The next table shows the types of hyposalivation treatment according to Turner & Ship (2007), treatment strategies include salivary replacement therapies, as well as use of statory, masticatory and pharmacological stimulants.

Gustatory and tactile sialogogues
Acid-tasting substances
Acidic (sugar-free) sweets
Acidic or effervescent drinks (lemon juice, citric acid, buttermilk)
Citric acid crystals
Cotton-wool gauze soaked in a citric acid and glycerine solution
Lemon pastilles
Lemon slices
Vitamin C tablets
Miscellaneous substances
Dried pieces of reed root (calami rhizome)
Sugar-free chewing gum
Sugar-free sweets
Vegetables or fruits
Anetholetrithione
Benzapyrone
Betanechol chloride
Carbachol
Cevimeline
Folia Jaborandi and tinctura Jaborandi
Neostigmine, neostigmine bromide, pyridostigmine bromide
Destigmine bromide
Nicotinamide and nicotine acid
Pilocarpine hydrochloridey, pilocarpine nitrate
Potassium iodide
Trithioparamethoxyphenylpropene

Table 5. Treatment of hiposalivation

3. Conclusion

Xerostomia is the main oral side effect associated with the various classes of drugs, particularly those used continuously. There is, however, not always a positive correlation between hyposalivation and xerostomia. This symptom may be the result of both diminished salivary secretion and an alteration in saliva composition. Nevertheless, when present, xerostomia may affect the patient's emotional well being, aggravate his/her general state of health, as well as affect his/her oral health, as other reactions such as dygeusia, candidosis, caries and stomatitis are reported as being the consequence of xerostomia. It is important to emphasize the dentists' role as regards patients that make use of medications, mainly for treating chronic diseases. It is their obligation to keep a detailed and updated medical history of their patients, in order to be alert to problems related to medication, and the impact of this on the diagnosis and treatment plan, as well as to prepare the most adequate and effective preventive programs possible. In order to determine whether or not the patient presents hyposalivation, the dentist can have a complementary exam, called sialometry (salivary flow speed measurement), may be performed. If there is any doubt about the composition of the saliva, there are biochemical tests that can reveal alteration in its composition. Communication between the doctor and dentist is extremely important, so that together, they re-establish the patient's general and oral health as far as possible.

4. Acknowledgment

The authors thank to Sonia Maria Del Vigna for technical support, and to Pontifícia Universidade Católica do Paraná for financial support.

5. References

American Dental Association [ADA]- Division of Communications. (2005). For the dental patient. How medications can affect your oral health. *Journal of the American Dental Association*, Vol.136, No.6, (June 2005), pp.831, ISSN 0002-8177

Anttila, S.; Knuuttila, M. & Sakki, T. (1999). Depressive symptoms favor abundant growth of salivary lactobacilli. *Psychosomatic Medicine*, Vol.61, No.4, (July-August 1999), pp.508-512, ISSN 0033-3174

Astor, F.; Hanft, K. & Ciocon, J. (1999). Xerostomia: a prevalent condition in the elderly. *Ear, nose, & throat journal*, Vol.78, No.7, (July 1999). pp.476-479, ISSN 0145-5613

Atkinson, J. & Baum, B. (2001). Salivary enhancement: current status and future therapies. *Journal of dental education*, Vol.65, No.10, (October 2001), pp.1096-1101, ISSN 0022-0337

Bardow, A.; Nyvad, B. & Nauntofte, B. (2001). Relationships between medication intake, complaints of dry mouth, salivary flow rate and composition, and the rate of tooth demineralization in situ. *Archives of oral biology*, Vol. 46, No.5, (May 2001), pp.413-423, ISSN 0003-9969

Barman Balfour, J. & Jarvis, B. (2000). Venlafaxine extended-release: a review of its clinical potential in the management of generalized anxiety disorder. *CNS Drugs*, Vol.14, No.6, (December 2000), pp.483-503, ISSN 1172-7047

Ben-Aryeh, H.; Miron, D.; Szargel, R. & Gutman, D. (1984). Whole-saliva secretion rates in old and young healthy subjects. *Journal of dental research*, Vol. 63, No.9, (September 1984), pp.1147-1148, ISSN 0022-0345

Bertini, F.; Costa, N.; Brandão, A.; Cavalcante, A. & Almeida, J. (2009). Ulceration of the oral mucosa induced by antidepressant medication: a case report. *Journal of medical case reports*, Vol.3, No.3, (November 2009), pp.98, ISSN 1752-1947

Bostwick, J. & Jaffee, M. (1999). Buspirone as an antidote to SSRI-induced bruxism in 4 cases. *The Journal of clinical psychiatry*, Vol. 60, No.12, (December 1999), pp.857-860, ISSN 0160-6689

Brow, E. & Hong, S. (1999). Antidepressant-induced bruxism successfully treated whith gabapentin. *Journal of the American Dental Association*, Vol.130, No.10, (October 1999), pp.1467-1469, ISSN 0002-8177

Brown, C. (1970). The parotid puzzle: a review of the literature on human salivation and its applications to psychophysiology. *Psychophysiology*, Vol. 7, No.1, (July 1970), pp.65-85, ISSN 0048-5772

Butt, G. (1991). Drug-induced xerostomia. *Journal of the Canadian Dental Association*, Vol.57, No5., (May 1991), pp.391-393, ISSN 0008-3372

Cho, M.; Ko, J.; Kim, Y. & Kho, H. (2010). Salivary flow rate and clinical characteristics of patients with xerostomia according to its aetiology. *Journal of oral rehabilitation*, Vol.37, No. 3, (March 2010), pp.185-193, ISSN 0305-182X

Christensen, L. & Somers, S. (1996). Comparison of nutrient intake among depressed and nondepressed individuals. *The International journal of eating disorders*, Vol.20, No.1, (July 1996), pp.105-109, INSS 0276-3478.

Ciancio, S. (2004). Medications' impact on oral health. *Journal of the American Dental Association*, Vol.,135, No.10, (October 2004), pp.1440-1448, ISSN 0002-8177

Coccaro EF, & Siever LJ (1985) Second generation antidepressants: a comparative review. *Journal of clinical pharmacology*, Vol.25, No.4, (May-June 1985), pp.241-260, ISSN 0091-2700

de Almeida, P.; Grégio, A.; Brancher, J.; Ignácio, S.; Machado, M.; de Lima, A. & Azevedo L,. (2008). Effects of antidepressants and benzodiazepines on stimulated salivary flow rate and biochemistry composition of the saliva. *Oral surgery, oral medicine, oral pathology, oral radiology, and endodontics*, Vol.106, No.1, (July 2008), pp.58-65, ISSN 1079-2104

Douglas, C. (2002) *Tratado de fisiologia aplicada à saúde* (5th ed), Robe Editorial, ISBN 8573630256, São Paulo, Brazil

Edgar, W. M. (1992) Saliva: its secretion, composition and functions. British dental journal Vol.172, No.8, (April 1992), pp. 305-312, ISSN 0007-0610

Elter, J.; Beck, J.; Slade, G. & Offenbacher, S. (1999). Etiologic models for incident periodontal attachment loss in older adults. *Journal of clinical periodontology*, Vol.26, No.2, (February 1999), pp.113-123, ISSN 0303-6979

Feighner, J. (1999). Mechanism of action of antidepressant medications. *The Journal of clinical psychiatry*, Vol.60, Suppl.4, (1999), pp.4-11, ISSN 0160-6689

Ferguson, M. (1993). Pilocarpine and other cholinergic drugs in the management of salivary gland dysfunction. *Oral surgery, oral medicine, oral pathology*, Vol.75, No.2, (Feburary 1993), pp.186-191, ISSN 0030-4220

Fox, P. (1998). Acquired salivary dysfunction. Drugs and radiation. *Annals of the New York Academy of Sciences*, Vol.842, (April 1998), pp.132-137, ISSN 0077-8923

Fox, P.; van der Ven, P.; Sonies, B.; Weiffenbach, J. & Baum, B. (1985). Xerostomia: evaluation of a symptom with increasing significance. *Journal of the American Dental Association*, Vol.110, No.4, (April 1985), pp.519-525, ISSN 0002-8177

Friedlander, A.; Friedlander, I. & Marder, S. (2002). Bipolar I disorder: psychopathology, medical management and dental implications. *Journal of the American Dental Association*, Vol.133, No.9, (September 2002), pp.1209-1217, ISSN 0002-8177

Friedlander, A. & Mahler, M. (2001). Major depressive disorder: psychopathology, medical management and dental implications. *Journal of the American Dental Association*, Vol.132, No.5, (May 2001), pp.629-638, ISSN 0002-8177

Friedlander, A. & Norman, D. (2002). Late-life depression: psychopathology, medical interventions and dental implications. *Oral surgery, oral medicine, oral pathology, oral radiology, and endodontics*, Vol.94, No.4, (October 2002), pp.404-412, ISSN 1079-2104

Goodnick, P.; Dominguez, R.; DeVane, C. & Bowden, C. (1998). Bupropion slow-release response in depression: diagnosis and biochemistry. *Biological psychiatry*, Vol.44, No.7, (October 1998), pp.629-632, ISSN 0006-3223

Greabu, M.; Battino, M.; Mohora, M.,; Totan, A.; Didilescu, A.; Spinu, T.; Totan, C.; Miricescu, D. & Radulescu, R. Saliva--a diagnostic window to the body, both in health and in disease. *Journal of medicine and life*. Vol.2, No.2 (April-June 2009), pp.124-132, ISSN 1844-122X.

Grégio, A.; Durscki, J.; Lima, A.; Machado, M.; Ignácio, S. & Azevedo, L (2006). Association of amityptiline and Diazepam on histomorphometry of rat parotid glands. *Pharmacologyonline*, Vol.2, (2006), pp.96-108, ISSN, 1827-8620.

Guggenheimer, J. & Moore, P. (2003). Xerostomia: etiology, recognition and treatment. *Journal of the American Dental Association*, Vol.134, No.1, (January 2003), pp.61-69, ISSN 0002-8177

Hopcraft, M. & Tan, C. (2010). Xerostomia: an update for clinicians. *Australian Dental Journal*, Vol.55, No.3, (September 2010), pp.238-44, ISSN 0045-0421

Hunter, K. & Wilson, W. (1995). The effects of antidepressant drugs on salivary flow and content of sodium and potassium ions in human parotid saliva. *Archives of oral biology,* , Vol.40, No.11, (November 1995), pp. 983-989, ISSN:0003-9969

Keene, J.; Galasko, G. & Land, M. (2003). Antidepressant use in psychiatry and medicine: importance for dental practice. *Journal of the American Dental Association*, Vol.134, No.1, (January 2003), pp.71-79, ISSN 0002-8177

Lamy, M. (1984). Drugs and oral health. *Journal of the Maryland State Dental Association*, Vol.27, No.3, (December 1984), pp.125-130, ISSN 0025-4355

Locker, D. (1995). Xerostomia in older adults: a longitudinal study. *Gerodontology*, Vol.12, No.1, (July 1995), pp.18-25, ISSN 0734-0664

Loesche, W.; Bromberg, J.; Terpenning, M.; Bretz, W.; Dominguez, B.; Grossman, N. & Langmore, S. (1995). Xerostomia, xerogenic medications and food avoidances in selected geriatric groups. *Journal of the American Geriatrics Society*, Vol.43, No.4, (April 1995), pp.401-407, ISSN 0002-8614

Mandel, I. & Wotman, S. (1976). The salivary secretions in health and disease. *Oral sciences reviews*, Vol.8, (1976), pp.25-47, ISSN 0300-4759

McClain, D.; Bader, J.; Daniel, S. & Sams, D. (1991). Gingival effects of prescription medications among adult dental patients. *Special care in dentistry*, Vol.11, No.1, (January-February 1991), pp.15-18, ISSN 0275-1879

Meskin, L. & Berg, R. (2000). Impact of older adults on private dental practices, 1988-1998. *Journal of the American Dental Association*, Vol.131, No.8, (August 2000), pp.1188-1195, ISSN 0002-8177

Messer, T.; Schmauss, M. & Lambert-Baumann, J. (2005). Efficacy and tolerability of reboxetine in depressive patients treated in routine clinical practice. *CNS Drugs*, Vol.19, No.1, (2005), pp.43-54, ISSN 1172-7047

Moss, M.; Beck, J.; Kaplan, B.; Offenbacher, S.; Weintraub, J.; Koch, G.; Genco, R.; Machtei, E. & Tedesco, L. (1996). Exploratory case-control analysis of psychosocial factors and adult periodontitis. *Journal of periodontology*, Vol.67, 10 Suppl, (October 1996), pp.1060-1069, ISSN 0022-3492

Murray Thomson, W.; Poulton, R.; Mark Broadbent, J. & Al-Kubaisy, S. (2006) Xerostomia and medications among 32-year-olds. *Acta odontologica Scandinavica*, Vol.64, No.4, (August 2006), pp.249-254, ISSN 0001-6357

Nagler, R. (2004). Salivary glands and the aging process: mechanistic aspects, health-status and medicinal-efficacy monitoring. *Biogerontology*, Vol.5, No.4, (2004), pp.223-233, ISSN 1389-5729

Närhi, T. (1994). Prevalence of subjective feelings of dry mouth in the elderly. *Journal of dental research*, Vol.73, No.1, (January 1994), pp.20-25, ISSN 0022-0345

Nederfors, T. (1996). Xerostomia: prevalence and pharmacotherapy. With special reference to beta-adrenoceptor antagonists. *Swedish dental journal*. Supplement, Vol.116, pp.1-70, ISSN:0348-6672

Nederfors, T.; Isaksson, R.; Mörnstad, H. & Dahlöf, C. (1997). Prevalence of perceived symptoms of dry mouth in an adult Swedish population – relation to age, sex, and pharmacotherapy. *Community dentistry and oral epidemiology*, Vol.25, No.3, (June 1997), pp.211-216, ISSN 0301-5661

Osailan, S.; Pramanik, R.; Shirodaria, S.; Challacombe, S. & Proctor, G. (2011). Investigating the relationship between hyposalivation and mucosal wetness. *Oral diseases*, Vol.17, No.1, (January 2011), pp.109-114, ISSN 1354-523X

Osterberg, T.; Landahl, S. & Hedegard, B. (1984). Salivary flow, saliva, pH and buffering capacity in 70-year-old men and women. Correlation to dental health, dryness in the mouth, disease and drug treatment. *Journal of oral rehabilitation*, Vol.11, No.2, (March 1984), pp.157-170, ISSN 0305-182X

Pajukoski, H.; Meurman, J.; Halonen, P. & Sulkava, R. (2001). Prevalence of subjective dry mouth and burning mouth in hospitalized elderly patients and outpatients in relation to saliva, medication, and systemic disease. *Oral surgery, oral medicine, oral pathology, oral radiology, and endodontics*, Vol.92, No.6, (December 2001), pp.641-649, ISSN 1079-2104

Perry, P.; Alexander, B. & Liskow, B. (1997). *Psychotropic drug handbook*. 7th ed, American Psychiatric Press, ISBN 0-88048-851-4, Washington, USA

Persson, R.; Izutsu, K.; Truelove, E. & Persson, R. (1991). Differences in salivary flow rates in elderly subjects using xerostomatic medications. *Oral surgery, Oral Medicine, and Oral Pathology*, Vol.72, No.1, (July 1991), pp.42-46, ISSN 0030-4220

Preskorn, S.; Ross, R. & Stanga, C. (2004). Antidepressants: past, present and future. Springer Verlag, ISBN 3-540-43054-7, Berlim, Germany

Rees, T. (1998). Drugs and oral disorders. *Periodontology 2000*, Vol.18, (October 1998), pp.21-36 ISSN 0906-6713

Rindal, D.; Rush, W.; Peters, D. & Maupomé, G. (2005). Antidepressant xerogenic medications and restoration rates. *Community dentistry and oral epidemiology*, Vol.33, No.1, (February 2005), pp.74-80, ISSN 0301-5661

Rodrigues, M.; Facchini, L. & Lima, M. (2006). Modifications in psychotropic drug use patterns in a Southern Brazilian city. *Revista de Saúde Pública*, Vol.40, No.1, (Feburary 2006), pp.107-114, ISSN 0034-8910

Rundegren, J.; Van Dijken, J.; Mörnstad, H. & Von Knorring, L. (1985). Oral conditions in patient receiving long-term treatment with cyclic antidepressant drugs. *Swedish dental journal*, Vol.9, No.2, (1985), pp.55-64, ISSN 0347-9994

Schou, M. (1999). Perspectives on lithium treatment of bipolar disorder: action, efficacy, effect on suicidal behavior. *Bipolar disorders*, Vol.1, No.1, (September 1999), pp.5-10, ISSN 1398-5647

Schubert, M. & Izutsu, K. (1987). Iatrogenic causes of salivary gland dysfunction. Journal of dental research, Vol.66, Spec No., (Feburary 1987), pp.680-688, ISSN 0022-0345

Scully, C. (2003). Drug effects on salivary glands: dry mouth. *Oral diseases*, Vol.9, No.4, (July 2003), pp.165-176, ISSN 1354-523X

Smith, R. & Burtner, A. (1994). Oral side-effects of the most frequently prescribed drugs. *Special care in dentistry*, Vol.14, No.3, (May-June 1994), pp.96-102, ISSN 0275-1879

Sreebny, L. & Schwartz, S. (1986). A reference guide to drugs and dry mouth. *Gerodontology*, Vol.5, No.2, (Autumn 1986), pp.75-99, ISSN 0734-0664

Sreebny, L. & Schwartz, S. (1997). A reference guide to drugs and dry mouth: 2nd edition. *Gerodontology*, Vol.14, No.1, (July 1997), pp.33-47, ISSN 0734-0664

Sreebny, L. & Valdini, A. (1987). Xerostomia: a neglected symptom. *Archives of internal medicine*, Vol.147, No.7, (July 1987), pp.1333-1337, ISSN 0003-9926

Stack, K. & Papas, A. (2001). Xerostomia: etiology and clinical management. *Nutrition in clinical care*, Vol.4, No.1, (March-April 2001), pp.15-21, ISSN: 1523-5408

Stahl, S. (1992). Neuroendocrine markers of serotonin responsivity in depression. *Progress in neuro-psychopharmacology & biological psychiatry*, Vol.16, No.5, (September 1992), pp.655-659, ISSN 0278-5846

Tenovuo, J. & Lagerlöf, F. (1994). Saliva. In: Textbook of clinical cariology, 2nd ed. Thylstrup, A. & Fejerskov, O. (Ed.), Munksgaard, ISBN 8716109163, Copenhagen, Denmark

Turner, M. ; Ship, J. (2007). Dry mouth and its effects on the oral health of elderly people. *Journal of the American Dental Association*, Vol.138, Suppl., (September 2007), pp. 15S-20S, ISSN 0002-8177.

Uher, R.; Farmer, A.; Henigsberg, N.; Rietschel, M.; Mors, O.; Maier, W.; Kozel, D.; Hauser, J.; Souery, D.; Placentino, A.; Strohmaier, J.; Perroud, N.; Zobel, A.; Rajewska-Rager, A.; Dernovsek, M.; Larsen, E.; Kalember, P.; Giovannini, C.; Barreto, M.; McGuffin, P. & Aitchison, K. (2009). Adverse reactions to antidepressants. *The British journal of psychiatry : the journal of mental science*, Vol.195, No.3, (September 2009), pp.202-210, ISSN:1472-1465

Ursache, M.; Grădinaru, I.; Nechifor, M. & Cherciu-Ciubotaru, B. (2006). Implications of xerostomia in oral dis-homeostasis. *Revista medico-chirurgicală a Societății de Medici și Naturaliști din Iași*, Vol.110, No.2, (April-June 2006) pp.432-437, ISSN: 0048-7848

Vivino, F.B., Al-Hasshimi, I.; Khan, Z.; Leveque, F.G.; Salisbury, P.L.; Tran-Johson, T.K.; Muscoplat, C.C.; Trivedi, M.; Goldlust, B.; Gallagher, S.C. Pilocarpine Tablets for the treatment of dry mouth and dry eye symptoms in patients with Sjogren syndrome: a randomized, placebo-controlled, fixed-dose, multicenter trial. P92-01 Study Group. *Archives of internal medicine*, Vol.159, No.2, (January 1999), pp.174-181, ISSN 0003-9926

Von Knorring, A. & Wahlin, Y. (1986). Tricyclic antidepressants and dental caries in children. *Neuropsychobiology*, Vol.15, No.3-4, (1986), pp.143-145, ISSN 0302-282X

Von Knorring, L. & Mörnstad, H. (1981). Qualitative changes in saliva composition after short-term administration of imipramine and zimelidine in healthy volunteers. *Scandinavian journal of dental research*, Vol.89, No.4, (August 1981), pp.313-320, ISSN 0022-0345

Von Knorring, L. & Mornstad, H. Saliva secretion rate and saliva composition as a model to determine the effect of antidepressant drugs on cholinergic and noradrenergic transmission. *Neuropsychobiology*, Vol.15, No.3-4, (1986), pp. 146-54, ISSN 0302-282X

Wellington, K. & Perry, C. (2001) Venlafaxine extended-release: a review of its use in the management of major depression. *CNS Drugs*, Vol.15, No.8, (2001), pp.643-669, ISSN 1172-7047

Wynn, R. & Meiller, T. (2001). Drugs and dry mouth. *General dentistry*, Vol.49, No.1, (January- Feburary 2001), pp.10-14, ISSN 0363-6771

Zaclikevis, M.; D'Agulham, A.; Bertassoni, L.; Machado, M.; de Lima, A.; Grégio, A. & Azevedo-Alanis, L. (2009). Effects of benzodiazepine and pilocarpine on rat parotid glands: histomorphometric and sialometric study. *Medicinal Chemistry*, Vol.5, No.1, (January 2009), pp.74-78, ISSN 1573-4064

Epidemiology of Dental Caries in the World

Rafael da Silveira Moreira

Centro de Pesquisas Aggeu Magalhães, Fundação Oswaldo Cruz, Recife, Pernambuco

Brasil

1. Introduction

The oral health of children 12 years old is the object of several epidemiological studies conducted around the world. According to the World Health Organization (WHO, 1997), the importance given to this age group is due to the fact that it is this age that children leave primary school. Thus, in many countries, is the last age at which data can be easily obtained through a reliable sample of the school system. Moreover, it is possible that at this age all the permanent teeth except third molars, have already erupted. Thus, the age of 12 was determined as the age of global monitoring of caries for international comparisons and monitoring of disease trends.

Even considering the large number of scientific evidence from several epidemiological studies in schoolchildren worldwide, the majority are regional studies. In addition, the information is too outdated for some countries, which does not make easy international comparison. The index that measures the number of permanent teeth decayed, missing and filled teeth (DMFT) is the common outcome for such studies.

Although there are differences in both the sampling plan and the types of individual attributes collected at different times in history, epidemiology has been developing epistemological and methodological tools that allow revisit both old and recent data in order to understand the influence of environmental characteristics on individual outcomes, seeking correct the effect of aggregate, also known as ecological fallacy (Moreira & Nico, 2010). At the same time, the use of Geographic Information Systems (GIS) and statistical methods have allowed a more sophisticated processing of data since the observations are given an adequate spatial analysis.

As for the health-disease process, perceiving it as a historical phenomenon, the health situation of a given society is the result of models of health care employees in the past.

The interest in developing appropriate methodologies for knowledge and monitoring of social inequalities health has grown around the world. Area until recently restricted to a few academic groups, now finds conditions of highest use by health system managers, as a powerful instrument for establishing priorities agendas and evaluate the impact of adopted policies.

The global oral health database is currently being developed as part of the WHO Global InfoBase and it provides for the outcome evaluation of national and community oral health promotion and disease prevention programmes. The data stimulate providers of oral health care in countries and health authorities to implement preventive oral care programmes by sharing experiences and ensures data for adjustment of ongoing programmes. Oral health status of target population groups is monitored worldwide and linked with selected chronic diseases and common risk factors.

High quality health statistics are essential for planning and implementing health policy in all country settings. The Infobase assembles, for the first time in one place, non-communicable disease (NCD) risk factor data collected from WHO Member States. NCD risk factor data are crucial for predicting the future burden of chronic diseases in populations and also for identifying potential interventions to reduce the future burden.

The aim of this study is to describe the dental caries status of countries that are part of the WHO regions.

2. Methods

This research can be classified as an ecological study (Costa & Nadanovsky, 2005), as it takes to investigate aggregate data. Ecological studies are those using measured values for population groups rather than individuals. In them, a description and analysis are referred to the mean exposure and the prevalence in geopolitical units considered. They have a lower cost, simplicity and easy analytical process in relation of the ethical aspects. It is extremely useful for the evaluation of policies, programs and interventions in health (Peres & Antunes, 2006). The unit of analysis were the WHO member countries. Analyses were performed in each of the six WHO regions: the Americas (AMRO), Africa (AFRO), South East Asia (SEARO), Europe (EURO), Eastern Mediterranean (EMRO) and Western Pacific (WPRO). Figure 1 shows the spatial distribution of the six WHO regions in the world.

We used data of dental caries, expressed by the DMFT index at 12 years-old. These data were provided by WHO Oral Health Country / Area Profile Programme (CAPP). The "CAPP" was established at the WHO Collaborating Centre for Education, Training and Research at the Faculty of Odontology, Malmö, Sweden, in 1995. Before that, extensive consultations had taken place with the WHO Noncommunicable Diseases Cluster, Geneva, and with several WHO Collaborating Centres, organizations and individuals around the world. The objective is to present information on dental diseases and oral health services for various countries/areas. The data are publicly accessed at the site http://www.mah.se/CAPP.

Thus, thematic maps were constructed to show the spatial distribution of the dental caries in the world. Measures of association such as Relative Risk (RR) and Population Attributable Risk (PAR) were made. The main results were presented through charts and graphs.

Relative Risk (RR) consists of a ratio between rates of each class variable and an arbitrary reference value. In the analysis was taken as reference value the average of the WHO regions, thus evaluating how much each country is away from the mean (values above 1 showed an excess and values below 1 showed a lack in relation to the regional average).

Population Attributable Risk (PAR) is the relative difference between each of the proportional units of analysis and an arbitrary reference value, which in this study refers to the average of each region. It is intended to measure the impact it would have on the indicator considered the reduction of inequality between each value and the reference value. It can also be taken as a goal to guide interventions.

WHO regional offices

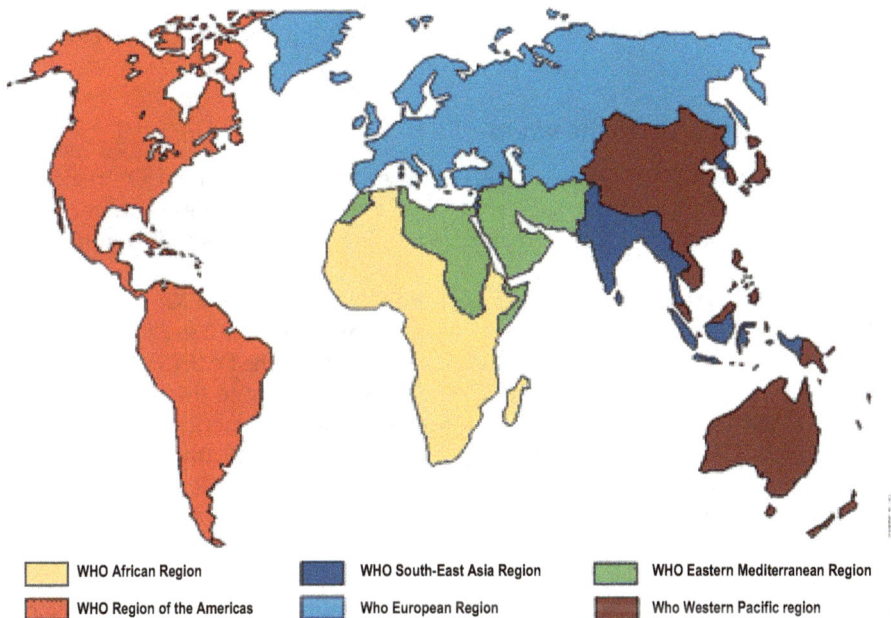

Fig. 1. Spatial distribution of the six WHO regions in the world.
Source: WHO (http://www.who.int/about/regions/en/index.html)

2.1 Measurement of the decay

To measure mouth disease in epidemiological studies, there is standardization of criteria according to WHO, using indexes. To diagnose coronary cavity (located at the crown of the tooth) in permanent teeth, the index used is the sum of the number of decayed teeth (component), missing (component) and restored / filled (component), called DMFT index. Subsequently we calculate the average population.

2.2 Caries

Dental caries is a complex disease caused by a physiological imbalance between fluid and mineral dental biofilm (microbial cells in a matrix, favoring the use of nutritional resources available, formerly known as plaque). It is recognized that microorganisms are not only sufficient to explain it, highlighting the important role of biofilm in its development (Fejerskov, 2004).

The mechanism of the cavity can be presented as follows: from the fermentation of carbohydrates, the bacteria produce organic acids such as lactic acid, the formic, acetic and propionic. These acids penetrate the dental tissues, dissolving the enamel (the outside of the tooth), dentin and cementum (tooth root). The dissolution may cause cavitation. In noncavitated lesions, demineralization can be reversed by calcium and phosphate, together with fluor, a result of new deposits on the remnants of crystals (tooth enamel). The new mineral crystal surface is much more resistant to acid when compared with the original hydroxyapatite (tooth enamel). The process of de-and remineralization cavitation occur daily, leading to cavitation, repair, reversal or maintaining the *status quo* (Featherstone, 2004).

3. Distribution of caries in the world

Was analyzed data on DMFT index in 190 countries that are part of WHO's regions. The year in which data were available showed that, on average, the studies were of 1997. Half of the studies was of 1998. Were seen studies ranging from the year 1973 until the year 2008.

With respect to the DMFT index, the average worldwide was 2.11 (± 1.32). Half the country had about 1.8 teeth decayed, missing or filled. Values ranged from 0.2 to 7.8. Figure 2 shows the distribution of countries according to the year of study and the DMFT index.

Figures 3 and 4 show, respectively, the RR and PAR according to the six WHO regions, with reference to the world average. It is observed that the American Region (AMRO) and the Europe Region (EURO) present a risk of 1.14 and 1.10 times higher than the average in the world, representing an average increase in PAR by 14% and 10%, respectively. AFRO region was with a 19% lower risk compared to the average of all countries surveyed.

Figure 5 shows the spatial distribution of caries at 12 years-old in the world according to quartiles. There were high DMFT indices in most countries of South America, Northern Europe and South Asia. Interestingly, a significant proportion of African countries have low rates of caries.

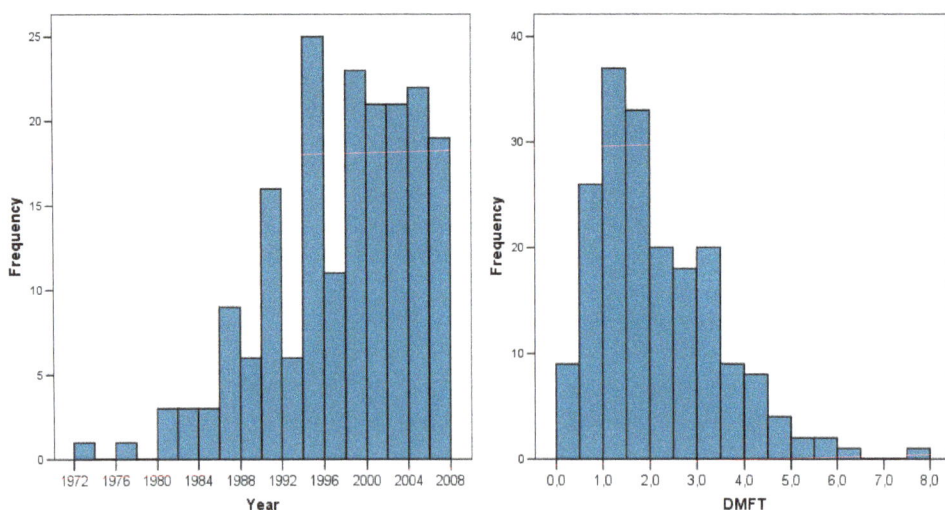

Fig. 2. Distribution of the world's countries according to the year of the study and the DMFT index

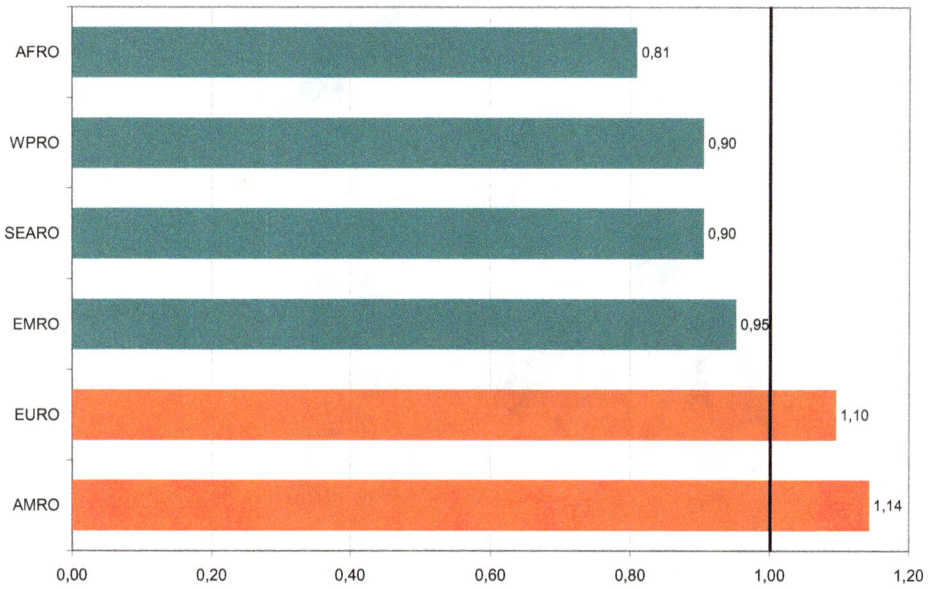

Fig. 3. Relative risk for dental caries according to WHO regions

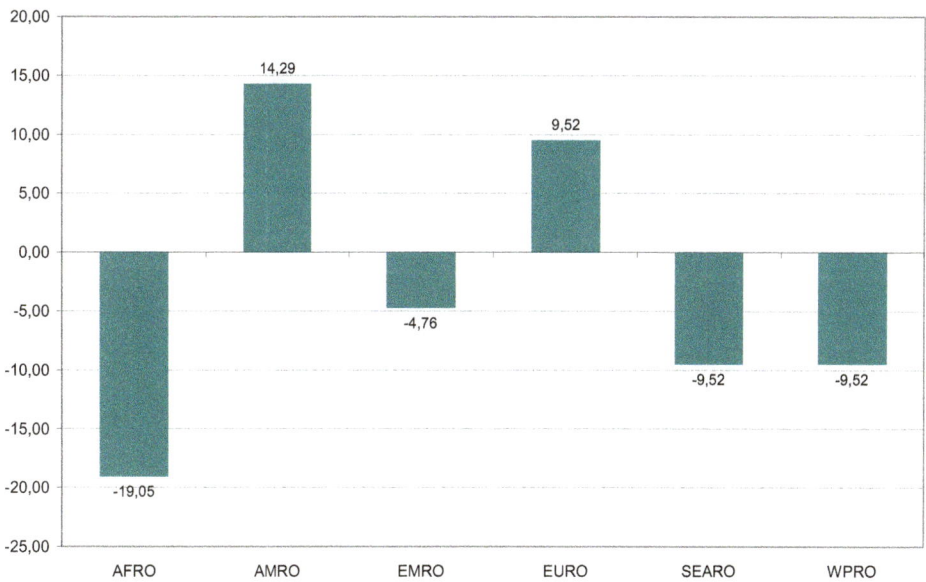

Fig. 4. PAR caries according to WHO regions

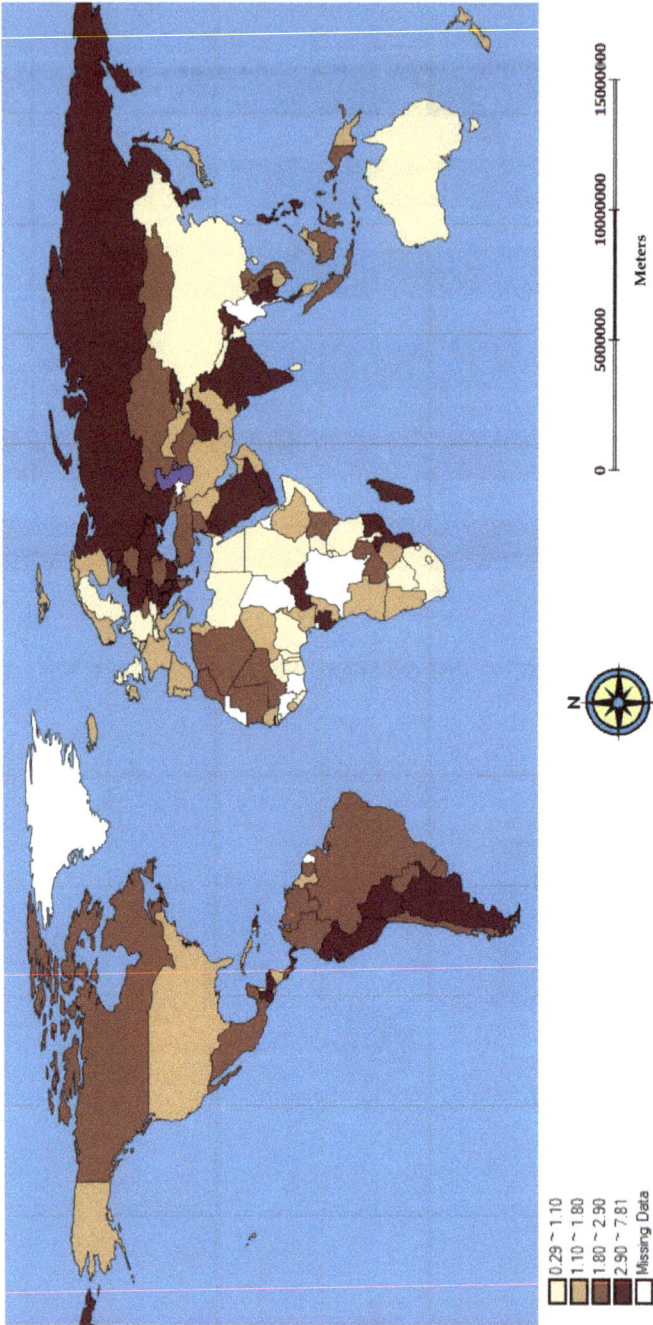

Fig. 5. Spatial distribution of the dental caries (12-years-old) in the world according to quartiles

4. Distribution of dental caries according to WHO regions

4.1 WHO African Region (AFRO)

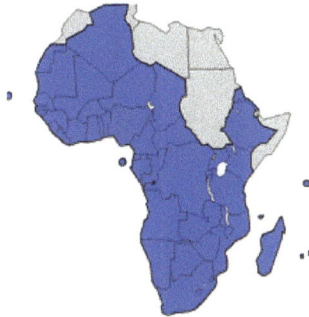

The WHO African region have 46 countries. However, it was possible to find oral health data for 40 countries. Analyzing the available studies regarding the year, there was a downgrade of the data. Half of the information was stemmed by the year 1992, also representing the average year of the surveys. The data ranged from 1977 to 2004.

Figure 6 shows the distribution of countries according to the year of study and the DMFT index. With respect to the DMFT index, there was an average of 1.7 (± 1.3). Considering the goals set by WHO and the Fedération Dentaire Internacionale (FDI, 1982) of a DMFT of three for the year 2000, it is observed that the African region achieved these results even before the deadline. In this way, at least with respect to decay, the region does not present a precarious scenario. The index ranged from 0.3 to 5.5. Half of the countries had a index of 1.3. Figure 7 shows the values of DMFT according to the countries of the African region.

Figure 8 shows the spatial distribution of Relative Risk of each country in relation to the regional average. Analyzing the RR, it was found that Mozambique had a risk 3.2 times higher than the average for the region. Tongo and Tanzania already had PAR 82.5% lower than the regional average.

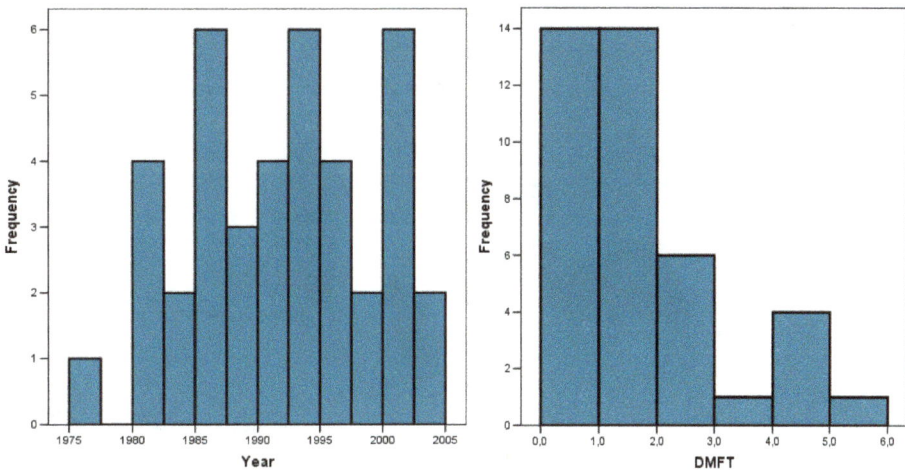

Fig. 6. Distribution of the AFRO countries according to the year of the study and the DMFT index

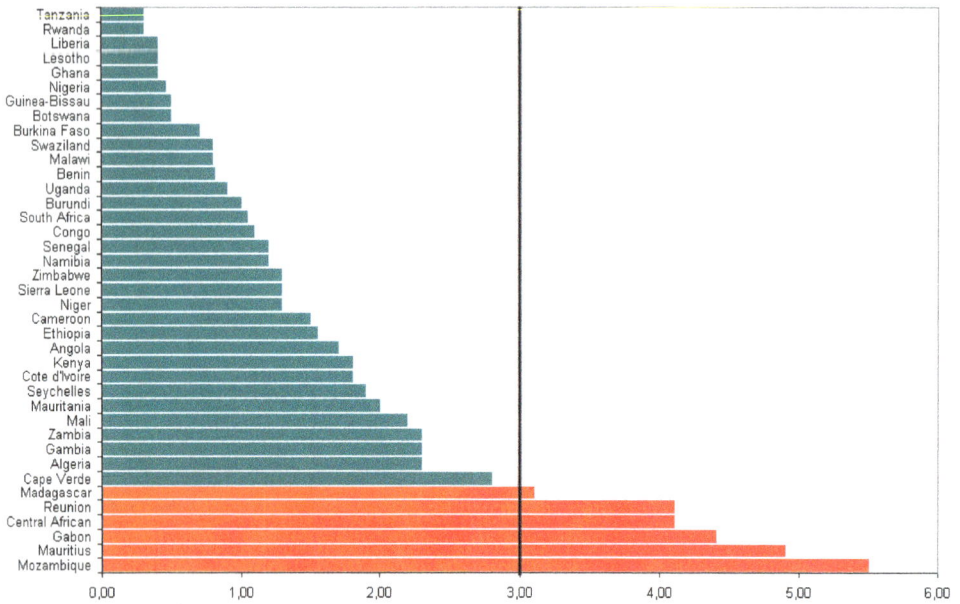

Fig. 7. Distribution of DMFT according to the countries of the African region

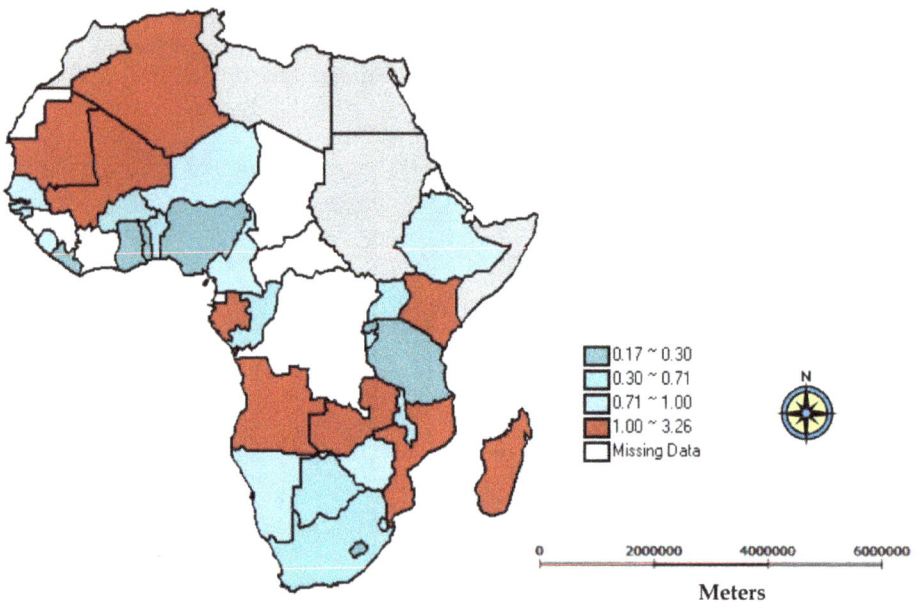

Fig. 8. Spatial distribution of Relative Risk of DMFT in relation to the average for the African region

4.2 WHO Region of the Americas (AMRO)

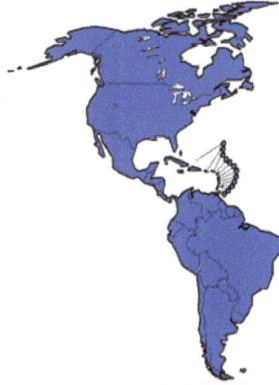

The regional of the Americas have 47 countries. However, only 40 countries had data on caries at 12 years-old.

Just as the average, half of the studies was available in 2000. Although more recent data than Africa, the results are given with more than 10 years, making it difficult to capture a more current data. The studies ranged from 1987 to 2008. Figure 9 shows the distribution of studies according to the year in which they were made and according to the DMFT index.

The DMFT index showed an average of 2.4 (± 1.4). Half of the countries had DMFT equal to 2.1. Figure 10 shows the ranking of countries according to the DMFT of the Americas. With the highest levels found in Ecuador and Martinique (6.3 and 5.2, respectively). Belize and Haiti had low (0.60 and 0.65 respectively). Figure 11 shows the spatial distribution of the countries of the Americas according to relative risk, with reference to the regional average.

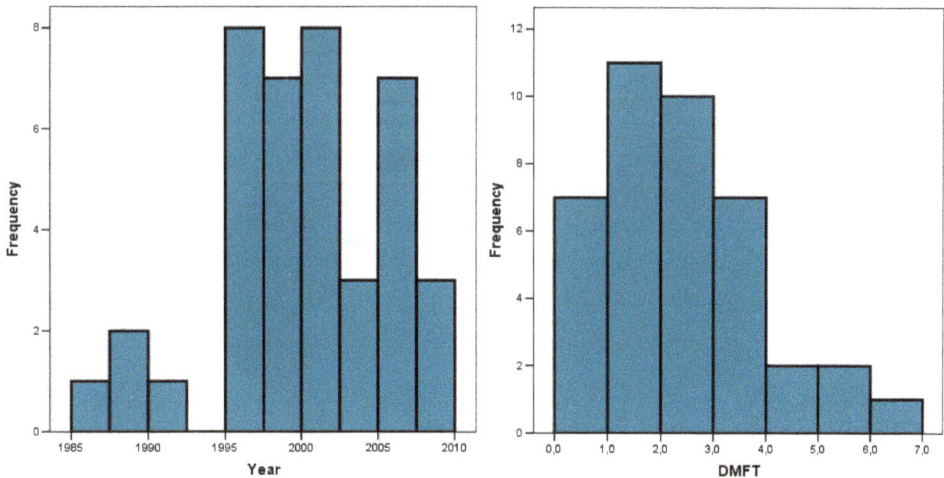

Fig. 9. Distribution of the AMRO countries according to the year of the study and the DMFT index

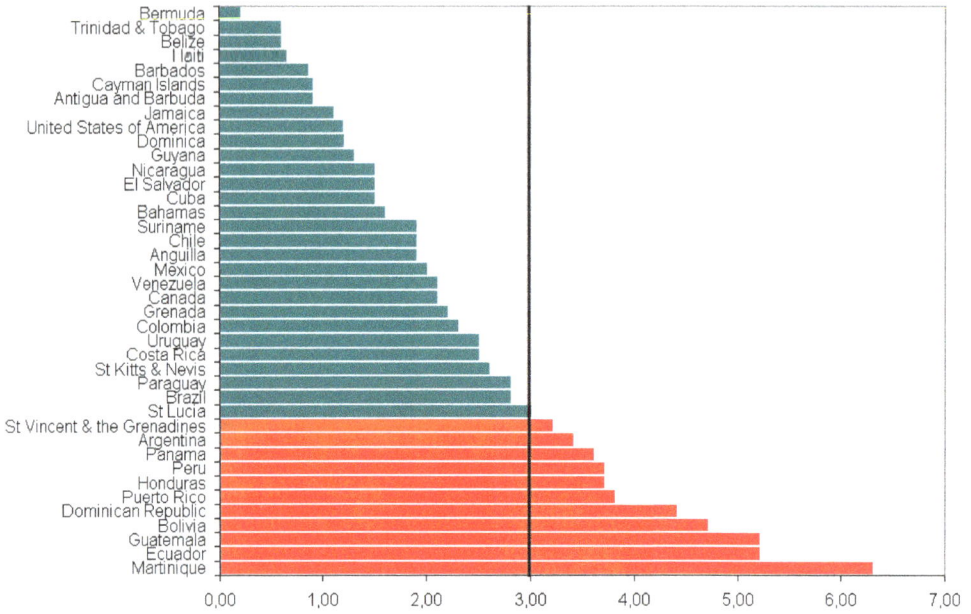

Fig. 10. Distribution of DMFT according to the countries of the Americas

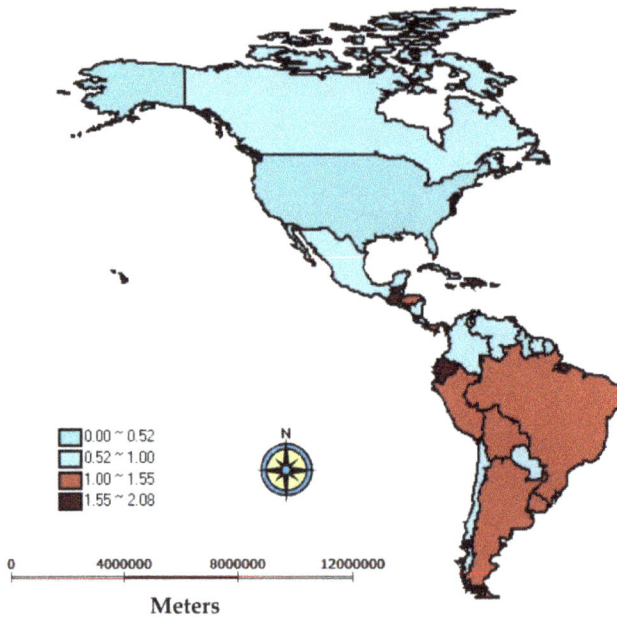

Fig. 11. Spatial distribution of relative risk of DMFT in relation to the average for the Americas

4.3 WHO Region of South East Asia (SEARO)

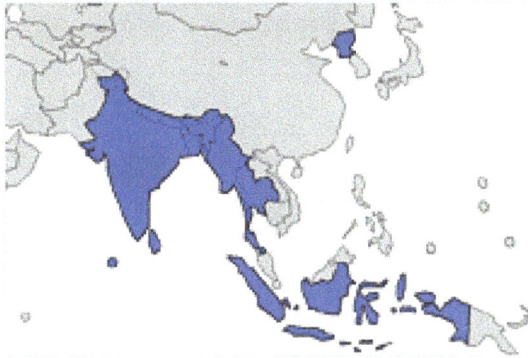

The Southeast Asian region consists of 11 countries. Only one country (East Timor) had no data on dental caries at 12 years-old.

The average years of studies completed was 1999. But half of the studies were of 2001. The studies ranged from 1984 to 2008. Figure 12 shows the distribution of studies according to the year in which they were made and according to the DMFT index.

The DMFT index showed an average of 1.95 (± 1.24) and a median of 1.65. The minimum and maximum values were 0.50 to 3.94, respectively.

Figure 13 shows the PAR of caries, with reference to the regional average. It was observed that India and Thailand respectively show a PAR of 101.84% and 89.55% more caries compared to the reference value. Nepal and Sri Lanka had the lowest risk being about 74% and 54% less in relation to the regional average, respectively.

Figure 14 shows the map with the RR of the region. It was observed that India, Thailand, Indonesia and Korea are in the categories of risk (RR> 1.00) for the highest DMFT.

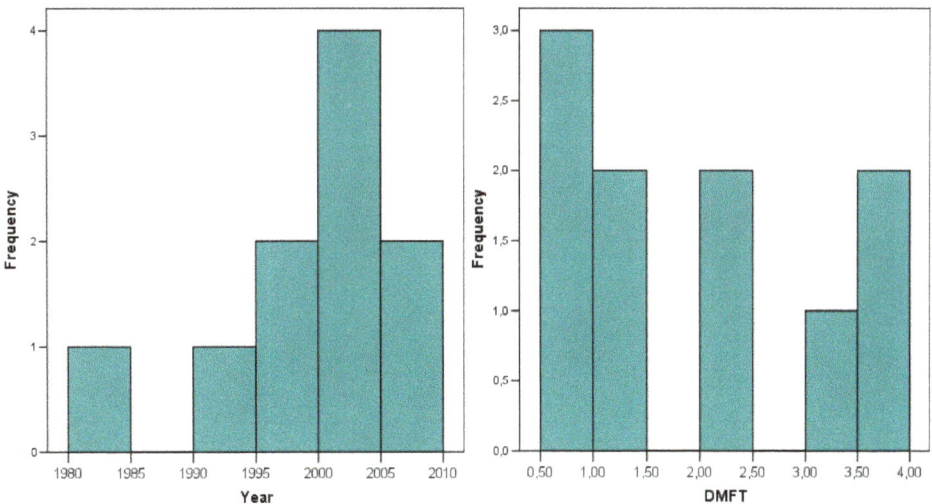

Fig. 12. Distribution of the SEARO countries according to the year of the study and the DMFT index

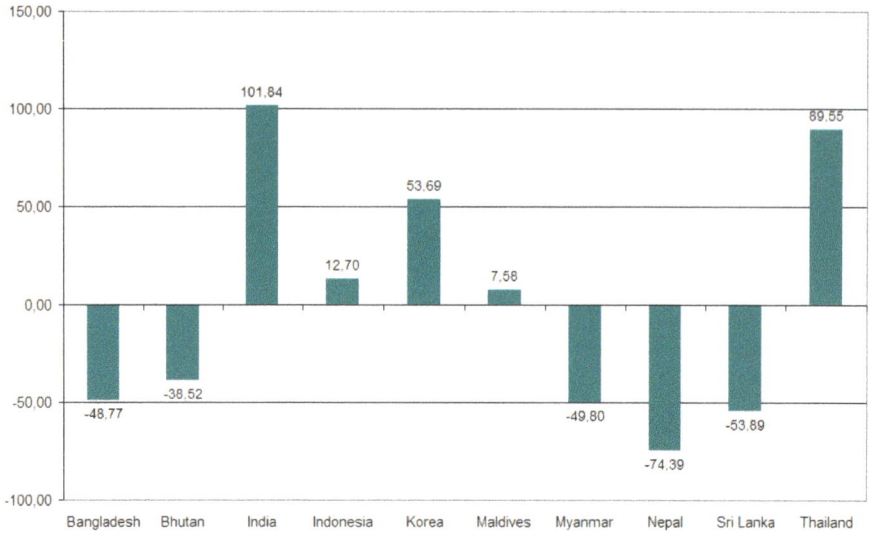

Fig. 13. PAR caries according to the countries in the SEARO Region

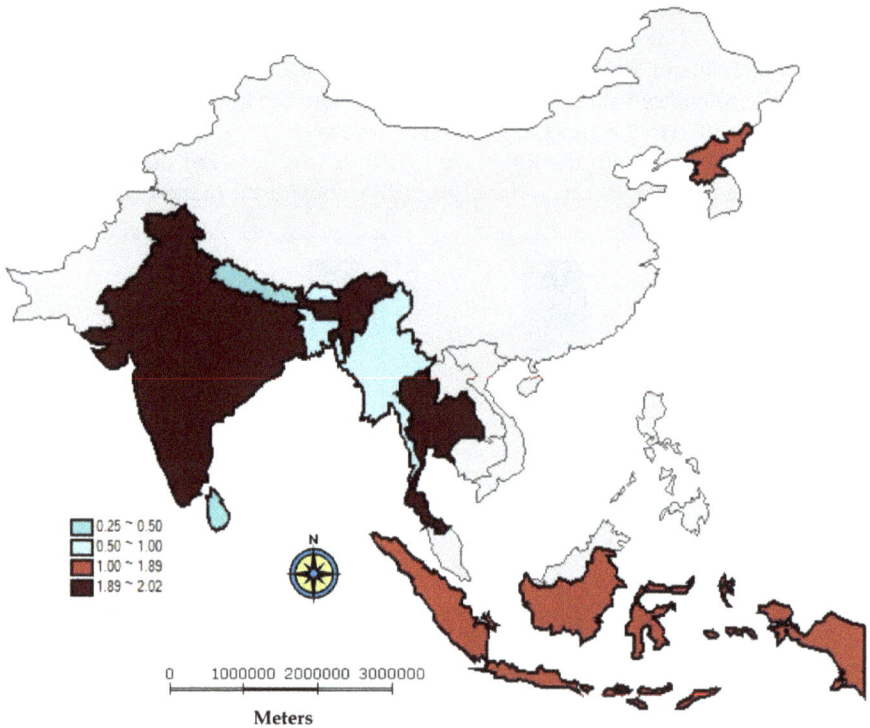

Fig. 14. Spatial distribution of relative risk of DMFT in relation to the average for the region SEARO

4.4 WHO European Region (EURO)

The European region comprises 53 countries. Data from 51 countries on dental caries in schoolchildren 12 years-old were available.

The average publication year was 1998. Half of the studies were of the year 2000. The surveys ranged from the years 1973 to 2008. The mean DMFT index was 2.3 (± 1.3). Half of the countries in the region of Europe had 2.2 teeth decayed, missing or filled teeth. The index ranged from 0.7 to 7.8.

Figure 15 shows the distribution of studies according to the year in which they were made and according to the DMFT index.

Figure 16 shows the distribution of countries according to the PAR. It was observed that most Western European countries have lower risks compared to the regional average.

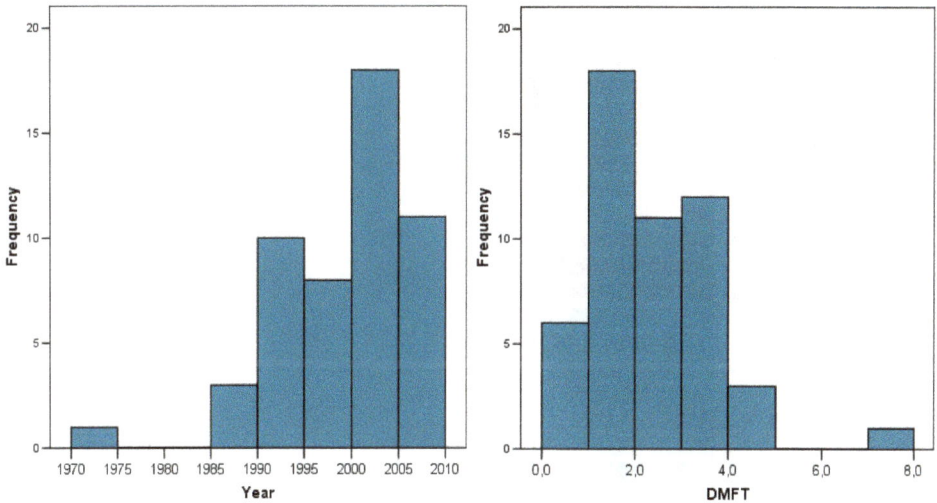

Fig. 15. Distribution of the EURO countries according to the year of the study and the DMFT index

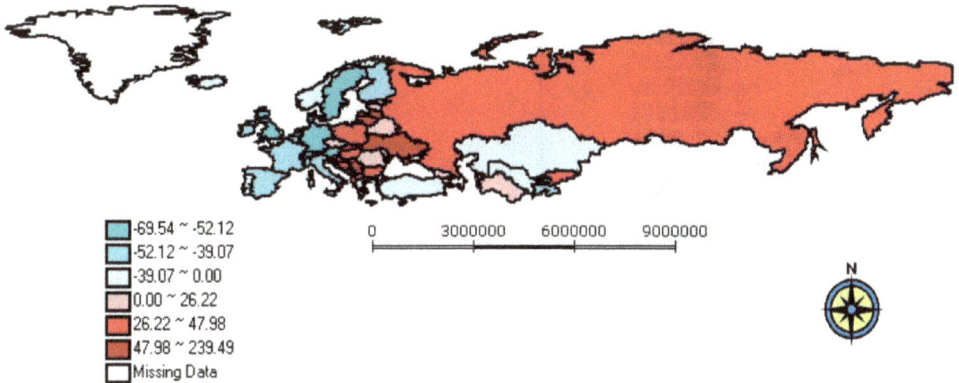

Fig. 16. Spatial distribution of PAR from the average for the Euro Region

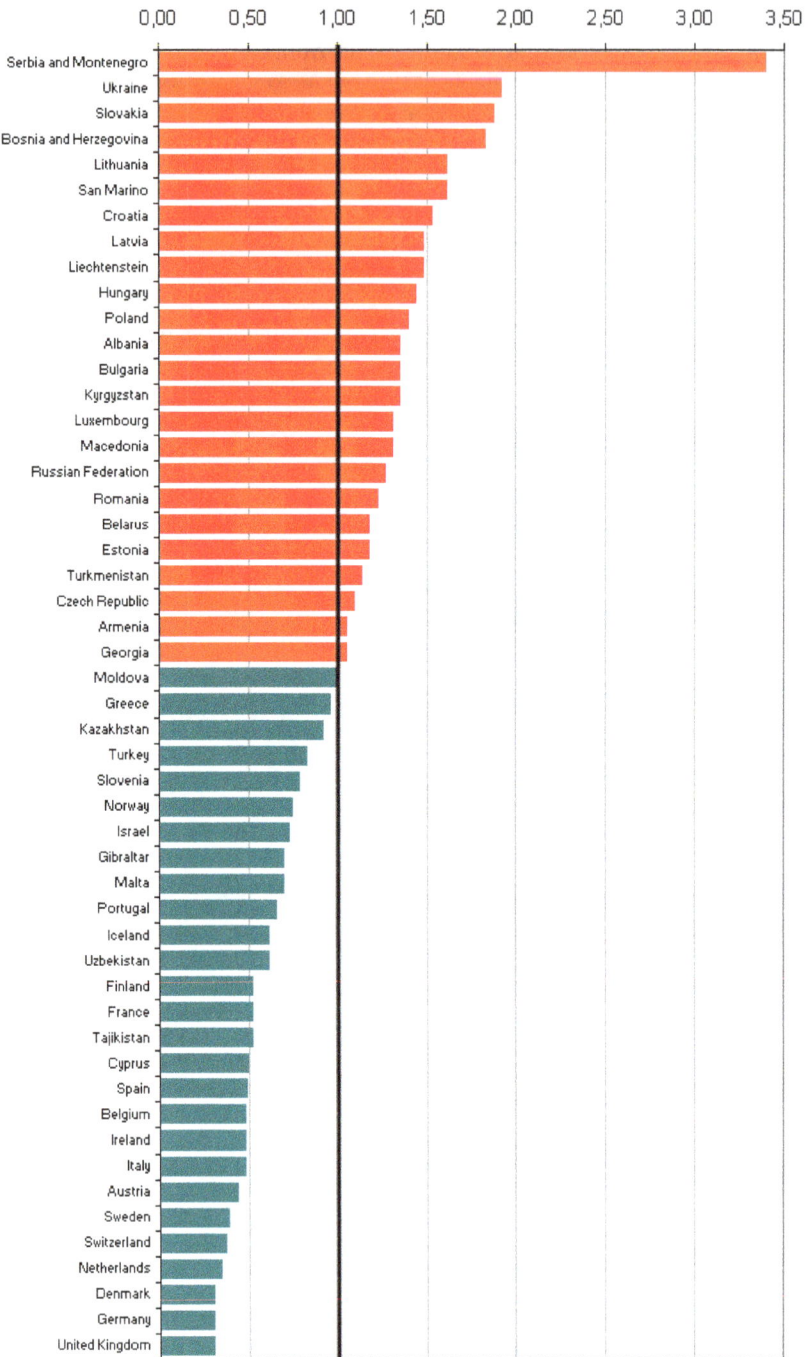

Fig. 17. RR caries according to the countries of the Euro Region

Regarding the relative risk observed in Figure 17, it was found 24 European countries with a rate of decay higher than the average for the region. Among them were Serbia, Montenegro and Ukraine, being the first two countries with risk of 3.4 and the last with a risk 1.9 times higher than the regional average. The countries with the lowest rates were United Kingdom, Germany and Denmark with a relative risk around 0.3.

4.5 WHO Eastern Mediterranean Region (EMRO)

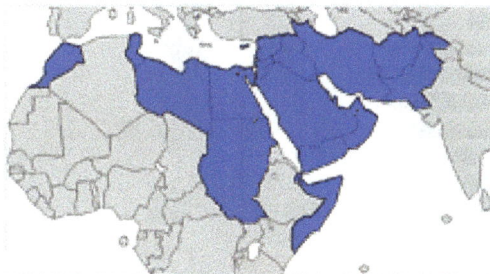

Comprising the EMRO region 21 countries. Data on caries was available for 20 countries, only Quatar did not provide data.

Both the mean and the median date of the studies was 1998. The researches ranged from 1987 to 2008. The average DMFT index found in the region was 2 (± 1.3). Half of the countries had a index of 1.6 and the values ranged from 0.4 to 5.9.

Figure 18 shows the distribution of studies according to the year in which they were made and according to the DMFT index. Figure 19 shows the ranking of countries according to the DMFT. It is observed that only four countries (20%) had higher values than the target recommended by WHO in 2000 (DMFT = 3). They are: Saudi Arabia, Lebanon, Jordan and Yemen.

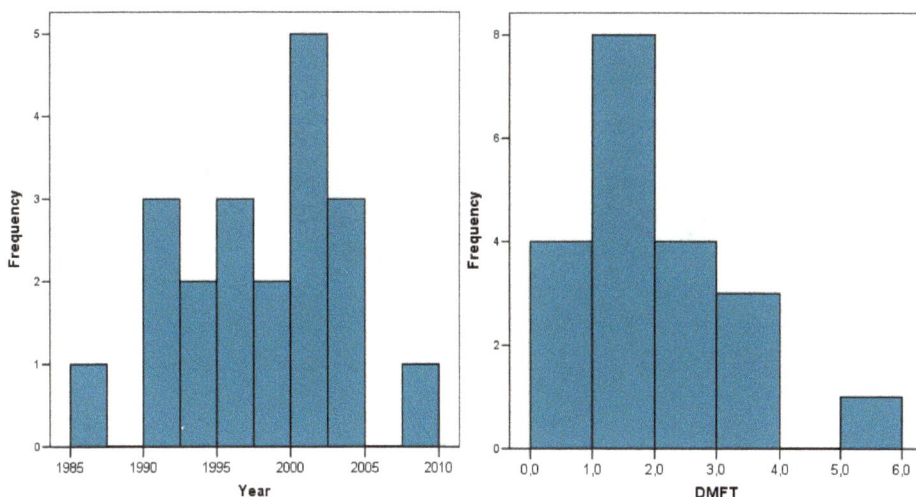

Fig. 18. Distribution of the EMRO countries according to the year of the study and the DMFT index

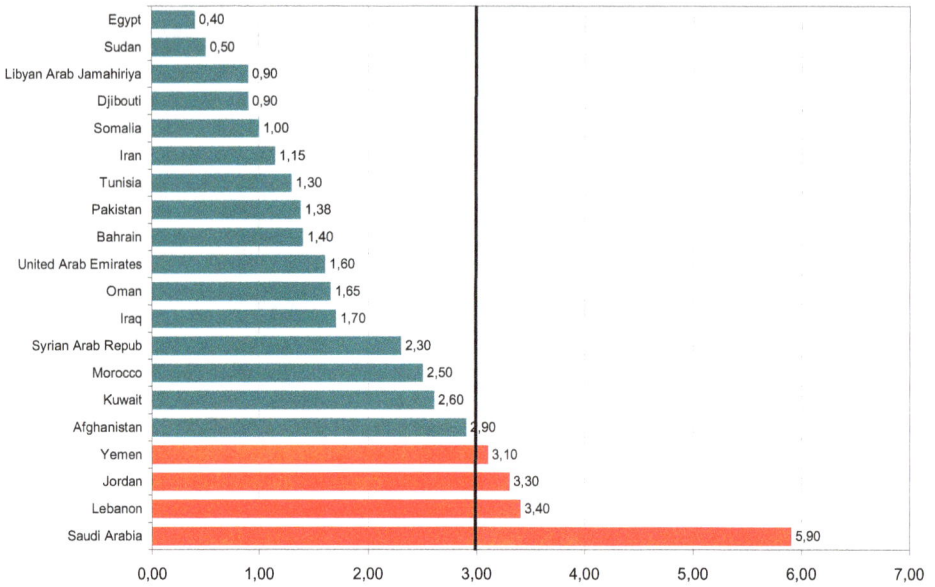

Fig. 19. Distribution of DMFT according to the countries of the EMRO region

Figure 20 shows the map of the spatial distribution of relative risk (RR) with reference to the regional average. Saudi Arabia presented a RR three times higher than the regional average, followed by Lebanon and Jordan with RR of 1.7. Egypt and Sudan appeared to countries with lower risks, respectively, 0.20 and 0.25 and Libya with RR of 0.45.

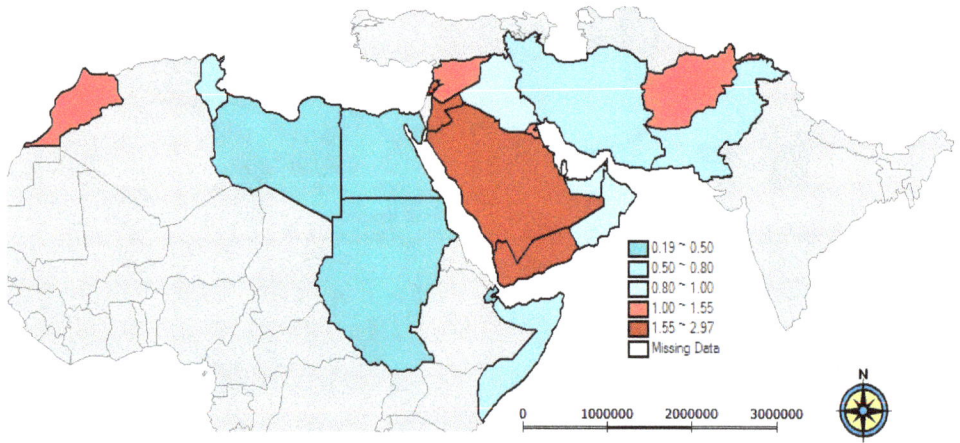

Fig. 20. Spatial distribution of RR in relation to the average DMFT for the EMRO region

4.6 WHO Western Pacific Region (WPRO)

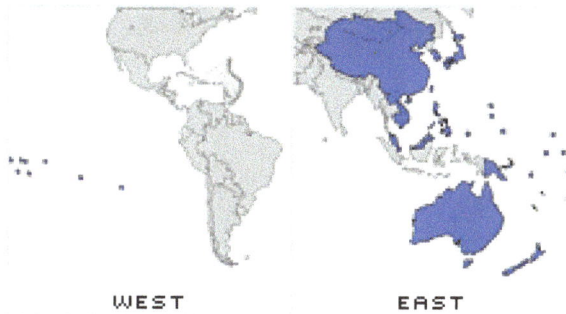

WEST   EAST

The WPRO comprises 27 countries. Data on caries was available for 24 countries in the region.

The studies, on average, were from the years of 1998 and half of them were developed in 1997. The researches ranged between 1984 and 2007. With respect to the DMFT index, the average for the region was 1.93 (± 0.9). Half of the countries had an index of 1.75. DMFT values ranged from 1 to 5.

Figure 21 shows the distribution of studies according to the year in which they were made and according to the DMFT index. Figure 22 shows the values of the PAR. It may be noted that six countries had a higher risk with reference to the regional average. Brunei Darussalam had an increase of 127% in the risk of caries, followed by the Republic of Korea and Tonga (both with an increase of 47%), Philippines (37%), Solomon Islands (28%) and Samoa (18%). Singapore, Kiribati, China and Australia showed a 52% lower risk compared to the reference value.

Figure 23 shows the map of the RR with reference to the regional average. There is more risk in the Philippines, Korea, Mongolia and Vietnam.

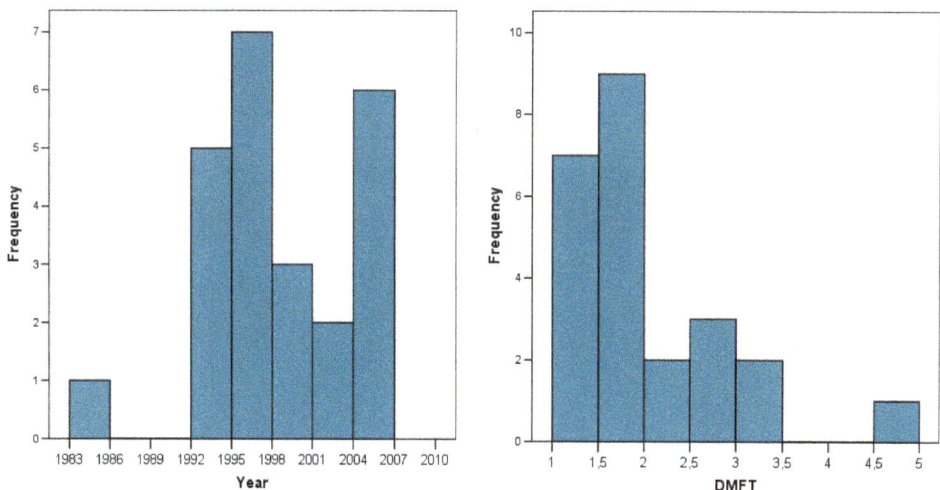

Fig. 21. Distribution of the WPRO countries according to the year of the study and the DMFT index

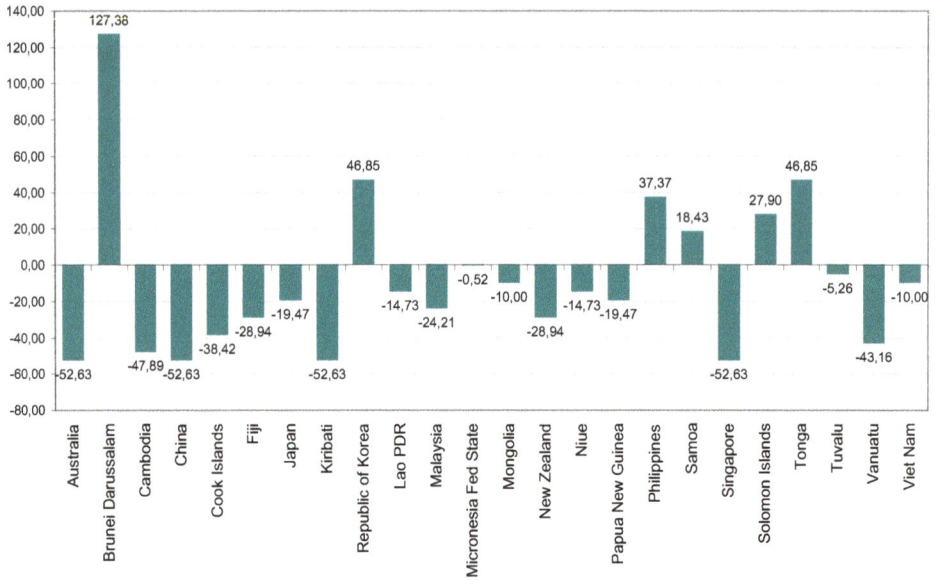

Fig. 22. PAR caries according to the countries of the WPRO Region

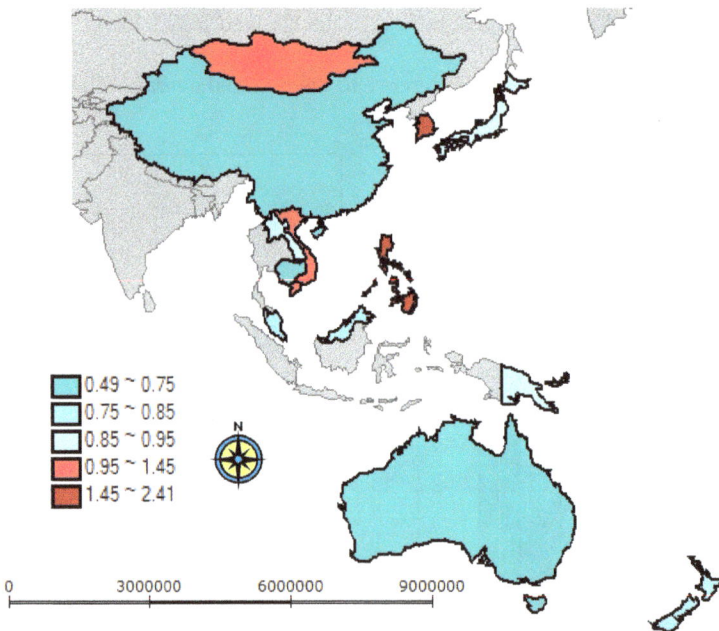

Fig. 23. Spatial distribution of relative risk of DMFT in relation to the average for the region WPRO

5. Discussion

The reduced level of caries in schoolchildren of 12 years-old is quite visible in the period and has been the subject of several other studies. This reflects the very recommendation of WHO to monitor the DMFT index at age 12. It is noteworthy, in this scenario, the traditionally history of the national oral health systems have on the public school.

The WHO Oral Health Program (Petersen, 2003) presented in its report on the global oral health conditions, a four-level scale for the classification of the DMFT index at 12 years-old. They are: very low (less than 1.2), low (1.2 to 2.6), moderate (2.7 to 4.4) and high (over 4.4). In this sense, it was established that all WHO regions had an average DMFT classified as low, since the change occurred between the values from 1.7 to 2.4. However, when you look at differentials between countries, this classification varies widely, with representatives in all categories of the index.

The Fedération Dentaire Internacionale (FDI), the International Association for Dental Research (IADR) and WHO set oral health goals for the year 2020 (Hodbell et al., 2003). Unlike the goals for the year 2000, which indicated a rate of not more than 3 DMFT at age 12, the target set was: "to reduce the DMFT at age 12, in particular the component 'D' on X%, with special attention for high-risk groups, considering both the average values as their distributions."

Antunes et al. (2006) make three observations about this statement. First, should be given special attention to high-risk groups. This indication is due to intensely unequal distribution of caries. Second, the idea of monitoring not only the average values, but also their distributions, which tries to correct the effect on the measurement of a disease with high inequality in its distribution. And third, there is not the establishment of absolute values, because they must adapt to local conditions regarding the availability of databases, priorities, current levels of prevalence and severity, socioeconomic status, available resources and characteristics of health systems.

It was observed that the more developed countries, especially in the EURO, presented DMFT index greater than the least developed countries, especially the AFRO region. This finding corroborates the fact that most of the twentieth century (the period when most studies were performed), the decay was seen as a disease of rich countries with low prevalence in the poorest countries. The most obvious reason for this is the standard diet. The high consumption of refined carbohydrates in the richer countries has led to a selective proliferation of cariogenic bacteria, unlike the poorest countries that had a diet based on hunting and subsistence agriculture, with low-carbohydrate diets (Burt & Eklund, 2005).

However this scenario is quite out of date due to data analyzed being old. There is strong evidence that this pattern is altered with marked reduction in caries experience in children and young adults in rich countries. Other factors are helping reverse this scenario within a context of a globalized world. The increased access to foods and the exclusive and selective oral health services offering are changing the global profile of caries. Recent studies are needed to evaluate such changes.

6. Conclusions

The existence of a database with information on tooth decay of 12 years-old favors the presentation of an epidemiological scenario of oral health in the world. Easy access to the data publicly available over the internet enables the analysis by the researchers favoring the transformation of data into information. Such information may serve to guide policy goals for oral health according to the different realities observed.

However, this analysis has some limitations. Besides being restricted to countries that are part of the regional offices of the WHO, some countries had no data available on oral health. Another factor was wide variations in the years to disseminate the studies. It was observed studies from 1973 to 2008. This distance of 35 years makes comparisons very weak and outdated. However, this evidence should be that the countries and regions where data are more outdated, especially countries in the AFRO, pay greater attention to the epidemiological diagnosis of the oral health of their populations.

The existence of information about the DMFT index for most WHO member states legitimize this indicator as a measure universally accepted and used for global comparisons. However, the lack of other oral health indicators reduces to only one face of its characteristics and consequences. Index that measure other dimensions, such as periodontal disease, tooth loss and access to oral health services should have the same range observed in the systematization of the DMFT index.

It was observed that all regions had an average of DMFT below 3, which represents the achievement of targets set by WHO for the year 2000. However, there was wide variation between countries. Moreover, it is noteworthy that this global ecological analysis, assuming the countries as units of analysis, it homogeneous areas with large heterogeneities in their local realities. Studies with smaller units, with increased geographic scale are needed to access the micro-realities concealed by means of their countries.

7. References

Antunes JLF, Peres MA, Frazão P. Cárie dentária. In: Antunes JLF, Peres MA (org). Epidemiologia da Saúde Bucal. Rio de Janeiro: Guanabara Koogan; 2006. p.49-67.

Burt BA, Eklund AS. Dentistry, Dental Practice, and the Community. 6th Ed. Missouri: Elsevier Saunders; 2005.

Costa AJL, Nadanovsky P. Desenhos de estudos epidemiológicos. In: Costa AJL, Nadanovsky P, Luiz RR. Epidemiologia e bioestatística na pesquisa odontológica. São Paulo: Atheneu; 2005. p. 215-43.

Featherstone JDB. The continuum of dental caries--evidence for a dynamic disease process. J Dent Res 2004;83 Spec No C:C39-42.

Fedération Dentaire Internacionale. Global goals for oral health in the year 2000. Int Dent J, 32 (1): 74-7, 1982.

Fejerskov O. Changing paradigms in concepts on dental caries: consequences for oral health care. Caries Res. 2004 May-Jun;38(3):182-91.

Hodbell M, Petersen PE, Clarkson J, Johnson N. Global goals for oral health 2020. International Dental Journal 2003; 53(5): 285-8.

Moreira RS; Nico LS. Aspectos contextuais da ausência de cárie em escolares de 12 anos no Brasil, em três períodos históricos. Rev Odonto UNESP 2010; 39(5): 263-70.

Peres MA, Antunes JLF. O metodo epidemiologico de investigacao e sua contribuição para a saude bucal. In: Peres MA. Fundamentos de Odontologia: epidemiologia da saúde bucal. Rio de janeiro, Guanabara Koogan, 2006, p. 8-9.

Petersen PE. The world oral health report 2003. Continuous improvement of oral health n the 21st century – the approach of the WHO Global Oral Health Programme. Geneva: World Health Organization, 2003.

World Health Organization. Oral health surveys: basic methods. 4 ed. Geneva: ORH/EPID, 1997.

Classical and Modern Methods in Caries Epidemiology

M. Larmas, H. Vähänikkilä, K. Leskinen and J. Päkkilä
University of Oulu
Finland

1. Introduction

In epidemiological research the focus is on the occurrence, causes, and modifying factors of diseases and thereby their prevention. During the last decades, the epidemiology of dental caries has not dealt with the prevalence of the disease, but is measuring the past and present caries experience in terms of past and present treatment need, which does not follow the practices in epidemiology. Therefore it would be important that dental research returns the rules of (medical) epidemiology.

The World Health Organization [WHO] has recommended that the International Statistical Classification of Diseases and Related Health Problems [ICD] must be followed in diagnoses by both physicians and dentist. Because of this legislation all dental patients must have one primary diagnosis and when necessary, one or multiple secondary diagnoses.

The primary diagnosis is not necessarily the most serious disease but it only means that the disease which needs most treatment in time or equipment during the emergency visit or normal treatment period. This practice is meant only for statistical purposes in dental care, and therefore, represents some overview of the prevalence of diseases in that community.

The same system has been used by dentists in the secondary care level in hospitals or other institutes. This WHO´s decision recombined medical and dental professions. At the same time it also revealed that some diverse practices occurred in the use of certain common terms (for example disease prevalence) or principles of making diagnoses between dentistry and medicine. WHO determines dental caries in two different ways as discussed recently (Larmas, 2010a): in ICD it is a disease (WHO, 1977, 1992), and in oral health surveys as a process (WHO, 1997), assessing also the treatment need at the same time. Early epidemiological surveys on dental caries assessed number of persons suffering from the disease, thus, following the normal medical practice (Morelli, 1924).The aim of this review is to shed light on these diagnostic or assessment practices for epidemiological purposes.

2. Diagnosis of dental caries and caries assessment

2.1 Caries diagnosis

As a disease dental caries is determined in the classifications of diseases [ICDs]. They are systematic classifications of diseases, subject to agreement by governments. They are widely used for national mortality and morbidity statistics. The diseases as described verbally are about the same in different revisions of the ICDs, but their codes vary. The codes of the ninth revision (ICD-9, WHO, 1977) are presently used in the USA, the tenth (ICD-10, WHO, 1992) in most other countries. ICD-10 is revised periodically.

The recommended use of ICD states that all diagnoses must be recorded at the appropriate level, meaning that when the disease codes are used, they are used as three, four, or five characters levels. Of the licensed health care personnel, who has the right to make diagnoses, physicians are educated to make the caries diagnosis at three character level i.e. "dental caries" (K02 in ICD-10 or 521 in ICD-9) whereas dentists must use the four character level, like "caries of cementum" (K02.2 in ICD-10).

Another recommendation in the use of ICD is the fact that diseases needing treatment only should be recorded in the list of diagnoses. Thus, in the case of "caries limited to enamel" (coded at four character level K02.0, ICD-10) it should be diagnosed only when needing intervention (not only treatment by a restoration but also, for example, fluoride or sealing treatments), otherwise this diagnosis is omitted from the list of diagnoses in the record.

In the case a dentist makes a special diagnosis of caries like "feeding bottle caries", or "caries due to hyposalivation", both diseases should be classified into the ICD category "other specified dental caries", the latter needing additionally a secondary ICD diagnosis as "disturbances of salivary secretion" or shortly "hyposecretion".

2.2 Caries assessment

In Oral Health Surveys (WHO, 1997) dental caries is determined "decayed" (code 1 for permanent teeth, code A for primary teeth) or "filled, with decay" (codes 2 or B, respectively). The "decay" codes caries at the dentinal level of involvement, requiring evidence of cavitations to record it. The F-component is classified as "filled, no decay" (codes 3 and D), and the M-component as "missing as a result of caries" under the age of 30 years and in older patient, the M is "missing, any other reason". These tooth-specific recordings are only tooth-specific diagnoses, but real diagnoses commit patients as a whole and therefore the real diagnosis of the patient is "dental caries in one or multiple teeth", as will be discussed in detail later.

When caries prevalence rose to close hundred percent in the population (even before the adulthood), more accurate measures of caries experience were needed. Attempts were made to measure mean number of teeth affected by caries in populations, until a standardized index of decayed (D), missing (M) or filled (F) teeth was defined (Klein et al., 1938). Originally it was meant to inform caries "prevalence and treatment need" in elementary school children, later its use was expanded to describe past and present caries experience also in adults.

The DMF index is still used in high number of scientific articles, which underlines its leading role in the present caries research. However, the term caries experience underlines that it does not describe caries prevalence in the epidemiological sense.

The discrepancy between caries diagnosis and caries assessment is vanished in practice, because caries, termed "decay" in oral health surveys has reached the level of caries (=dentine) needing restoration and all its previous stages (white or chalky spots; discolored or rough spots; stained pits or fissures etc.) are omitted from the list of diagnoses in ICD (WHO, 1992) or are recorded as "sound" in oral health surveys (WHO, 1997).

A relatively new system for caries detection and assessment has lately developed [ICADS] to facilitate caries epidemiology, research and appropriate clinical management to grapple with some of the problems of caries assessment (Pitts, 2004). This system records both enamel and dentine caries and explores the measurement of caries activity (Pitts, 2004).

However, ICADS does not follow the normal epidemiological practice in that sense that the patient has one or multiple diseases in one or multiple organs, which means that the number of patients (not that of teeth) is the number of cases in the statistics.

A patient with carious lesions in three teeth is not three times more sick than a patient with caries in one tooth, both are simply "carious", whereas subjects with multiple restorations or dental implants are "healthy"in the ICD. The same concerns any cancer: a patient with for example an epithelial cancer in any organ with multiple metastases is simple one "cancer" patient, the number of diseased organs or metastases does not change the diagnosis, nor the mean number of lesions or metastases in the population is counted. The severity and treatment need of the patient will increase with the number of lesions, but not the number of that disease.

3. Prevalence of a disease

In epidemiology, prevalence of a disease may be defined as the proportion of population that has disease at a specific point in time (Rothman and Greenland, 1988). Textbooks in epidemiology use also terms "point prevalence", "prevalence proportion" and "prevalence rate", meaning the same thing. The prevalence pool is the subset of the population with the disease (Rothman and Greenland, 1998). Lifetime prevalence is the proportion of a population that has had the disease in question at some time during their lives.

In epidemiology a subject is either healthy or has one or numerous different diseases. The prevalence(s) of disease(s) varies in a community, as does the number of lesions / restorations / fractures in a patient, but one patient has one ICD-category of dental caries in one or multiple teeth. Then the single patient with dental caries increases dental caries prevalence by one in the population, or else, increases first maxillary and mandibular molar caries cases by four (if all first molars have caries). In the latter case, the caries prevalence is one (patient) with four carious lesions in the first molars, or else one patient with caries in the first maxillary and mandibular, right and left molars, i.e. four different caries diseases, which, however, does not follow the ICD.

In medicine/dentistry, for example, there are two possible diagnostic approaches when the locations of diseased organs are studied. "General diseases" like "osteoporosis" may concern the whole skeleton although some parts of the skeleton are more vulnerable for other osteoporosis-connected diseases, like fractures of bones. Some bones may have fractures more frequently than the other bones of the same osteoporotic patient. The ICD sub-classification of "osteoporosis with fractures" is based on its aetiology, like "postmenopausal", "malabsorption", etc., not the location or number of fractured bones. Dental caries (as a disease in enamel, dentine etc.) can be classified similarly as a "general disease", although some teeth/surfaces are more vulnerable than others, and patients are caries prone or resistant.

"Local diseases" like injuries or fractures of bones/teeth occur in certain sites of the body due to external reasons. Fractures of skull and facial bones, maxilla and mandible, fractures of teeth, etc. are examples of local diseases in ICD. Each bone or tooth has its own fracture, or even many fractures, and the subject may have multiple fractures. Dental caries can be classified also as a "local disease". In this case caries in canines is not the same disease which commits caries in molars, although the aetiology is (about) the same, like is the aetiology of fractures.

ICD classifies dental caries as a general disease, like osteoporosis, and one patient with caries may have carious lesions in one or multiple teeth. This results in a hierarchical nature of the disease data, in which carious teeth are clustered within patients. This complicates the statistical analysis of the observed differences of caries in cohorts in epidemiological or experimental studies.

This may be avoided when each tooth, primary or permanent, is treated as having its own "caries" resulting in a possibility of 32 different caries onsets in permanent and 20 in primary teeth, or else, even five more lesions on different surfaces of each tooth (Larmas et al., 1995). However, this type of classification is not possible following the ICD in the disease prevalence studies, but it is possible when the severity and treatment need of the disease is determined. We may count that each tooth have five surfaces (incisal edges of incisors and cuspal tips of canines being a surface), though many epidemiological surveys count each tooth having different numbers of "missing" surfaces, basing on their mean caries occurrence values. All dentists agree with our "anatomical" system when counting the treatment fees, and therefore we recommend that practice also in research.

4. Epidemiological research

In epidemiology, the focus is on the occurrence of disease. If the subject has a disease or diseases, he/she is a "case" in statistics, a "patient" in medicine/dentistry, with the rest of the population being healthy (Rothman and Greenland, 1998). Both ICD-10 and-9 (the latter with different codes) determine different types (enamel, dentine, cementum etc.) of dental caries as diseases, which may occur in one or multiple locations determining thereby the prevalence of these diseases in patients (not in teeth) in that population. If caries commits many teeth, the disease is more severe, but still the same "single" disease in that patient.

This medical/dental principle is followed only rarely in dental statistics: each tooth or restoration is treated as its own "case", which does not follow the principles of clinical epidemiology where the patient is always the "case" (=N). Another possibility, which, however, does not follow the present ICD system, is to consider each carious tooth/surface as its own disease in the patient. This quantitative approach is followed when the efficacy of caries preventive measures is scientifically (meaning by calibrated examiners) determined in caries research, but should not be followed when the possible reduction of caries prevalence after a clinical trial is determined.

5. Evidence-based [EBD] vs. practice-based dentistry [PBD]

Systematic clinical reviews demonstrating causality normally evolve from laboratory studies through animal studies to case series and thereafter to controlled clinical trials (Niederman and Leithch, 2006). These studies demand strict scientific rules (good laboratory practice, good clinical practice, cross-over study design etc.) for providing information for each of these steps. The evidence-based approach to create knowledge may not be enough: translational research (know how) is also needed in addition to the classical laboratory and clinical studies to show how science works in practice (Niederman and Leithch, 2006, Mjör, 2008, Larmas, 2010b).

Same statistical methods are always used in analyzing the EBD and PBD study results, the research protocols having only different aims and principles. All drugs are carefully tested applying EBD protocol before the registration for use, their efficacy should be very high, often almost 100%, or at least significantly more effective than the older ones. Their practical effectiveness is another issue: Is a drug with an efficacy of 100 % to cure the disease truly

100% effective if it is used as prescribed only by 50 % of the patients? Restoration certainly eliminates caries, but is not effective when not used.

The real effectiveness of the use of an effective drug or treatment in everyday practice can be studied applying PBD study design. Because non-calibrated clinicians (in this case also examiners) are providing information on the efficacy of different treatments in practice, the possibility of use the huge longitudinal study material with sophisticated statistical methods created in the course of normal dental practice would provide more statistical power in analyzing possible differences between different treatment protocols with the same effective treatment, and thereby the effectiveness in real life conditions. When the research protocol is not standardized and non-calibrated researchers are conducting them, more sophisticated statistical methods can overrule some of the flaws in calibration and standardization.

6. Recording events in the dentition

During the patient examination, a dental chart (tooth and surface specific data) for research purposes in EBD and for patient care in PBD is created and thereafter the treatment is recorded by the progress notes. The life cycle of a tooth can be visualized in a lexis diagram as follows (Fig. 1): On the x-axis the dates from the birth of a subject (which actually is the first "observation") to a series of dental examinations (E_1 to E_n) that provided observations of dental health in the dental chart along with separate treatment visits for restorations of observed lesions as progress notes (F_1 to F_n), form a series of events in the dental record in a chronological order. This information is available in countries were regular dental visits, for example by the recall system, is the practice. Unfortunately, in many countries such data is unlikely to be available.

Some of the events, excluding for example (primary) tooth exfoliation, sealant treatments, extractions, implant placements and replacements, during the life-cycle of tooth are illustrated on the y-axis in Fig. 1. If the tooth is recorded to have emerged through the gingiva (at point GE) at the examination time E_2 and observed as un-erupted at the previous examination time E_1, the gingival perforation may have occurred at any time between E_2 and E_1, illustrated as grey in the picture.

Because caries never develops in an un-emerged tooth, the initiation of caries will not be recorded in an un-erupted tooth. In our example enamel caries (EC) is recorded for the second examination time (E_2) when gingival emergence (GE) was also recorded to have happened. The diagnosis of dentine caries (DC) was made at the third examination time (E_3). The restoration of the tooth was recorded to have been performed at the point F_1 in the progress notes thereafter. The onset of caries in the dentine may have happened any time between EC and DC and thus are marked as grey in the picture.

If an "event" is a long-lasting one, like is the incubation time of an infectious disease like dental caries, or the disease itself, again like caries, which is chronic in its nature, its exact timing of onset is not possible in the normal cross-sectional analyses of its prevalence. The normal practice then is that the prevalence of the disease is recorded on the day of examination when the diagnosis is made, regardless its duration.

The variables, such as the date of birth, the date of examination and the dates of individual treatment procedures are exact. On the other hand, tooth eruption, and the progression of dental caries from initiation on the enamel surface into dentin/pulp are long-lasting events, may cease, and may be even reversible, especially in the enamel and may halt in dentine.

STAGE OF TOOTH

RE-RESTORED

RESTORED

DENTIN CARIES

ENAMEL CARIES

Carious   EC   DC   C F_2 F_1

FULLY ERUPTED

GINGIVAL EMERGENCE

Erupting   GE

UNERUPTED

BIRTH OF SUBJECT

EXAMINATIONS E_1 E_2 E_3 E_4 E_n TIME

VISITS FOR TREATMENTS F_1 $F_2 F_n$

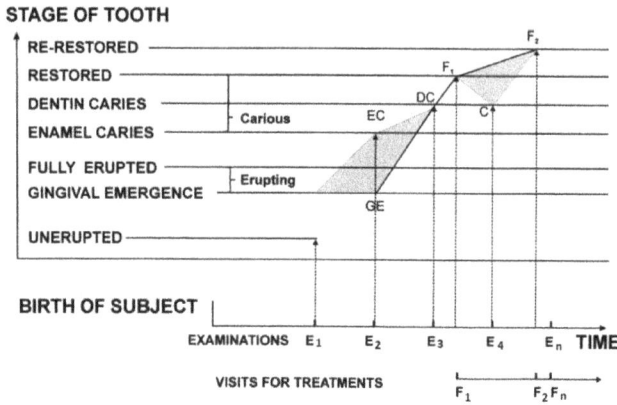

Fig. 1. Schematic presentation of the life cycle of a tooth (y-axis) as a function of time (x-axis) There are exact dates separately for clinical examinations, E_1, E_2…E_n (dental chart) and treatment visits (progress notes), F_1, F_2…F_n. The eruption process is a long-lasting event and marked as grey in the picture. Carious process is also long lasting event (two grey areas)

Tooth eruption from the time of emergence into the oral cavity to full occlusion could last as long as 5.5 years for permanent canines and 2.6 years for the first permanent molar teeth (Pahkala et al., 2002). The estimate of the average times from the stage of incipient lesion to the clinical caries lesion was 18 + 6 months in children (Parfitt, 1956). Therefore, observations in dental record cannot give an accurate picture of the exact date of tooth emergence or the exact date of the onset of carious lesion on enamel surface but certain time limits can be determined retrospectively from the dental charts and progress notes of the record (Bogaerts et al., 2002).

7. Cross-sectional and longitudinal studies of mean prevalence or -index values

The mean caries prevalence (or the mean DMF) value is counted as the number of diseased patients (or DMF-teeth or –surfaces) of a cohort of all subjects, e.g. all subjects born in a certain year or students of a school grade. They form the cohort A (encircled with standard deviation in the example), one year older cohort form cohort B, etc. (Fig. 2A). When these figures or means (+ SD) are retrospectively combined to a summary line of repeated cross-sections, they form steps to inform that they are not longitudinal means.

In a clinical trial the cohort A will be followed for the next consecutive years and the mean values (± SD) in each year will be determined (Fig. 2B). At the end of the follow-up this A cohort makes the longitudinal study cohort in which the annual caries increments can be determined. Similarly, another longitudinal cohort from the original cohort D can be created and followed for consecutive years during which time the longitudinal information of caries increment is available. Different mean values on the same age of the subjects between these two longitudinal cohorts, at points A_4 and D_1, show the difference which exists between longitudinal and repeated cross-sectional studies (Fig. 2B). These observations are longitudinal and therefore may be reported as continuous lines without any steps.

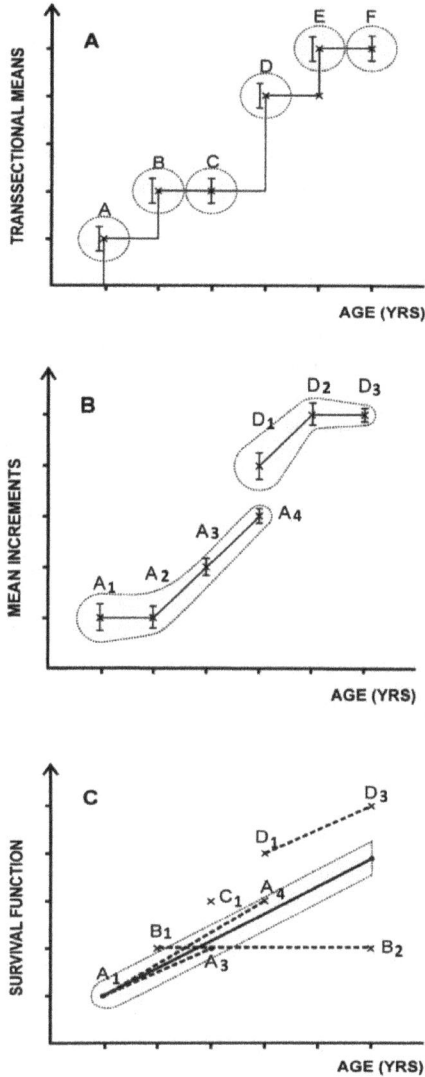

Fig. 2. Principles of trans-sectional (A) and longitudinal (B) studies as well as survival analysis (C)

A. Repeated cross-sections of the means ($\pm$ SD) of a group of subjects (e.g. born on year A, B, C or else, for example a school grade A, B, C etc) form the mean prevalence or index curve.

B. The group A is followed for three consecutive years from A_1 to A_4 and group D is followed for two years from D_1 to D_3. The difference between step A_4 and D_1 shows the difference between longitudinal and trans-sectional analyses.

C. All observations of the examinations of age cohorts (2A) and longitudinal (dotted lines) study groups (2B) are combined as a summary survival estimate (solid line) as long as information is available. There are numerous statistical methods to model this

When the examinations of the cohorts A, B, C, D etc. from the cross-section (Fig. 2A) and the examinations of the two longitudinal cohort studies (Fig. 2B) are combined, a summary line can be created applying similar methods which are used in survival analysis: each individual is indicated by lines or points as long as information is available, from one day to several years. These lines and points can be combined to mean values per subject at different ages. This system has been recently used in Finland where digital patient records have been used for more than ten years in many health centres resulting in a digital dataset with annual examinations with many patients but only with one examination with some other patients. An automatic data-mining system was develop and used for the determination of mean DS, MS, and FS, for all ages with varying number of subjects during the follow-up (Korhonen et al., 2007).

Mean or median values of the prevalence of diseases have certain pros and cons: they are very simple and commonly used. But in caries research problems arise. Caries is an infectious but chronic disease and therefore it is suitable for an analysis of a cross-section of a lengthy time period. But on the other hand, its later forms are irreversible and the body itself can not cure those forms. Treatment by a dentist does this, but then the disease disappears even from the ICD, but not from dental indices, unless used separately for each parameter (Korhonen et al., 2007).

8. Principles of time to event [TTE] analyses

When the dots and lines (Fig 2A, and 2B) are used as a dataset for time to event (TTE) analyses, they can also be combined with numerous survival analysis methods into a summary curve (Fig. 2C). Survival analysis system as such is only a complimentary to the traditional ones and in a way more accurate statistical method for the prediction of events and analysis of statistical differences between cohorts. These methods can be used in analyzing the irreversible transitions from e.g. sound to (first) caries onsets, which covers mainly children and adolescents in practice, but also survival from first carious attack to second caries onsets of the same teeth, restorations, re-restorations and even the presence of tooth in the oral cavity, survival of restorations, crowns, bridges, implants etc, not shown in the picture.

During last years the development of statistical methods has advanced so that many of the problems with the classical methods, like determining the mean and median values in groups of subjects with normal or skewed distributions or when (prospective) longitudinal cohort design is followed, the information of censored observations cannot be incorporated in the analysis, if traditional caries increment studies are conducted. In the latter case, the lost of subjects during the trial is the major problem, because it reduces the number of subjects and if there is a systematic pattern in who is lost it may bias the findings. Survival analysis system may provide tools to make the analyses more informative.

To produce meaningful information of the survival time of a tooth or the whole dentition remaining caries-free, and how these vary between patients, or observing dentists, the standard methodology can be applied, like estimating the mean cumulative intensity curves of the events for each individual and/or for each tooth and surface. When the mean values are replaced by survival curves, this can lead to the problem of a large number of curves, one for each patient and/or each tooth/surface. A more compact and integrated picture is preferred for a group of teeth or patients.

Fig. 3 represents an example of survival times of five different individual teeth or five different carious patients (A, B, C, D, E). Tooth emergence is recorded (interval censored) at points of A_1, B_1, C_1, D_1, E_1 and first caries attack (interval censored) by arrows at points A_2, B_2, C_2, D_2, E_2 according to the chronological age. Tooth coded with A is emerged at A_1 and diagnosed carious at A_2, tooth coded with B from B_1 to B_2. This leads to a mixture of lines with different slopes A_1 – A_2, B_1 – B_2 ... one for each 32 permanent tooth or 160 for each permanent tooth surface. As stated earlier the latter figure follows the anatomy of a 5-surface tooth. This results in a group of lines for a subject. When the emergence times are combined together and marked as zero on the x-axis (tooth age), the picture is more clear because the starting point of the individual curves is the same and takes into account the large variation of the emergence times of permanent teeth (Fig. 3B).

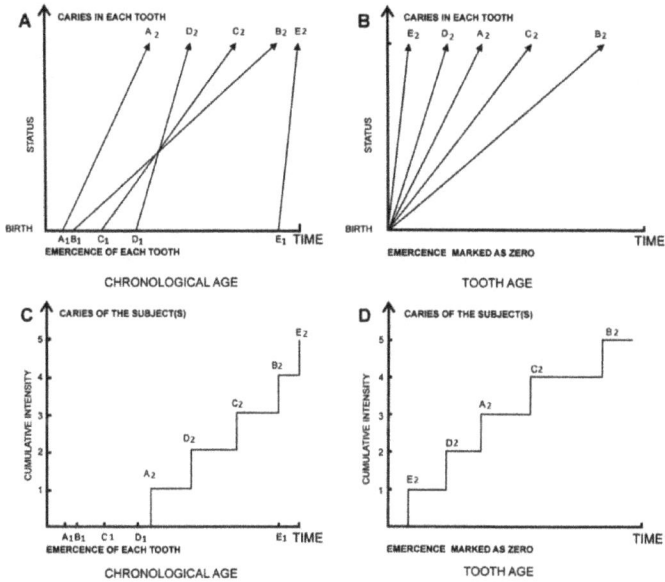

Fig. 3. The principle of time to event analysis
A. Survival measures the time between two events (y-axis). The first event may represent the emergence of the tooth and could be marked on the chronological age at points A_1, B_1, C_1 D_1 etc. The second event may represent caries, restoration, etc. and are marked with A_2, D_2, C_2 etc. The picture shows e.g. that tooth B was erupted early but became carious late whereas the tooth E erupted late but became carious soon. This picture shows the chronological age-scale.
B. When A_1, B_1, C_1, D_2, E_1 are turned to the origin, the survival times can be represented as a function of tooth age. The shortest survival time is shown with the tooth E and the longest with the tooth B.
C. The same events of different teeth (A_2. B_2...) as presented in Fig. 2A above are combined together as a cumulative curve of the subject. Because the time scale is the chronological age of the subject the timing of tooth emergence is also indicated although only the failure (caries) is shown in the cumulative curve.
D. The same events of different teeth (A_2, B_2...) are combined together as a cumulative curve as a function of the tooth age. Note that the shapes of the curves of the same events are now different from the curve following the chronological age (3C)

When these five lines of timing of caries onsets are combined as a cumulative summary curve for each carious tooth (or five patients with caries), a curve with five steps (one for each tooth/patient) is obtained as a function of chronological age (Fig. 3C) or tooth age (Fig. 3D). Although the caries onset curves describe the same five teeth of the same patient and event, or else, five different carious patients, the slopes of these curves vary and differ from each other. These summary lines represent the events in the chronological or tooth age.

TTE of any tooth is the time from birth of the subject to the event in the chronological age-scale of the subject. When the age-scale is the "tooth age", it is from tooth emergence into the oral cavity to the event. In our example of tooth life cycle, the time without enamel caries is zero in the tooth age scale (Fig. 1) because tooth emergence (GE) and enamel caries onset (EC) is observed at the second examination (E_2) after the first examination (E_1) when the tooth was recorded as unemerged.

Time between the irreversible events can be statistically described as "survival times" between these two occasions. The statistical term "event" may mean the first appearance of a tooth into a mouth, which is also called "tooth emergence".

Biologically the real tooth "eruption" is the movement of tooth from its position in bone to full occlusion. For example, the eruption time of first permanent molars covers the time from birth to 11-12 years of age, but their tooth emergence time is their out-coming, around 7 years.

Standard survival analysis requires independent data for significance testing. Because each tooth in the oral cavity is dependent on each other, independence is a special problem in dental research. In recent years it has been recognized that survival analysis could also be applied to dependent data, for example in repeated observations of the same individual (Aalen et al., 1995).

9. Survival analysis

9.1 Models of survival analysis

There are many types of models that have been used for survival analysis also in dental research, as discussed recently (Stephenson et al., 2010a). Some terms used in the context may still demand verbal description (statisticians give equations only): first (1) the survival function gives an estimate of the probability that the time of "death" is later than some specified time. The survival function is also called the survivor function or survivorship function in problems of biological survival, and the reliability function in mechanical survival problems. In the latter case, the methods of estimating survival functions are non-parametric in which no assumption is made about the underlying distribution, whether it is skewed (they are biased) or bell-shaped. A variety of methods (non-, semi-, and fully parametric) of survivorship analysis have been developed. Second (2) the hazard function is defined as the event rate at a certain time conditional on survival until the same time or later. Quantities derived from the survival distributions are (3) future lifetime at a given time is denoted by the time remaining until death. The expected future lifetime represents this.

Survival models can be usefully viewed as (ordinary) regression models in which the response variable is time. However, computing the likelihood function (needed for fitting parameters or making other kinds of inferences) is complicated by the censoring. The likelihood function for a survival model, in the presence of censored data, is the joint probability of the data given the parameters of the model. It is customary to assume that the data are independent given the parameters. Then the likelihood function is the product of the likelihood of each datum.

It is convenient to partition the data into four categories: uncensored, left-censored, right-censored, and interval-censored, as will be discussed later. In the context of caries data analysis, the initial state, in addition to the birth of the subject, might represent un-erupted or sound tooth/surface in primary or permanent tooth, and the end state might represent a carious, exfoliated, restored, or extracted tooth/surface. Because oral cavity contains high number of primary and permanent teeth/surfaces, this results in clustering of data within children/subjects and thereby at least two different approaches in statistical survival analyses: (1) a subject specific time-dependent analysis tries to cover eventualities where units are subject to potential failure from multiple causes. This, however, results in quantification of caries in the individual and this, on the other hand, a variety of distributions of events in the oral cavity. (2) a tooth specific approach, in which a carious patient has different caries onsets in different teeth.

Clustering is inherent in caries data, for example with surfaces clustered within teeth and teeth clustered within subjects. Many survival analyses also involve repeated observations of the same individual. Repeated observations on the same unit comprise a dependency in the same way that dependency arises through clustering.

There are numerous statistical methods which take into account the dependence problem when caries is regarded as quantitative terms in the oral cavity as the research unit. When caries in each tooth is regarded as a different disease and comparisons between patients are performed between these individual teeth, some of the dependence problems are avoided, but a clinical problem arises from the fact that this approach does not follow the principles of ICD, because caries as a disease commits the dentition, not individual teeth.

In short, survival analysis involves the modelling of time to event data; in this context, death or failure is considered an "event" in the survival analysis literature. The flexibility of a counting process is that it allows modelling multiple (or recurrent) events. This type of modelling fits very well in many situations (e.g. people can have caries multiple times even in the same teeth/surfaces, and restorations can be re-restored multiple times). The most important benefit of that system is the possibility of use retrospectively all the (huge) information available in real life conditions [PBD] and/or else problems due to loss of subjects during longitudinal trials [EPD].

9.2 Censoring in the statistical treatment

The observed timing of the event is not always exact which leads to "censoring" in the statistical analysis of longitudinal data (Lindsey and Ryan, 1998). Each subject is followed for a certain period of time, and the event must be censored if it did not occur at the completion of the follow-up or had happened before the follow-up. Though the term "censoring" has a negative meaning in the scientific sense, in statistics it only means that the observation time is not exact or that the event did not occur during the follow-up.

If the tooth has already erupted or restored at the first examination, no exact date can be recorded for these events before that time. In statistical analyses such survival data are normally "left-censored". If the observation period is terminated at certain point, the failure times of those teeth are "right-censored" after that. They may happen later but are not included in the analysis. If a series of examinations are conducted over a lengthy time "interval-censored" observations can be recorded as having occurred at the first examination following the event or alternatively, at the midpoint of the two last examinations (Aalen et al., 1995).

Interval censored events are those that occur between two points. If the event is interpreted as having occurred at the first examination following the event, then information relating to the previous observation has been lost, and this lost of information may be significant. This approach is analogous to treating left-censored data as failures at the time of the first examination, which approach occurs in cross-sectional studies on the disease prevalence, or mean values of DMF-index.

In a sense all caries related data cannot be left-censored as tooth emergence does not happen at birth. Interval censoring at the first examination after the event is the appropriate approach, unless the event of interest is tooth emergence itself. Also then, interval censoring to the first examination after age of two years for primary molars and after six years for any permanent teeth (but left censoring after age 8 years for incisors and first molars, and 14 years for the rest permanent teeth, excluding wisdom teeth) seems to be scientifically acceptable in that sense that clinical experience gives some limits for tooth emergence (and primary tooth exfoliation) which "window" can be taken into account in recording dental observations.

Thus, all caries experience studies should be interval-censored on the day of examination as the onset of caries. The time between examinations affects the observed and real occurrence times. If the interval between examinations of sound-carious or unerupted-erupted events is about 1 year, interval censoring at the first examination after the event seems appropriate, so that if a tooth was unerupted at age 6 and emerged at age 7, the observed emergence time can be considered to be 7 years on that subject. However, the real event has happened any date between 6 and 7 years, the midpoint being 6 ½ years. Both 6 ½ and 7 years are very close to the date reported in textbooks.

If the examination interval is one year, a deduction of six months should be performed in the interval censored date/data to obtain the most probable real date on the onset of the event. Interval censoring to that "most probable" date is commonly used for tooth emergence, but as we stated above, we recommend interval-censoring at the first examination after the event, because both tooth eruption and caries initiation are long-lasting events, and in this case the "relative truth" is closer than the "absolute truth" on the correct timing of caries initiation: If the examination interval is one year, in the determination of caries onset, a deduction of half a year should be performed both from the tooth emergence time and onset of caries. This deduction is unnecessary if caries onset is determined from the tooth emergence. Exfoliation or extraction of any primary or permanent tooth should result in right censoring of any event in these teeth after their exfoliation/extractions.

9.3 Patient specific failure intensities

The failure rate may vary between patients, but also between teeth, some having a high failure rate and others a lower one. For each patient or tooth an intensity of failure or hazard rate can be defined. To obtain a picture of the intensity, it is useful to estimate the cumulative intensity (cumulative hazard rate). The hierarchical nature of the caries data inside the oral cavity results in clustering within children and can be accounted for by formulating the model as performed recently by Stephenson et al. (2010a). Hierarchical model structures of analyzing caries data, in which surfaces are assumed to be nested within individuals, have been observed to be appropriate (Burnside et al., 2006).

The interpretation of these plots is that the intensities of failure can be estimated from the slopes of the curves. Some of them rise/fall rapidly, (depending on whether they are drawn upward or downward), indicating a high failure rate while others rise/fall more slowly, indicating a lower failure rate. The plots for some individuals are flat, meaning that no failures have been observed.

The direction of the curve depends on the function it represents and the data being modeled, but mathematically the direction of the curve is insignificant. Because the hazard function often increases but the survivor function decreases over time, the direction of hazard rate is normally drawn upward, while survival function downward, with the exception of the expected future lifetimes, which are normally drawn upward.

9.4 Survival analysis in evidence-based dentistry

The first study utilizing survival analysis methods by calibrated examiners is the classic study of Carlos and Gittelsohn (1965). Their report was based on a clinical trial of children aged 4-18 years at baseline and conducted in two towns in the state of New York, USA in the 1940's. They applied life table estimates of logarithmic failure intensities separately to different teeth. Some of their results can be questioned: First, the follow-up time was divided into four-month computational intervals, in which interval-censored occurrence times were denoted to have taken place at the mid-points of the dental examination interval, but left-censoring so that all permanent teeth that had erupted before the first clinical examination, was conducted leaving only 2104 children out of 7400 to be analyzed in the data set. This resulted in systematic biases (Härkänen et. al., 2002), because many caries-prone teeth were left-censored.

Since then, survival analysis methods have been applied to reanalyzing the longitudinal caries data in many other clinical trials, too (Hannigan et al., 2001, Hujoel et al., 2003, Baelum et al., 2003). All these large-scale time dependent analyses of caries data have employed fully parametric tooth-specific methods in permanent dentitions. Recently, multivariate multilevel parametric survival models were also applied at tooth surface level to the analysis of the sound-carious and sound-exfoliation transitions to which first and second primary molar surfaces were subject (Stephenson et al., 2010a). The highest rate of occurrence and lowest median survival times were observed to be associated with occlusal surfaces of children from poor socio-economic class in non-fluoridated areas.

Survival analysis methods have also applied to the analysis of how rapidly dental caries progresses (Shwartz et al., 1984a,b) as also seen in prospective radiographic studies (Mejare et al., 1999) or oral health surveys by calibrated examiners (Leroy et al., 2005a,b). When more sophisticated survival analyses are conducted e.g. with clinical trials in which different variables and cofactors are determined in the EBD-fashion, multivariate survival methods, like the semiparametric Cox-regression are conducted. In these cases the variables and their impact and timing is carefully determined. In addition to the complexity of modeling multivariate survival data, the disease itself (dental caries) further complicates the analysis because of the causality.

Fully parametric regression models are widely used for the sound- carious transitions inside the oral cavity, where tooth surfaces are clustered within children, and such methods are preferred in many caries data analyses (Hannigan et al., 2001, Baelum et al., 2003, Leroy et al., 2005a,b, Stephenson et al., 2010). In particular for the interval-censored data, parametric modeling is preferred to non-fully parametric models such as the Cox proportional hazards model (Leroy et al., 2005a), and parametric models may lead to more precise inferences than those arising from semiparametric methods (Baelum et al., 2003).The log-logistic distribution selected for the parametric competing risk models was parameterized in an accelerated failure time setting and was found to describe caries data well in permanent dentition (Hannigan et al., 2001).

Leroy et al., (2005a,b) used multivariate survival analysis for the identification of factors, like caries in primary molars, with cavity formation of first permanent molars in a follow-up study with the EBD-fashion. Stephenson et al (2010a) reported that socio-economic class, fluoridation status and surface type (occlusal vs. all other) were found to be the strongest predictors of caries in primary molars. They applied multilevel competing risks methodology to identify factors associated with caries occurrence in the presence of concurrent risk of exfoliation, but not the effect of different emergence times between the first and second primary molars. The concurrent risk of exfoliation was shown to reduce the distinction in survival experience between different types of surfaces and children in different socio-economic class or fluoridation status. All these studies used multiple teeth as indicators or predictors but Stephenson et al., (2010a) fund that clustering of data had little effect on inferences of parameter significance. They also reported that treatment by restoration was found to be significantly associated with survival with respect to extraction, with survival rates of over 80% at 14 years, double those of untreated teeth (Stephenson et al 2010b). However, only a few, if any, primary molars are in the oral cavity on that age.

Is dental caries a general disease (=dental caries with cavities in different teeth is like osteoporosis with fractures in different bones) or a local disease like are fractures (due to external breaks) in different bones. If it is a "local disease", it is a microbial disease in molars, incisors, canines, and/or in fissures, smooth surfaces, etc, perhaps by different microbes. If caries is a "general disease", host factors (like salivary secretion rate, resistance of dentition to caries, and developmental status of different teeth) may be the primary aetiological factors. To compare these possibilities, sophisticated statistics may determine the modeling of the hazard function or the survivor function. Interpretation of the shapes of the curves may even help in the determining the nature of caries disease: general or local, which is not fully analyzed yet.

9.5 Survival analysis in practice-based dentistry

Today, the use of digital dental records, in which the observations are made on tooth surface level, and the interval of examinations is predetermined to be, for example, one year, automatically creates huge datasets, which can be used for prospective scientific analyses, too. In these datasets the problem is the registration of caries: it does not meet the requirement of calibrated observations though observations of especially amalgam restorations and missing teeth are very accurate, but unfortunately, the "past caries experience" leading to either restoration or extraction is, again, un-exact, because they are always conducted by uncalibrated examiners and they may change over time, as discussed previously (Larmas, 2010a).

An example of this kind of arbitrary is the observation of Korhonen et al., (2009) who reported that practicing dentists (N= more than 100) found regularly significantly more carious lesions in their new patients than in their old patients (N= more than 100.000) after the age of 20 years during the 10-15 years follow-up time, which was the digital era of the

Finnish public dental. This difference between old and new patients was so distinct that even the mean values revealed it, but more sophisticated statistical methods are needed when the effect of various cofactors on un-calibrated caries assays are reliably analyzed. Nobody really knows how much the variation of caries diagnosis of new and old patients has effect on the present DMF values.

The tooth-specific system has been used in longitudinal (retrospective) analyses of caries onsets as seen in normal dental records i.e. in PBD. In these studies one tooth (only) is treated as an indicator of dental health of that oral cavity and these teeth are compared to their counterparts in other subjects (Larmas et al., 1995, Virtanen and Larmas, 1995, Suni et al., 1998, Härkänen et al., 2000, Ollila and Larmas, 2007). All these studies used the non-parametric Kaplan-Meier method or Bayesian analysis for comparing the tooth-specific survival data.

The non-parametric methods have been used for the determination of the survival time of each tooth remaining caries-free, either from the tooth emergence (Virtanen and Larmas, 1995, Suni et al., 1998) or from the birth of the subject up to 20 years of age (Leskinen et al., 2008a). The results show that onset of caries occurs immediately after tooth emergence in first and second molars, equally on left and right sides (probably indicating that caries commits these two molar teeth at the same time on the left and right sides), but caries onsets on maxillary and mandibular molars differ (significantly), mandibular molars being more caries prone. All canines and mandibular incisors do not commit caries under 20 years of age (Korhonen et al., 2003), whereas maxillary incisors and all premolars commit caries, but only some years (termed lag phase) after the tooth emergence (Virtanen and Larmas, 1995).

A summarized curve of teeth erupting during the first and second phases of tooth emergence is also obtained in order to reveal if carious prone circumstances exist during the whole transitional phase of permanent tooth eruption. Teeth that emerged at the first transitional phase (incisors and first molars) at 6 – 8 yrs of age may have different shapes of survival curves than those teeth that emerge during the second mixed dentition period (premolars and second molars) four-five years later (Korhonen et al., 2003). This explains why the DMF-index ages of the WHO are 12 years old (end of the first mixed dentition period), 15 years (end of second mixed dentition period), and in adults, but in the latter case with a very large age scales, 35-55, and 65-74 years (WHO, 1997).

Comparison on caries onsets in sealed and unsealed fissures revealed that the onset of caries in sealed fissures was less than that of unsealed molars, but not in premolars, and sealing of first molars of very caries active subjects (caries in first permanent molars before age 8 years) was not enough for the prevention of caries in other (non-sealed) first molars, but restoration was performed in these unsealed molars before age 10 years (Leskinen et al., 2008b).

The variation of intensities between patients can be analyzed by means of the "frailty" type model also in non-parametric models (Clayton and Cuzick, 1985). The intensity of frailty of a particular individual can be determined by a frailty or mixing variable that is a random variable for the population of individuals. Hence any given individual has a specific frailty. Those with a large value have a high rate of failure (they are caries prone) while those with a small value have a small rate of failure (are caries resistant). The idea is that individuals or even different tooth types may have different frailties, and caries prone/active subjects/teeth will have more caries than caries resistant.

Härkänen et al., (2000) applied Bayesian analysis and frailty model so that the baseline intensity functions were modeled non-parametrically, and the frailty component was introduced by using cross-validation techniques by assuming a hierarchical gamma prior especially to find the ages at which the intensity model can provide better predictions than the simple models using DMFS-index values.

Later it appeared that it was necessary to relax the time-independence assumption of the individual frailties due to changes of habits related to oral health and oral environment, presence vs. absence of open cavities which factors can affect the infection process, and changes in the ways of actions of dentists who treated the patients (Härkänen et al., 2000). They observed that the most difficult age interval appeared to be from 8 to 10 years and they believed that the most obvious reason for that is the fact that first molars erupt around 7 years and the high risk surfaces of these teeth are soon after their emergence, and therefore very few surfaces of high risk are left after age 8 years. This novel observation contradicts that textbook information by Carlos and Gittelsohn (1965) that molar teeth (as most other teeth) are most vulnerable to caries 2- 2½ years after tooth emergence, which probably is due to the heavy left-censoring of the data as discussed before.

9.6 Advantages of survival analysis

As Hannigan (2004) stated in her excellent review of TTE methods of the use of survival time as the outcome measure in caries, the additional statistical system provides an approach that can be understood easily by everyone. She stated that the most common approaches to modeling multivariate survival data scientifically include: 1) using the time to the first event in the patient as the survival time while ignoring the multiplicity, 2) conditional models, such as the frailty model, which include a random per-subject effect, and 3) the marginal models approach.

When the methodology proposed here is either subject or tooth (surface) based, it uses all the data collected during the clinical treatment of the patient during his/her lifetime in the PBD, or calibrated data in clinical trials or prevalence studies [EBD]. It includes data collected at the clinical examinations and data from subjects in intermediate examinations as long as the subjects are visiting that dental office or attended the trial, but censoring can be accounted, too. The results of the analysis are easily interpreted with the use of survival curves and median survival times.

Survival modeling has mainly used in the renewed statistical treatment of the findings of previous caries trials, the results showing that the differences existed also when using more sophisticated survival analysis. Hujoel et al., (2003) established the benefits of xylitol with Poisson regression models and Hannigan et al., (2001) who reanalyzed the effect of diet and tooth brushing habits by the log-logistic distribution selected for the parametric competing risk models, showed a good fit to the caries data. She concluded that the marginal model approach may be more suitable than the frailty model for multivariate survival data from caries clinical trials, since most of the source of variability is due to different anatomic susceptibilities of the tooth surfaces (caries may be regarded as a local disease in different teeth) rather than to the specific subject – specific frailty (caries is a general disease in caries prone subjects, like is osteoporosis with fractures).

Computationally, the marginal model approach is easier to implement with standard software packages.

The results of sophisticated TTE studies on caries onsets in different teeth can be summarized: caries commits erupting molar teeth especially immediately after tooth emergence (even in months), all other teeth have a "lag-phase" of several years after their emergence (Virtanen and Larmas, 1995), the length of which in all canines and mandibular incisors is not known in any country, however, more than 15 years. Is the different behavior of individual teeth due to their different time independent "frailties" and/or must the time-independence of the individual frailties relaxed so that teeth during primary dentinogenesis have different "frailty" than the same teeth during the secondary dentinogenesis. In this case the statistical "frailty" may be connected to the biological "young" odontoblast versus "old" odontoblast context, or odontoblast/ odontocyte terminology, as discussed recently (Larmas, 2008).

The survival analysis is usually time consuming and the most modern frailty-based approach supplemented with empirical estimates demands plenty of computer capacity, and is thus suitable for scientific analyses of longitudinal clinical trials in evidence based dentistry [EBD]. A simplified empirical approach for the determination of lifetime of sound tooth and tooth surfaces should be developed for the clinical practice [PBD], which could be fully automatically been performed when digital dental records are available. For that purpose either subject-specific or tooth-specific approach seems appropriate from the statistical point of view. When the cumulative values are used (separately for D, M, or F) survival analysis principles (instead of dividing the subjects afterwards into age cohorts) are recommended for counting the means of the different dental index values of the subjects as a function of age fully automatically from the digital dental records (Korhonen et al., 2007) or survival of teeth caries-free in different health centres (Korhonen et al., 2003). Thereby modern TTE analyses have a link to previous epidemiological observations on mean and median values as well as results of clinical trials.

10. Conclusions

The most serious problem in caries epidemiology today is the use of certain index values, which try to combine (1) the past and present at the same time, which is impossible, (2) treat dental caries, but also restorations and extractions as "diseases" due to caries, which is also impossible , and (3) try to determine the seriousness of the disease inside the patient in quantitative terms, all of which procedures do not follow the practices in epidemiology: subjects are either healthy or have one or many different diseases, but never many diseases with the same ICD-classification. This dental practice has left the real caries prevalence un-determined all over the world, though mean DMF-index values are reported worldwide in thousands of publications.

11. References

Aalen OO, Bjertness E, Sonju T. (1995). Analysis of dependent survival data applied to lifetimes and amalgam fillings. *Stat Med*;14:1819-1827.

Baelum V, Machiulskiene V, Nyvad B, Richards A, Vaeth M. (2003). Application of survival analysis to carious lesion transitions in intervention trials. *Community Dent Oral Epidemiol*;31:252-260.

Bogaerts K, Leroy R, Lesaffre E, Declerck D.(2002). Modelling tooth emergence data based on multivariate interval-censored data. *Stat Med* ; 21:3775-3787.

Burnside G, Pine CM, Williamson PR (2006). Statistical aspects of design and analysis of clinical trials for the prevention of caries. *Caries Res*; 40:360-365.

Carlos JP, Gittelsohn AM. Longitudinal studies of the natural history of caries – II.(1965). *Arch Oral Biol*;10:739-751.

Clayton D and Cuzick J (1985). Multivariate generalizations of the proportional hazards model (with discussion). *J Royal Stat Soc* Ser A;148:82-117.

Espelied I, Treit AM, Mejare I, Sundberg H, Hallonsten AL.(2001). Restorative treatment decisions on occlusal caries in Scandinavia. *Acta Odontol Scand*;59:21-27.

Hannigan A. Using survival methodologies in demonstrating caries efficacy. (2004). *J Dent Res*:83:C99-C102

Hannigan A, O'Mullane DM, Barry D, Schafer F, Roberts AJ (2001). A re-analysis of a caries clinical trial by survival anaysis. *J Dent Res*;80:427-431.

Härkänen T, Larmas MA, Virtanen JI, Arjas E.(2002). Applying modern survival methods to longitudinal dental caries studies. *J Dent Res*;81:144-148.

Härkänen T, Virtanen JI, Arjas E. (2000). Caries on permanent teeth: a non parametric Bayesian analysis. *Scand J Stat;* 27:577-588.

Hujoel PP, Isokangas PJ, Tiekso J, Davis S, Lamont RJ, Derouen TA, Mäkinen KK.(2003). A re-analysis of caries rates in a preventive trial using Poisson regression models. *J Dent Res*; 73:573-579.

Hujoel PP, Löe H, Anerud A, Boysen H, Leroux BC. (1998). Forty-five-year tooth survival probabilities among men in Oslo, Norway. *J Dent Res*; 77:2020-2027.

Klein H, Palmer CE, Knutson JW. (1938). Dental status and dental needs of elementary school children. *Public Health Reports*; 53:751-755.

Korhonen M, Käkilehto T, Larmas M. (2003). Tooth-by-tooth survival analysis of the first caries attack in different age cohorts and health centers in Finland. *Acta Odontol Scand*; 61:1-5.

Korhonen M, Salo S, Suni J, Larmas M. (2007). Computed online determination of life-long mean index values for carious, extracted, and/or filled permanent teeth. *Acta Odontol Scand*; 65:214-218.

Korhonen M, Gundogar M, Suni J, Salo S, Larmas M (2009). A practice-based study of the variation of diagnostics of dental caries in new and old patients. *Caries Res*; 43: 339-344.

Larmas M. (2008). Pre-odontoblasts, odontoblasts, or odontocytes. *J Dent Res* ; 87: 198-199.

Larmas M. (2010a). Has dental caries prevalence some connection with caries index values in adults? *Caries Res*; 44: 81-84.

Larmas M. (2010b). End of cross-over designs for studies on the effect of sugar substitutes? *Caries Res* ; 44:169.

Larmas MA, Virtanen JI, Bloigu RS. (1995). Timing of first restorations in permanent teeth: a new system for oral health determination. *J Dent*; 23:347-352.

Leroy R, Bogaerts K, Lesaffre E, Derclerck D. (2005a;). Effect of caries experience in primary molars on cavity formation in the adjacent first permanent molars.*Caries Res* ; 39:342-349.

Leroy R, Bogaerts K, Lesaffre E, Derclerck D. (2005b). Multivariate survival analysis for the identification of factors associated with cavity formation in permanent first molars. *Eur J Oral Sci*; 103:145-152.

Leskinen K, Ekman A, Oulis C, Forsberg H, Vadiakas G, Larmas M. (2008a). Comparison of the effectiveness of fissure sealants in Finland, Sweden, and Greece. *Acta Odontol Scand.;* 66:65-72.

Leskinen K, Salo S, Suni J, Larmas M. (2008b). Comparison of dental health in sealed and non-sealed first permanent molars: 7 years follow-up in practice-based dentistry. *J Dent.;*36: 27-32.

Lindsey JC, Ryan LM. (1998). Tutorial in biostatistics – methods for interval-censored data. *Stat Med;*17: 219-238.

Mejare I, Källestål C, Stenlund H. (1999). Incidence and progression of approximal caries from 11 to 22 years of age in Sweden: a prospective radiographic study. *Caries Res;*43: 93-100.

Morelli MG. (1924). The introduction of a quantitative caries index for teeth. *Dent Cosmos;* 66:1068-1075.

Mjör I.(2008). Conrolled clinical trials and practice-based based research in dentistry. *J Dent Res;* 87:605.

Niederman R, Leithch J. (2006). "Know what and "know how"! Knowledge creation in clinical practice. *J Dent Res;*85:296-297.

Ollila P, Larmas M. (2007). A seven-year survival analysis of caries onset in primary second molars and permanent first molars in different caries risk groups determined at age of two years. *Acta Odontol Scand;* 65: 29-35.

Pahkala R, Pahkala A, Laine T. (1991). Eruption pattern of permanent teeth in a rural community in northeastern Finland. *Acta Odontol Scand;* 49:341-349.

Parfitt GJ. (1956). The speed of development of a caries cavity. *Br Dent J;* 100:204-207.

Pitts N. (2004). ´ICADS´ - an international system for caries detection and assessment being developed to facilitate caries epidemiology, research and appropriate clinical management. *Community Dent Health;* 21:193-198.

Rothman KJ, Greenland S. (1998). Measures of disease frequency. in: *Modern epidemiology,* Rothman KJ, Greenland S. (Eds). Philadelphia, Lippincott-Raven Publishers, , pp.42-43.

Shwartz M, Pliskin JS, Grondahl HG, Boffa J. (1984a). Use of the Kaplan-Meier estimate to reduce biases in estimating the rate of caries progression. *Community Dent Oral Epidemiol;* 12:103-108.

Shwartz M, Pliskin JS, Grondahl HG, Boffa J. (1984b). Study desing to reduce biases in estimating the percentage of caries lesions that do not progress within a time period. *Community Dent Oral Epidemiol;* 12:109-113.

Stephenson J, Chadwick BL, Playle RA, Treasure ET. (2010a). Modelling childhood caries using parametric competing risks survival methods for clustered data. *Car Res* ‚44:69-80.

Stephenson J, Chadwick BL, Playle RA, Treasure ET. (2010b). A competing risk survival analysis model to assess the efficacy of filling carious primary teeth. *Car Res.;* 44:285-93.

Suni J, Helenius H, Alanen P. (1998). Tooth and tooth surface survival rates in birth cohorts from 1965, 1970, 1975 and 1980 in Lahti, Finland. *Community Dent Oral Epidemiol;*26:101-106.

Virtanen JI, Larmas MA. (1995). Timing of first fillings on different permanent tooth surfaces in Finnish schoolchildren. *Acta Odontol Scand;*53:287-92.

World Heath Organization. (1977). *International Statistical Classification of Diseases and Related Health Problems*. Ninth revision, Geneva, WHO,.

World Heath Organization. (1992). *International Statistical Classification of Diseases and Related Health Problems*. Tenth revision, vol 1, Tabular list, Geneva, WHO,.

World Heath Organization. (1997). *Oral Health Surveys*, Basic Methods, ed 4, Geneva, WHO,

Part 3

Public Health Dentistry and Epidemiology

Probiotics and Oral Health

Harini Priya Vishnu
Department of Pedodontics and Preventive Dentistry,
Vydehi Institute of Dental Sciences and Research Centre, Bangalore
India

1. Introduction

All great thoughts have already been thought; what is necessary is only to try to think them again....
Johann Wolfgang

Man is the most intelligent animal on the earth, as he is the only species gifted with the power of thinking and reasoning. He always manages to come up with solutions for *most problems* on earth. Ironically, most problems on earth are directly or indirectly created by Man himself. That's the reason he is most often referred to as an *intelligent fool*.

The man-made problem prevailing across the field of medicine is the development of *antibiotic resistance,* largely contributed by us, the health professionals. The indiscriminate and reckless use of antibiotics has led to the emergence of multi-resistant strains of bacteria. This unfortunate development has led scientists to seek other means of fighting infections. [1]

The good-old but forgotten concept of *bacteriotherapy* seem to offer innovative tools for the treatment of infectious diseases. Hence, rightly quoted "All great thoughts have already been thought; what is necessary is only to try to think them again".

Bacteriotherapy is the administration of naturally occurring bacteria of human origin as a therapeutic manipulation of the bacterial microenvironment in the patient's body. [1] The Basic principle is to use good bacteria to compete against pathogenic bacteria. Bacteriotherapy has been studied and tested to control infectious diseases, particularly in the GI tract. Recent studies have shown that this therapeutic method may be used to influence body function in other systems too, beyond the intestine. [1, 2, 3]

2. History

It was in the first decade of 1900, the beginning of the 20th century when the Ukrainian-born Nobel prize laureate Elie Metchnikoff observed the positive beneficial effect of some bacteria on the human health and suggested that these beneficial bacteria can be used to replace harmful microbes in the body. He reported that Bulgarians lived longer than other population which was due to their consumption of Bulgarian yoghurt which contained lactic acid bacteria.[4] Metchnikoff worked at the Pasteur Institute in Paris and had discovered Lactobacillus bulgarius, a strain he later introduced into commercial production of sour-milk products in France and throughout Europe. He devoted the last decade of his life to the study of lactic-acid producing bacteria as a means of increasing human longevity. [5] He developed a theory stating that senility is caused by poisoning of the body by the products of some of the bacteria for which he proposed a diet containing milk fermented by lactobacilli producing lactic acid to prevent the multiplication of these organisms. [6] The concept of probiotics was thus born and a new field of microbiology came into light.

The first clinical trials were performed in the 1930s on the effect of probiotics on constipation. Ever since then, different microorganisms have been used for their ability to prevent and cure diseases. [7]

In 1994, the WHO deemed probiotics to be the next-most important immune defence system when commonly prescribed antibiotics are rendered useless by antibiotic resistance. The use of probiotics in antibiotic resistance is termed as *microbial interference therapy*. [7]

The literature on the possible role of probiotics on oral and dental health is scarce and the studies on probiotics v/s oral health are still in their cradle. [6]

3. What are Probiotics?

The term probiotic means 'for life', was first coined by Lilly and Stillwell. [8]

4. Definition

[Adopted by the International Scientific Association for Probiotics and Prebiotics term]
Probiotics are defined as "Live microorganisms, which when administered in adequate amounts, confer a health benefit on the host" (Guarner et al 2005) [9]

5. Oral probiotic organisms [7]

The most common probiotic strains belong to the genera Lactobacillus and Bifidobacterium. Bacterial strains that have been tested for probiotic action in the oral cavity include:

LACTOBACILLI SPECIES	BIFIDOBACTERIUM SPECIES	OTHERS
• L. acidophilus	• B. bifidum	• S. salivarius
• L. rhamnosus GG	• B. longum	• W. cibaria
• L. johnsonii	• B. infantis	•
• L. casei	• Bifidobacterium DN-173 010	•
• L. rhamnosus		
• L. gasseri		
• L. reuteri		
• L. paracasei		

Table 1.

L. rhamnosus GG, ATCC 53103 (LGG) is the most widely studied probiotic bacterium. Named after the discoverers, Sherwood Gorbach and Barry Goldin, produces a substance with potential inhibitory activity against different bacterial species including cariogenic Streptoccus species. [1]

6. Vehicles for probiotic administration for oral health purpose

The various means of administration of probiotics for oral health purpose that has been studies are:

- Lozenges
- Tablets
- Cheese
- Yoghurt
- Mouth rinse
- Capsule, Liquid

7. Mechanisms of probiotic action on oral health

An essential requirement for an organism to be "an oral probiotic" is its ability to adhere to and colonize surfaces in the oral cavity. Microorganisms generally considered as probiotics may not have oral cavity as their inherent habitat, so their possibility to confer benefit on oral health is then questionable. [6]The suggested mechanisms of probiotic action are drawn entirely from gastrointestinal studies. Since, mouth is the gateway of the GI tract, there is every reason to believe that atleast some probiotic mechanisms may play a role in the oral cavity. [1]
Some of the hypothetical mechanisms of probiotic action in the oral cavity are:

- Lactobacilli play an important role in maintaining the microecological balance in the oral cavity.[11]
- Direct interaction in dental plaque
- Involvement in binding of oral micro-organisms to proteins [interference in formation of acquired pellicle]
- Action on plaque formation and on its complex ecosystem by competing and intervening with bacterial attachments.
- Involvement in metabolism of substrate and production of chemicals that inhibit oral bacteria.[12, 13]

Indirect probiotic actions are also featured such as

- Modulating systemic immune function.
- Effect on local immunity.
- Effect on non-immunologic defense mechanisms.
- Regulation of mucosal permeability.
- Probiotics as an antioxidants and produce antioxidants.
- Prevent plaque formation by neutralizing the free electrons. [14, 15, 16]

Immune inductive sites in the oral cavity are within the diffuse lymphoid aggregates of the Waldeyer's ring. Lingual and pharyngeal tonsils and adenoids contain most of the lymphatic tissue. Dentritic cells in the mucosal surfaces play vital role in antigen presentation and in activating T-cell responses. Depending on the signals from dendritic cells either immune tolerance or active immune response toward a specific antigen may occur. [6] However, more studies investigating the role probiotics on activation of the oral immune inductive sites are required before further conclusions are drawn.

Probiotic bacteria

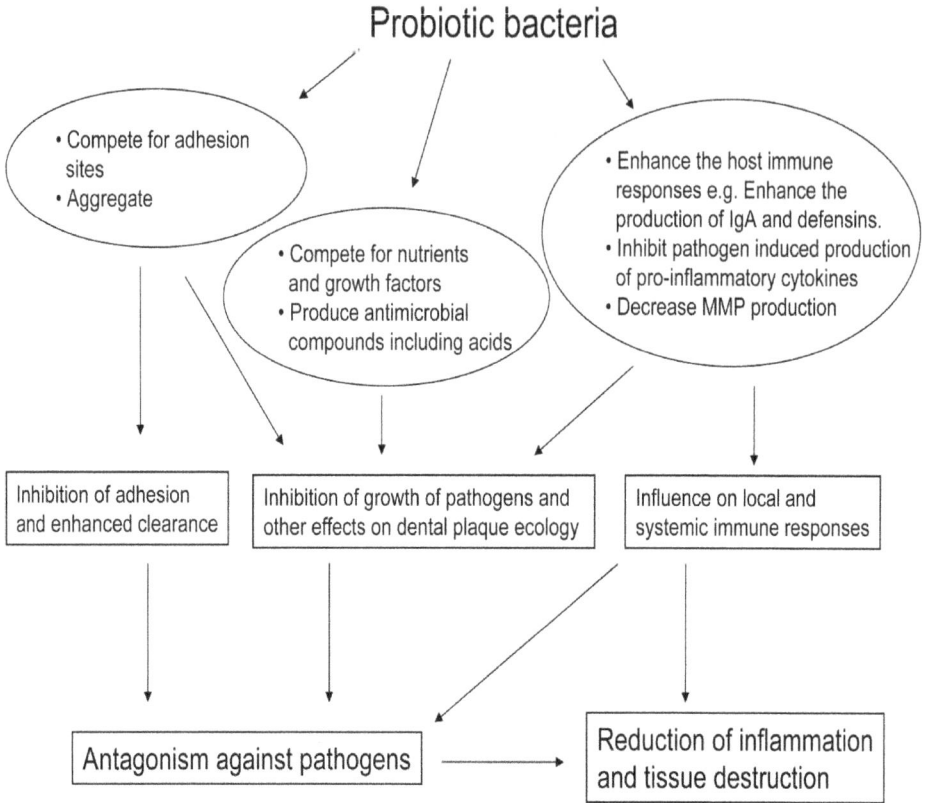

- Compete for adhesion sites
- Aggregate

- Compete for nutrients and growth factors
- Produce antimicrobial compounds including acids

- Enhance the host immune responses e.g. Enhance the production of IgA and defensins.
- Inhibit pathogen induced production of pro-inflammatory cytokines
- Decrease MMP production

| Inhibition of adhesion and enhanced clearance | Inhibition of growth of pathogens and other effects on dental plaque ecology | Influence on local and systemic immune responses |

| Antagonism against pathogens | ⟶ | Reduction of inflammation and tissue destruction |

Fig. Possible Mechanisms of Probiotic Action in the Oral Cavity [10]

8. Action of probiotics on oral health

8.1 Action on organisms associated with dental caries

Several investigations have shown reduction in the number of mutans streptococci in saliva after consumption of various probiotic products, [17 – 25] however such an effect has not been observed in all studies. [26]

Náse et al, 2001 showed that supplementing 1-6 year old children with L. rhamnosus for 7 months significantly reduced the risk of dental caries. [17]

Comelli EM et al (2002) studied 23 dairy bacterial strains for the prevention of dental caries and reported that only two strains namely Streptococcus thermophilus and Lactcoccus lactis were able to adhere to saliva-coated hydroxyapatite and were further successfully incorporated into a biofilm similar to the dental plaque. Furthermore, they could grow together with five strains of oral bacterial species commonly found in supragingival plaque. In this system, Lactobacillus lactis was able to modulate the growth of the oral bacteria, and in particular to diminish the colonization of Streptococcus oralis, Veillonella dispar, Actinomyces naeslundii and of the cariogenic Strep.sobrinus. [27]

Chung et al, 2004 showed that the probiotic strain L. fermentum found in the saliva of healthy children significantly inhibited the formation of the insoluble glucan produced by S.mutans. It did not affect the multiplication of this pathogenic strain, but it completely inhibited the adherence onto cuvette walls. [28]

Koll-Klais et al (2005) used various lactobacilli strains in their study and stated that 69% of these strains inhibited S. mutans, 82% inhibited P. gingivalis. [29]

An increase in the number of salivary lactobacilli has also been seen in some studies. [18, 26] The products containing probiotic LGG bacteria may have beneficial effects on the dental health. The LGG bacteria had been shown not to ferment lactose or sucrose. [30]

Stamatova et al, in their study that was in conducted in 2007 stated that L. rhamnosus & Lactobacillus bulgaricus produced inhibitory effects against P. gingivalis, Fusobacterium nucleatum & streptococcal species. [31]

Strahnic et al, 2007 conducted a study using probiotic strains L. salivarius & L. fermentum and both strains showed antagonistic activity on the growth of S. mutans and Streptococcus pneumonia. L. salivarius was able to survive an environment of low pH as that produced by a high number of S. mutans. [32]

N.S.H. Mehanna et al (2009) investigated the effect of plant meswak and some probiotic bacteria on Streptococcus mutans and Porphyromonas gingivalis isolated from human oral cavity as most common oral pathogenic strains. The results of the study indicated that lactobacillus rahmonosus had a marked decreasing effect on the colonization of both Streptococcus mutans and Porphyromonas gingivalis. [33]

A recently published review article by Anna Haukioja in 2010 does not give a conclusive statement about the effect of probiotics on dental caries or caries related organisms since the study groups have been relatively small and of fairly shorter duration. [10]

8.2 Action on periodontal diseases

Encouraging results have been obtained in studies investigating the role of probiotics for the treatment of various periodontal diseases, gingivitis, plaque levels, and periodontitis.

Reduction in the number of periodontopathogens in the plaque has also been observed. Again, most studies have been fairly short. [10]

Koll-Klais and team (2005) found a prevalence of Lactobacillus gasseri and L. fermentum in the oral cavity of healthy individuals compared to those with chronic periodontitis. Further to this, the same researchers have found that lactobacilli inhibit the growth of periodontopathogens, demonstrating the influence of lactobacilli in the oral cavity of a healthy individual. [29]

Riccia, et al (2007) recently studied the anti-inflammatory effects of Lactobacillus brevis in a group of patients with chronic periodontitis. The treatment, which involved sucking on lozenges containing L. brevis over a period of 4 days, led to improvements in the targeted clinical parameters (plaque index, gingival index, bleeding on probing) for all patients. In that study, a significant reduction in salivary levels of prostaglandin E2 (PGE2) and matrix metalloproteinases (MMPs) was also observed. The authors suggested that the beneficial anti-inflammatory effects of L. brevis could be attributed to its capacity to prevent the production of nitric oxide and, consequently, the release of PGE2 and the activation of MMPs induced by the nitric oxide. However, L. brevis may also be antagonistic, leading to a reduction in the quantity of plaque and therefore an improvement in the gingival index. [34]

Shimazaki and colleagues (2008) used epidemiological data to assess the relationship between periodontal health and the consumption of dairy products such as cheese, milk and yogurt. The authors found that individuals, particularly nonsmokers, who regularly consumed yogurt or beverages containing lactic acid exhibited lower probing depths and less loss of clinical attachment than individuals who consumed few of these dairy products. A similar effect was not observed with milk or cheese. By controlling the growth of the pathogens responsible for periodontitis, the lactic acid bacteria present in yogurt would be in part responsible for the beneficial effects observed. [35]

Harini PM and Anegundi RT 2010 found that probiotic mouth rinse was effective in reducing plaque accumulation and gingival inflammation in 6-8 year old children. [36]

8.3 Halitosis

There are a number of reasons for the onset of halitosis (bad smelling breath) –consumption of particular foods, metabolic disorders and respiratory tract infections – but commonly it is associated with an imbalance of the commensal microflora of the oral cavity. [37]

An unbalanced oral microflora has been associated with the production of malodorous substances called volatile sulphur compounds (VSCs). These are by-products of microbial degradation of proteins, blood, mucins found in saliva, and traces of food retained on oral surfaces. Kazor and team (2003) looked at the species of bacteria found on the tongue of patients suffering from halitosis and compared the findings with subjects who were considered healthy. The species found to be most associated with halitosis were Atopobium parvulum, Eubacterium sulci, Fusobacterium periodonticum. In the same study, Streptococcus salivarius was found to be the most prevalent in the healthy subjects, and this is thought to be due to the capability of S. salivarius to produce bacteriocins which could contribute to reducing the number of bacteria that produce VSCs. [38]

Probiotics are marketed for the treatment of both mouth and gut associated halitosis.

8.4 Probiotics and Candida albicans

C. albicans is a leading cause of infection in oral cavity; it is particularly common in the elderly and in immunocompromised patients. Hatakka et al (2007) showed a reduced prevalence of C. albicans after taking probiotics in cheese containing L. rhamnosus GG and Propionibacterium freudenreichii. [39]

Results obtained by Koll et al (2008) when assessing the effects of various Lactobacillus strains in oral cavity were markedly different; most strains suppressed growth of periodontal pathogens, including actinomycetemcomitans (60 out of 67 tested strains); Porphyromona gingivalis (35 out of 42 strains), P. intermedia (26 out of 42 strains), and cariogenic S. mutans (37 out of 67 strains). No inhibition was found, however, for C.albicans growth. [40]

Hasslöf P et al (2010) investigated the ability of a selection of lactobacilli strains, used in commercially available probiotic products, to inhibit growth of oral mutans streptococci and C. albicans in vitro by agar overlay method. At concentrations ranging from 109 to 105 CFU/ml, all lactobacilli strains inhibited the growth of the mutans streptococci completely with the exception of L. acidophilus La5 that executed only a slight inhibition of some strains at concentrations corresponding to 107 and 105 CFU/ml. All the tested lactobacilli strains reduced candida growth but the effect was generally weaker than for mutans streptococci. The two L. plantarum strains and L. reuteri ATCC 55730 displayed the strongest inhibition on Candida albicans. [41]

8.5 Probiotics and HIV

Recently it has been postulated that the probiotic bacteria may slow down AIDS progression. Lin Tao and his colleagues (2008) screened hundreds of bacteria taken from the saliva of volunteers. The results showed that some Lactobacillus strains had produced proteins capable of binding a particular type of sugar found on HIV envelope, called mannose. The binding of the sugar enables the bacteria to stick to the mucosal lining of the mouth and digestive tract, forming colonization. One strain secreted abundant mannose-binding protein particles into its surroundings, neutralizing HIV by binding to its sugar coating. They also observed that immune cells trapped by lactobacilli formed a clump. This configuration would immobilize any immune cells harboring HIV and prevent them from infecting other cells. [42]

9. Residence time of probiotics in oral cavity

Residence time of probiotics in oral cavity after treatment withdrawal was studied by Çaglar et al (2006) A reduced S. mutans level was shown after a two-week use of a L. reuteri-enriched yogurt; effects were observed during use and for a few days after discontinuation. [43]

A loss of L. reuteri colonization was observed by Wolf et al (1995) two months after having discontinued probiotic use. [44] L. rhamnosus GG administration and oral cavity colonization was studied by Yli-Knuuttila et al in 2006. The authors concluded that permanent colonization in oral cavity was unlikely (although possible in some cases) and suggested the probiotic to be used on a regular basis. [45]

Binding strength of 17 Lactobacillus strains and 7 bifidobacteria strains to saliva and oral mucous membrane was variable in different strains, according to a study by Haukioja et al in 2006, such a strength variation caused an increased residence time of probiotic in oral cavity.[46] Latency time of probiotic S. salivarius K12, 4 tablets/day for 3 days, was assessed in several oral cavity areas in a 35-day follow-up, by Horz et al (2007) probiotic could be found on oral mucous membrane, tongue and in stimulated saliva for more than 3 weeks, with a gradually reduced S. salivarius K12 level being detected beginning 8 days after treatment withdrawal. [47]

The findings of the studies on oral colonization of probiotics did not suggest that a permanent installation can take place. However, one needs to bear in mind that most studies were conducted in adults and it may be questioned if a permanent installation readily can occur in persons with an already established microflora.[1] Therefore, it seems especially important that further research needs to be carried on infants because it is very likely that the chance of a permanent colonization of probiotics increases with a regular exposure from early childhood. [3]

10. Conclusion

The oral cavity with its diversity of microbial species has been shown to harbor strains also distinguished as probiotics as such. Further studies identifying resident probiotics in the mouth, and their eventual effect on the oral environment are required.

Probiotics are a new and interesting field of research in oral microbiology and oral medicine. Bacteriotherapy in the form of probiotics seems to be a natural way to maintain health and protect oral tissues from diseases. But, this area of research in relation to oral health is still in its infancy and further long term randomized controlled studies are required before definite conclusions are drawn regarding their effective action on oral health.

11. References

[1] Meurman JH. (2005). Probiotics: do they have a role in oral medicine and dentistry? Eur J Oral Sci, 113: 188-196.

[2] Noordin K & Kamin S. (2007). The effect of probiotic mouthrinse on plaque and gingival inflammation. Annal Dent Univ Malaya, 14: 19-25.

[3] Twetman S & Stecksen-Blicks C. (2008). Probiotics and oral health effects in children. Int J of Pead Dent, 18: 3-10.

[4] Metchnikoff E. (1907). Lactic acid as inhibitory intestinal putrefaction. In Chalmers Mitchell P, ed. The prolongation of life: optimistic studies. London: Heinemann, 161-183.

[5] The Columbia Encyclopedia, (2001). 6th Ed. New York: Columbia University Press. Available at http://www.bartleby.com/65/me/Metchnik.html.

[6] Meurman JH & Stamatova I. (2007) Probiotics: contributions to oral health. Oral Diseases, 13: 443-451.

[7] Parvez S et al. (2006). Probiotics and their fermented food products are beneficial for health. J of Appl Microbiol, 100: 1171-1185.

[8] Lilly DM & Stillwell RH. (1965) Probiotic growth promoting substances produced by microorganisms. Science, 147: 747-748.

[9] FAO/WHO. (2001). Evaluation of health and nutritional properties of powder milk and live lactic acid bacteria. Cordoba, Argentina: Food and Agriculture Organization of the United Nations and World Health Organization Expert Consultation Report, 1-34.

[10] Haukioja A. (2010). Probiotics and Oral Health. Eurp J of Dent, 4: 348-355.

[11] Koll-Klais P et al. (2006) Oral lactobacilli in chronic periodontitis: species composition and antimicrobial activity. IADR Congress, Dublin, 13-16 Sept (Abstract 0081)

[12] Isolauri E et al. (1993). Lactobacillus casei strain GG reverses increased intestinal permeability induced by cow milk in suckling rats. Gastroenterology, 105: 1643-1650.

[13] Vanderhoof JA et al. (1999) Lactobacillus GG in the prevention of antibiotic associated diarrhea in children. J Ped, 135: 564-568.

[14] Suvarna VC & Boby VG. (2005). Probiotics in human health - A current assessment. Current science, 88: 1744-48

[15] Izumita D. (2001). A new approach in dentistry. Clinical and Basic Medical Research on EM-X--A Collection of Research Papers, 2:77-81.

[16] Minna KS, et al. (2002). Lactobacillus bacterium during a rapid increase in probiotic use of L. Rhamnosus GG in Finland. CID, 35:1155-60.

[17] Nase L et al. (2001). Effect of long-term consumption of a probiotic bacterium, Lactobacillus rhamnosus GG, in milk on dental caries and caries risk in children. Caries Res, 35: 412-420.

[18] Ahola AJ et al. (2002). Short-term consumption of probiotic-containing cheese and its effects on dental caries risk factors. Arch Oral Biol, 47: 799-804.

[19] Nikawa H, et al. (2004). Lactobacillus reuteri in bovine milk fermented decreases the oral carriage of mutans streptococci. Int J Food Microbiol, 95:219–223.

[20] Caglar E, et al. (2005). Effect of yoghurt with Bifidobacterium DN-173010 on salivary mutans streptococci and lactobacilli in young adults. Acta Odont Scand, 63:317–320.

[21] Caglar E, et al. (2006). Salivary mutans streptococci and lactobacilli levels after ingestion of the probiotic bacterium Lactobacillus reuteri ATCC 55730 by straws or tablets. Acta Odontol Scand, 64:314–318.

[22] Caglar E, et al. (2007). Effect of chewing gums containing xylitol or probiotic bacteria on salivary mutans streptococci and lactobacilli. Clin Oral Investig, 11:425–429.

[23] Caglar E, et al. (2008). Short-term effect of ice-cream containing Bifidobacterium lactis Bb-12 on the number of salivary mutans streptococci and lactobacilli. Acta Odontol Scand, 66:154–158.

[24] Caglar E, et al. (2008). A probiotic lozenge administered medical device and its effect on salivary mutans streptococci and lactobacilli. Int J Paediatr Dent, 18:35–39.

[25] Cildir SK,et al. (2009). Reduction of salivary mutans streptococci in orthodontic patients during daily consumption of yoghurt containing probiotic bacteria. Eur J Orthod, 31:407–4011.

[26] Montalto M, et al. (2004). Probiotic treatment increases salivary counts of lactobacilli: a double-blind, randomized, controlled study. Digestion. 69:53–56.

[27] Comelli EM, et al. (2002). Selection of dairy bacterial strains as probiotics for oral health. Eur J Oral Sci, 110(3):218-24.

[28] Chung J, et al. (2004). Isolation and characterization of Lactobacillus species inhibiting the formation of Streptococcus mutans biofilm. Oral Microbiol Immunol, 19(3): 214-6.

[29] Koll-Klais P, et al. (2005). Oral Lactobacilli in chronic periodontitis and periodontal health: species composition and antimicrobial activity. Oral Microbiol Immunol, 20(6): 354-61.

[30] Meurman J, et al. (1994). Recovery of Lactobacillus strain GG (ATCC 53103) from saliva of healthy volunteers after consumption of yoghurt prepared with the bacterium. Microb Ecol Health Dis, 7:295-298.

[31] Stamatova I, et al. (2009). In vitro evaluation of yoghurt starter lactobacilli and Lactobacillus rhamnosus GG adhesion to saliva-coated surfaces. Oral Microbiol Immunol. 24:218–223.

[32] Strahinic I, et al. (2007). Molecular and biochemical characterizations of human oral lactobacilli as putative probiotic candidates. Oral Microbiol Immunol, 22(2): 111-7.

[33] N.S.H. Mehanna et al. (2009). Effect of some probiotic strains and meswak plant on certain oral pathogenic strains. Int J of Academic Res, 1(2): 128-132.

[34] Riccia DN, et al. (2007). Anti-inflammatory effects of Lactobacillus brevis (CD2) on periodontal disease. Oral Dis, 13(4):376-85.

[35] Shimazaki Y et al. (2008). Intake of dairy products and periodontal disease: the Hisayama Study. J Periodontol, 79(1): 131-7.

[36] Harini PM & Anegundi RT. (2010). Efficacy of a probiotic and chlorhexidine mouth rinses: A short term clinical study. JISPPD, 28(3):179-182.

[37] Scully G & Greenman J. (2008). Halitosis (breath Odor). Periodontology 2000, 48: 667-75.

[38] Kazor CE, et al. (2003). Diversity of bacterial populations on the tongue dorsa of patients with halitosis and healthy patients. J. Clin. Microbiol, 41(2): 558-563.

[39] Hatakka K, et al. (2007). Probiotics reduces the prevalence of oral candida in the elderly-a randomized controlled trial. J Dent Res, 86:125-30.

[40] Kõll P,ct al. (2008). Characterization of oral lactobacilli as potential probiotics for oral health. Oral Microbiol Immunol, 23:139-47.

[41] Hasslöf P et al. (2010). Growth inhibition of oral mutans streptococci and candida by commercial probiotic lactobacilli - an in vitro study. BMC Oral Health, 10:18.

[42] Lin T. (2008). Current opinion in HIV and AIDS, 3:599-602.

[43] Caglar E, et al. (2006). Salivary mutans streptococci and lactobacilli levels after ingestion of the probiotic bacterium Lactobacillus reuteri ATCC 55730 by straws or tablets. Acta Odontol Scand, 64:314-8.

[44] Wolf BW,et al.(1995). Safety and tolerance of Lactobacillus reuteri in healthy adult male subjects. Microb Ecol Health Dis, 8:41-50.

[45] Yli-Knuuttila H, et al. (2006). Colonization of Lactobacillus rhamnosus GG in the oral cavity. Oral Microbiol Immunol, 21:129-31.

[46] Haukioja A, et al. (2006). Oral adhesion and survival of probiotic and other lactobacilli and bifidobacteria in vitro. Oral Microbiol Immunol, 21:326-32.

[47] Horz HP, et al. (2007). Distribution and persistence of probiotic Streptococcus salivarius K12 in the human oral cavity as determined by real-time quantitative polymerase chain reaction. Oral Microbiol Immunol, 22:126-30.

Oral and Dental Health in Pregnancy

Eftekharalsadat Hajikazemi and Fatemeh Haghdoost Osquei

Tehran University of Medical Sciences (TUMS), Center for Nursing Care Research,
Iran

1. Introduction

1.1 The role of oral and dental in physical, psychic and social healthy

Oral health is an important part of any individual health. Therefore preventing oral diseases are essential. Hygiene and prevention plays an important role in human health in many aspects (Jones et al, 1989). In fact trying to protect health is more valuable than recover it and early detection and treatment of gum disease can help and preserve teeth and smile for life. Millions of people don't know they have this serious infection that can lead to tooth loss if not treated (AAP, 2011)

Some consequences of oral and teeth diseases are pain, anxiety and fear of the treatment, limitation in food alternative and fear of having unpleasant and disturbing appearance.

Infection in the mouth can play havoc elsewhere in the body. For a long time it was thought that bacteria was the factor that linked periodontal disease to other infection in the body; however more recent research demonstrates that inflammation may link periodontal disease to other chronic condition. Research has shown, and experts agree that there is an association between periodontal disease and other chronic inflammatory condition such as diabetes, cardiovascular disease, and Alzheimer's disease. (AAP, 2011). It is also a potential source of infection of parathyroid gland and respiratory system, heart attack, stroke and diabetes In this case, the tongue is affected and become thick and even sore, thus the person doesn't feel the taste of food as a result problems such as malnutrition happens (Dugas,1991).

Every tooth in your mouth plays an important role in speaking, chewing and in maintaining proper alignment of other teeth. People with dentures or loose and missing teeth often have restricted diets since biting into fresh fruits and vegetables are often not only difficult, but also painful. This likely means they don't get proper nutrition. Gum and teeth have an important role in having a good appearance as well. A beautiful smile with well ordered teeth will make you much more beautiful. (AAP, 2011) Also teeth and gum protect facial muscles. Pulling each tooth disorders this situation and makes face ugly. The lack of teeth, especially the former teeth, increases wrinkles and changes appearance in an unpleasant way and speaking condition.

Considering the importance of appearance in personality and body image, dental problems can lead to social and psychological consequences, so that individual connections with others are impaired. Gingivitis also leads to Halitosis (bad smell of the mouth) that disrupts social interaction. So prevention is serious from childhood. World Health Organization, called year 1994, "oral health for healthy life" and announced, having a healthy mouth and teeth, helps to health promotion, comfortable and self steam in any person.

Mouth and teeth disorders also affect nutritional status and health of a pregnant woman. As tooth decay is the focus of infection, it may put a mother and her fetus's life in dangers (, AAP, 2011; Ogunboded, 1996). Sometimes one's sleeping is impaired by dental pain and this issue is harmful to pregnant women.

High percentage of children and adolescent do not treat their teeth and gum problem well, and married girls get pregnant without any special attention to their teeth health condition. Even such as pregnancy, menstruation and menopause in women affect physically on the oral health, so women should be more careful about their mouth and teeth health (AAP, 2011). It is necessary to note that the during the pregnancy Hormonal changes, particularly increased progesterone level in pregnancy lead to congestion and swelling gums that need special attention to provide their health. After pregnancy this congestion and swelling disappear and the gums return to the ordinary situation (Glliser, 1998; Yiping &et al, 2004).

2. The characteristics of healthy gum

The gums are as the holders' tissues for the teeth and protect them. The healthy gum has pink color and is strong in their place, without any swelling, redness or inflammation and spots. During brushing and dental examinations do not bleed.

Periodontal disease is often silent, meaning symptoms may not appear until an advanced stage of the disease (AAP, 2011).

3. How plaque and calculus form?

If hygiene of mouth and teeth do not consider gums and teeth will have serious problems.The lace of hygiene for mouth and teeth and not cleaning the teeth and the mouth environment cause the existed mouth bacteria's to form the thin, colorless layer and sticky plaque on the gum and teeth with the remaining food particles in coordination with saliva, These plaques can be removed with regular oral hygiene that includes in daily brushing and flossing. However, it is the onset of teeth decadence and gums diseases in the future, and gradually cause more stickiness of plaque upon the teeth that cannot be easily washed by water and each day increases its thickness(Jonson, 1985).

The toxins from the bacteria's in plaques gradually cause harms and destruction the tissue of gums, in addition to residue the gained mineral materials on plague helps hardness to the extent that reform's into white, yellow or dark colored stones that no longer can be taken off by brush and they are called calculus or germs (lime-stone masses). The calculus after its formation due to the rough and uneven surface cause more concentration upon the teeth and also while brushing or eating food especially while biting hard fruits cause contact with gums injuring and bleeding of it, this situation is called gingivitis. Gingivitis is first stage of periodontal disease. So removal of calculus is necessary, because, the calculus in addition for causing gum diseases is a suitable place for growth of bacteria's and for this reason in the major cause of halitosis. Removal the germs with especial dental equipments has been carried out, if cleaning germs does not take in time, the germ will extend the bon around teeth and this factor causes looseness of the teeth and ultimately losing them(Jonson, 1985).

Removal the germs do not harm the teeth and gums and doesn't cause sensitivity of the teeth towards coldness and hot conditions. Of course some minor sensitivity temporarily and will be removed. It is clear that are once cleaning germs and good oral and dental health may some time to make needless for new germ cleaning. Of the special saliva compound and the rate of secretion the probability for the formation of germs in some persons is more than others, so that this groups must take more care in oral health and sequential visit by the dentist in case for the need of germ cleaning within the shorter times. Some persons avoid germs cleaning for the fear of the pain or its complications, while this action does not have any particular complications and is not painful. The use of toothpaste for the elimination of germs has no effects because the germs are harder than to be taken by the toothpaste. Removal of germ for pregnant women has no dangers. The pregnant women must not be worry about it (Randy, 2005; Jeffcoat, 2000) .

4. Periodontal disease

Periodontal (gum) diseases, including gingivitis and periodontitis, are serious infections that, left untreated, can lead to tooth loss. The word *periodontal* literally means "around the tooth." Periodontal disease is a chronic bacterial infection that affects the gums and bone supporting the teeth. Periodontal disease can affect one tooth or many teeth. It begins when the bacteria in plaque (the sticky, colorless film that constantly forms on your teeth) causes the gums to become inflamed (AAP, 2011).

The gingivitis is common form of inflammation of the gum tissue (the first stage of periodontal disease) it has observed in all ages, but studies indicate that older people have the highest rates of periodontal disease and need the to do more to maintain good oral health (AAP, 2011).

The some effective factors in the gingivitis are bacterial plaque due to the poor oral hygiene; in the absence of treatment gingivitis may progress to Periodontitis. Consumption of tobacco, recent studies have shown that tobacco use may be one of the most significant risk factors in the development and progression of periodontal disease. Other factors are unnatural habit such as clenching or grinding teeth, poor nutrition, obesity and the consumption of some medicines, stress, genetic, puberty, pregnancy and menopause in women, diabetes and other systematic disease (AAP, 2011).

The plaques contain some number of bacteria's and sugars in foods are effective to bacteria's growth and enzymes activities, so the continuance of plaques in mouth and don't eliminations them in addition to their destruction of teeth, cause swelling and inflammation of the gum tissue, it is important that the gum-diseases in the beginning to be cured, because the cure of the disease of tissues in the final stages does not have good results. The bleeding of gums is the sign of gingivitis that must consult with the dentist and cleaning to be done, the consumption of some medicines can also be necessary the dentist will give some guide lines in this issue. Even in the cases of intensive surgery of the gums it is also necessary, sometimes massage the gums with finger-tips is useful. In the absence of treatment gingivitis may progress to periodontitis in this condition the teeth become loose and in addition of losing them and the Halitosis is created. The Halitosis is common symptom; According to the data about 40 percent of the world population suffers from the Halitosis. The cause of Halitosis is various reasons such as the poor health of mouth and teeth, the decay-teeth, gingivitis, the dryness of mouth, systematic diseases such as lung infections, uncontrolled Diabetes, the situation of nose and throat and sinuses of the jaws, the consumption of tobacco, hard regimes, and the consumption of food such as onion garlic. it must be noted that the Halitosis be dependent on time such as in the morning wake-up that according to the decrease amount of saliva during the night and could be removed by the consumption of breakfast and teeth brushing.

5. Signs and symptoms of gingivitis

Periodontal disease is often silent, meaning symptoms may not appear until an advanced stage of the disease. However, warning signs of periodontal disease include the following:
- Red, swollen or tender gums or other pain in your mouth
- Bleeding while brushing, flossing, or eating hard food
- Gums that are receding or pulling away from the teeth, causing the teeth to look longer than before
- Loose or separating teeth
- Pus between your gums and teeth
- Sores in your mouth
- Persistent bad breath
- A change in the way your teeth fit together when you bite
- A change in the fit of partial dentures (AAP, 2011).

The lack of hygiene for oral and dental in pregnant women cause the formation of inflammation in gums among the teeth of one or two teeth that is called pregnancy tumor, this increase volume of the swelling of teeth contains capillary and tissues that their colors according to the amount of blood vessels is from light red to unsettled Blue, it has soft constitution and pain less this inflammation in the event of smallest touch and finger – touching bleeds (Baum, 1994). There is a wrong belief: "pregnant woman normally will lose some teeth". This is dangerous and causes lack of paying attention to the issue that is avoidable. Statistically large number of developed tooth decays is reported. This is because of carelessness of mother to her oral health due to the pressure of new responsibilities after birth. Mothers should become convinced that oral problems are avoidable in case of daily attention to their teeth health while a safe and routine dental treatment during pregnancy is strongly recommended (Marjorio, 2006; Jeffcoat, 2006).

Hormonal changes, particularly increased progesterone level in pregnancy lead to congestion and swelling gums, so if there was a gum infection prior pregnancy this leads to gum inflammation. In these conditions, gum bleeding is inclined. Some women see bleeding of gums during brushing or using floss, so they stop cleaning their mouth, while in this condition, oral hygiene should be continued as soon as possible to cure the infection, because gum infection for mother and fetus can be harmful (Hajikazemi et al; AAP, 2006).

Studies have shown that sever gingival inflammatory disease in pregnant women is an important risk factor for preterm delivery and low birth weight. This conclusion has been confirmed by previous experiments on animals too. The research conducted by (Collins, 1994; Ogunboded ,1996). On laboratory mice to assess the effects of periodontal infection on pregnancy outcome, showed that gum infection in mice is associated by increasing the incidence of fetal growth retardation, fetal death and preterm labor (Lopez, 2005; AAP, 2006). Incidence of nausea in pregnant women can be another cause of their refusal of oral hygiene. On the other hand, women think if they take a few foods the oral and teeth care is not necessary, while it is a wrong belief; if plaque doesn't get removed by cleaning the mouth during 9-21days, it will lead to gum infection.

Sometimes pregnant women desire to eat the unusual material such as soil or ice, this is called "longing of pregnant women". Sometimes increase of sugar consumption is observed, this is harmful too. In case of frequent vomiting, tooth and gum problem will increase. These problems are preventable by washing the mouth after vomiting.

6. Preventing of the gingivitis

Gingivitis can be prevented by regular oral hygiene to reach purpose training different groups of community can be the best and easiest way. In fact the difficulties and diseases that today need the cure with high expenditure require great times, had been preventable yesterday. Usually the low income groups in the society due to the high expenditure of dental treatments do not visit dentist or it is too late, this cause serious harms to them, while with carrying out simple precautions such as daily brushing and flossing can remove the teeth from plaques. Saline normal or color hex dine mouth washes also are helpful. Consideration for the nutrition could prevent many of the problems and high cost.

Gingivitis can be prevented through regular oral health that includes correct brushing, flossing; interdentally brushes are also useful in cleaning the teeth from plaque. Incorrectly brushes do not only clean the plaque completely and from the other side can cause the injury in gums tissue, bleeding and erosion to the teeth. for brushing must not use hot water, when brush gets wet nearly one-third of its hardness is lost, so it is better to damping the brush to use the ordinary water. The brush life more with the style is dependent that the time of its usage, but the average life of brush normally is three month, if the brush hairs after six month is still straight are the sign of incorrect style of brushing. The duration of brushing is maximum ten minutes,

The importance of brushing before sleeping for all is great because the bacteria's of mouth have more opportunity for effecting upon the remains of food in the mouth and the probability of teeth destruction gets higher, it is necessary that before going to sleep to brush. This issue in the pregnant women that inflicted with some kind of inertia and sleepiness is more important.

Brushing is better to be done consciously and without mental engagements, because causes forgotten of the dean sing of some parts (Mathewson, 1994). The toothpaste has a helpful role in cleaning the teeth and mouth and is aromatic. Brushing singularly is not able to clean the teeth surface, so flossing helps the cleaning of teeth, because the onset of gum diseases is often from this area (Sharon,1994). Whatever the distance of teeth is closer to each other a thinner dental floss must be used. It is better that each time offer brushing to use the dental floss The dental floss removes the plaque between teeth, also causes the reduction of Halitosis. The usage of other tools such as pins, matches instead of dental floss to be used for teeth, because harms to the teeth. Washing the mouth with Saline normal for the cleansing of mouth and gums cause the strength of gums and reduces the bleeding. The focus of treatment for gingivitis is removal of the etiologic agent plague, aim is reduction of oral bacteria's and may take the form of regular periodic visit to dental professional together with adequate oral hygiene.

The pregnant women must be educated for oral health. A Upon a study conducted in Riyadh in 1994, a lack of awareness in pregnant women about their oral and dental care in pregnancy and regularly visiting dentist was observed. Prime porous women knowledge was lower than others (Al-Tammie, 1998).

The pregnant women after each vomiting wash the mouth with mouth washes because the vomiting is acidic and cause harms to the teeth and mouth, and is better to use the brushes with small head and medium roughness, that reduces the vomiting while using, and teeth cares must after pregnancy to be continued. And incase for the need of diagnoses in the third till seventh months for the carrying out of therapies are suitable. In some countries, it is over half century that special attentions are paid to oral care during pregnancy. In these countries, dental services during pregnancy up to one year after delivery are free. In these countries women treat their oral and dental diseases before they got decided for pregnancy. Recently, some activities in Iran, especially for at risk groups such as women and children, have been conducted. The integration of oral and dental hygiene into "primary health care" is one of such activities. According to the regulations of "Health Ministry" on November 1995, along with prenatal care of pregnant women, their mouth and teeth must also be examined at each visit, and the correct way of oral health must be taught to them. Their oral status in third, fifth and seventh month of pregnancy are recorded in their family record, and if any problem was observed, they got referred to the dentist of health center. Also examination and record of their oral status at three months and one year after delivery occurs. But statistics showed that women don't use of these services enough. In most countries, pregnant women don't take enough oral care. Considering statistics presented in 1991 Birmingham; UK, it showed that although dental services were completely free of charge, only 61% of women had referred to the dentist.

Sometimes the dentists also avoid doing some treatment for pregnant women. Studies on (non-specialist) dentists of their knowledge about the importance of dental treatment in pregnant women showed that they avoid doing some therapeutics for pregnant women, because they believe that, some women's have low awareness and negative attitudes about the oral and dental treatment and effects of dental materials on fetus, so dentists believe that, this may cause legal problems for them. So only economic barriers are not causes of not receive oral and dental care in pregnant women, but also awareness, believes and insight of women in this field have an important role. Nowadays science believes that: oral and dental disease is a behavioral disorder. Therefore it is needed that women prior to pregnancy meet the dentist and take the necessary information about oral and dental care during pregnancy and use those treatment services and facilities. Education and change of attitude of pregnant women in this field will be beneficial to maintain their oral health.

7. Nutritional and prevention

Today the world faces two kinds of malnutrition, one associated with hunger or nutritional deficiency and the other with dietary excess. Urbanization and economic development result in rapid changes in diets and lifestyles. Market globalization has a significant and worldwide impact on dietary excess leading to chronic diseases such as obesity, diabetes, cardiovascular diseases, cancer, osteoporosis and oral diseases. Diet and nutrition affects oral health in many ways. Nutrition, for example, influences cranio-facial development, oral cancer and oral infectious diseases. Dental diseases related to diet include dental caries, developmental defects of enamel, dental erosion and periodontal disease (WHO, 2011).

Proper Nutrition has a positive role in prevention of the oral disease. The use of all groups of food, suitable with the needs of budge considering the age and sex and particular conditions such as pregnancy, the consumption of fresh vegetables and fruit especially vitamin C and A for the generating Collagen tissue is necessary. Collagen tissue is the main protein of the tissues such as the gums. Vitamin A strengthens the weakness of gums against penetration of bacteria. The results of studies show that the decrease consumption of vitamins A and C causes gums bleeding, inflammation of gums, the decrease mineral of the bones and loosening the teeth. Also the consumption of low- fat milk, cheese, mustard seeds, cabbage, cauliflower, fish cans of fish with bones, the consumption of fluoride such as tea, and salmon fish is also in prevention of the diseases of mouth and teeth are effectual.

The consumption of kinds of cola is harmful for the health of teeth and mouth, because phosphor which is abundant in the cola causes the decrease amount of calcium in the bones some of the researcher believe that the calcium initially from the bones of jaws are removed that cause the loosening of teeth. The high consumption of sugar in addition to the speeding destruction of teeth also harms the gums tissue because the sugar cause the feeding of bacteria's that generate gingivitis, however this part must be studied more. The use of sugar sticky materials such as chocolates are harmful, because of their stickiness to the teeth for long times in the mouth. Consumption of high sugar materials and taking it more time during the day between main meals is not good; this point is important and must be emphasized. The WHO reports emphasized that despite great improvements in the oral health of populations in some countries, problems still persist. Dental caries remains a major public health problem in most high income countries, affecting 60-90% of schoolchildren and the vast majority of adults. It is also the most prevalent oral disease in several Asian and Latin American countries the World Oral Health Report 2003 anticipates that in light of changing living conditions and dietary habits, the incidence of dental caries will increase in many of that continent's low income countries. The principal reasons for this increase are growing consumption of sugars and inadequate exposure to fluoride (WHO, 2006).

8. References

American Academy of Periodontology. (2011). assess your risk of gum disease.
    URL: *http://www.perio.org/consumer/4a.htm*
American Academy of Periodontology. (2011Mouth-Body Connection.
    URL: *http://www.perio.org/consumer/mbc.top2.htm.*
American Academy of Periodontology.(2011). How to Keep a Healthy Smile for Life
    URL:.*http://www.perio.org/consumer/smileforlife.htm.*
American Academy of Periodontology. (2011). Gum Disease and Pregnancy Problems.
    URL: *http://www.perio.org/consumer/mbc.baby.htm*
American Academy of Periodontology. (2011). Protecting Children's Oral Health.
    URL: *http://www.perio.org/consumer/children.htm*
American Academy of Periodontology. (2011). Symptoms of Gum Disease.
    URL: *http://www.perio.org/consumer/gum-disease-symptoms.htm*
American Academy of Periodontology. (2011). Causes of Gum Disease.
    URL: *http://www.perio.org/consumer/gum-disease-causes.htm*
American Academy of Periodontology. (2011). protecting Your Oral Health.
    URL: *http: //www.perio.org/consumer/protect.htm*
American academy of periodontology.(2006). Baby steps to a healthy pregnancy and on –
    time delivery. URL: www.perio.org.
Al-Tammie S, Peterson P. 1998. Oral health situation of school children' mothers and school
    teachers in Saudi Arabia, *International Dental Journal* 43(3): 180-185.
American academy of periodontology.(2006). Protecting oral health throughout your life.
    URL: www.perio.org.
Baum p. (1994), *Text book of the operative dentistry.*UK Sanders's co.
Collins JG, Winley HW, Arnold RR, Offenbacher S. (1994) Effect of a prophyromonas
    gingivitis infection on inflammatory mediator response and pregnancy outcome in
    hamster, *Infection and Immunity*, 62(10): 4356-61
Dugas,B.(1991). *Introduction to patient care*. London Sanders Co.

Gleicher, N. (1998). *Principles & Practice of Medical Therapy in Pregnancy.* USA: Plenum Company.

IIajikazemi E,Oskouie F, Hossain Mohseny SH, Nikpour   S,Haghany H.(2008).The Relationship between Knowledge, Attitude, and Practice of Pregnant Women about Oral and Dental Care *European Journal of Scientific Research,* Vol.24 No.4 pp.556-562.

Jones, H., Mason, j. & David, K. (1998). *Oral Manifestation of systematic Disease.* philadelphia: WB.sunders.

Jahonson, A. (1985). Dental care during pregnancy. *Nursing time,* 11. 30-31.

Jeffcoat, A. (2000). Research presented today provides further evidence on the importance of good oral health in pregnant women. URL:*www.perio.org*

Lopez, N. (2005). Periodontal therapy protects preterm birth. *Journal of   periodontology,* 76, 2144-53.

Marjorio, s. (2003). Dental procedure may reduce risk of premature birth.
    URL: *www.perio.org*

Mathewson,RJ;et al.(1994). Fundamental of dentistry for children. London:quintessence.

Ogunboded, E. (1996). Socio economic factors and dental health in an Obstetric Population. *West African Journal of medicine,* 15, 158-62.

Ogunboded, E. (1996). Socio economic factors and dental health in an Obstetric Population. *Journal of medicine,* 15, 158-62.

Randy, M. (2005). Health-study: X-Ray may harm fetus. URL:*Wsbtv.com*

World Health Organization2011).Risks to oral health and intervention. Diet & nutrition. URL: *www.who.int/oral health/action/risk/en.*

World Health Organization. (2006). Global consultation on oral health Through   Fluoride. WHO in collaboration with the World Dental Federation and The International Association for Dental Research.
    URL:*www.who.int/oral_health/event/Glob_consultation en.index.html*

Yiping W et al. (2004). Fusobacterium nucleatum induces premature and term stillbirths in pregnant mice: Implication of oral bacteria in preterm birth, *journal of Infection and Immunity,* 72(4): 2272-2279.

11

The Determinants of
Self–Rated Oral Health in Istanbul Adults

Kadriye Peker

Department of Basic Sciences, Faculty of Dentistry, Istanbul University
Turkey

1. Introduction

No studies have been published on a comprehensive appraisal of the full range of factors that may affect Turkish adults' perceptions of their oral health status, as measured by a single item. Understanding the local context of self–rated oral health (SROH) and its determinants within Turkish culture will be important to develop oral health policy and to design oral health promotion programs for adults. Oral diseases, primarily dental caries and periodontal diseases, are major public health problems in Turkey (Gökalp et al., 2010). Oral health care resources are primarily allocated to curative care without an underlying oral health policy. The government's oral health care budget and the existing oral health services are inadequate to meet increasing oral health needs and demands of the adult population (Kargul & Bakkal, 2010). Utilization of oral health care services is low, and the oral health visits are usually problem-oriented (Gökalp et al., 2010; Kargul & Bakkal, 2010).

In Turkey, most studies of adults have focused dominantly on biological, clinical and behavioral health risk factors of oral diseases (Akarslan et al., 2008; Gökalp et al., 2010; Namal et al., 2008; Oztürk et al., 2008; Unlüer et al., 2007). In the past decade, few studies using validated subjective oral health measures have been conducted to verify the impact of different oral disorders and prosthodontic treatments on oral health quality of life in Turkish patients groups (Arslan et al., 2009; Baran & Nalcaci, 2011; Caglayan et al., 2009; Geckili et al., 2011). To the best of your knowledge, there is one published study that investigated the relationships among oral health beliefs, oral health behaviors, socio-demographic factors and SROH (Peker & Bermek, 2011).

SROH is an assessment of the functional, psychological, and social impact of oral disease and disorder on overall well being (Locker & Gibson, 2005). Although different approaches are available for evaluating self-perceived oral health, single-item indicators have frequently been used because they represent a valid and simple measure for evaluating oral health–related outcomes and summarizing oral health status (Dolan et al., 1998; Locker & Gibson, 2005). Most studies have been conducted with samples of adults, and findings indicate this measure is fairly stable over time (Peek et al., 1999), and positively associated with clinical assessment of oral health status (Gilbert et al., 1998; Kim et al., 2010; Pattussi et al., 2010; Peek et al., 1999). Over the past two decades there has been growing interest in examining individuals' SROH (Atchison & Andersen, 2000; Gilbert et al., 1998; Locker et al., 2005,

2009), mostly in adult and elderly populations in different countries. A single-item global self-rating is a valid, reliable measure of oral health (Pinelli & de Castro Monteiro Loffredo, 2007) and a good predictor of the use of oral health services (Abelsen, 2008; Araújo et al., 2009; Camargo et al., 2009; Gilbert et al., 2003; Locker & Miller, 1994; Matos &Lima-Costa, 2006; Maupomé & et al., 2004; Okunseri et al., 2008b; Pavi et al., 2010; Petersen et al., 2000; Thomson et al., 2010; Woolfolk et al. 1999; Wu et al., 2011). Nowadays, SROH has been widely used in nationwide and community-based surveys in many countries (Baker, 2009; Borrell & Baquero, 2011; Finlayson et al., 2010; Kim et al., 2010; Martins et al., 2010; Matos & Lima-Costa, 2006; Pattussi et al., 2010; Okunseri et al., 2008a, 2008b; Sanders & Spencer, 2005; Wu et al., 2011) and in the first and second International Collaborative study of Oral Health Outcomes (Arnljot et al., 1985; Chen et al., 1997). In many studies, SROH have been used to assess the perceived need for dental care and dental treatment outcomes (Jones et al., 2001; Lundegren et al., 2011; Martins et al., 2009,2010; Seremidi et al., 2009) and to estimate the effect of oral conditions on people's quality of life and well-being (Benyamini et al., 2004; Dahl et al., 2011; Jones et al., 2001; Kieffer & Hoogstraten, 2008; Locker et. al., 2005; Locker, 2009; Locker & Miller, 1994; Martins, 2009; Ostberg & Hall-Lord, 2011).

There are several reasons for investigating lay peoples' perceptions of their oral health. First, self-reported information has the advantage of being easier to gather in population-based samples compared to collecting data by clinical examinations. It also may be useful for estimating the resources needed to care for a specific population (Atchison & Gift, 1997; Jones et al., 2001; Pinelli & de Castro Monteiro Loffredo, 2007; Wu et al., 2011). SROH is used frequently in many national health surveys when clinical evaluations are too costly and has been shown to be a valid and useful summary indicator of overall oral health status (Locker & Miller, 1994). Secondly, it can be a useful tool for planning and monitoring health services and health promotion interventions. It also could provide benefits to health care providers in monitoring outcomes and evaluating treatments. (Locker, 1996). Thirdly, SROH is an assessment of the functional, psychological, and social impact of oral disease and disorder (Gilbert et al., 1998). Self-perceived oral health provides more information about how a certain disease affects an individual's life, rather than the objective measurements of this disease (Jones et al., 2001; Kim et al., 2010; Martins et al., 2009).

In Turkey, dental care for the adults needs to be improved and the identification of their self-perception of oral health could be the first step towards the development of oral health promotion programs aiming to increase awareness of oral health and to improve the oral health of Turkish adults (Gökalp et al., 2010; Kargul & Bakkal, 2010; Peker & Bermek, 2011). No studies have been published on a comprehensive appraisal of the full range of factors that may affect Turkish adults' perceptions of their oral health status, as measured by a single. Therefore, the aim of the study is to investigate the main factors associated with good SROH in Istanbul adults.

1.1 Conceptual framework

This study used a multidimensional model of oral health for measuring the association of tooth pain and dental problems with SROH (Locker, 1988) and an expanded version of the Andersen's Behavioral Model of Health Services Utilization (Andersen & Davidson, 1997; Baker, 2009).

A multidimensional model of oral health is comprised of five dimensions: namely - oral disease and tissue damage, oral pain and discomfort, oral functional limitation, oral disadvantage, and self-rated oral health (Gilbert et al., 1998; Locker, 1988). The Andersen's Behavioral Model consists of variables distributed into four levels: exogenous variables, primary determinants of oral health, health behaviors, and oral health outcomes. This model proposes that a person's characteristics, beliefs, and behaviors will predict one's perceptions of oral health (Andersen, 1995). These models as conceptual framework were used to assess differences in the multitude of factors influencing oral health and to explain population-based oral health behaviors and outcomes (Atchison & Gift, 1997; Baker, 2009; Gilbert, 2005; Martins et al., 2010, 2011).

In this study, these models were used to help develop the survey instrument and to guide data analysis, including the selection of variables for the logistic regression models. A set of independent individual-level variables were identified that may influence SROH: (1) exogenous variables (age, gender); (2) personal characteristics of primary determinants of oral health (predisposing socio-demographic and health beliefs factors - education, marital status, oral health locus of control (LOC) beliefs, perceived general health status; enabling characteristics - socio-economic status, having dental insurance; need factors - perceived dental treatment need, self-reported number of teeth, self-reported dental pain and dental problems, and (3) oral health behaviors (frequency of tooth brushing, dental attendance pattern, use of dental floss).

A number of studies showed that demographic and socio-economic variables such as gender, age, income and marital status have been associated with SROH (Borrell & Baquero, 2011; Finlayson et al., 2010; Kim et al., 2010; Okunseri et al., 2008a; Patussi et al., 2010; Ugarte et al., 2007; Wu et al., 2011).

Previous studies showed that individuals who perceive better oral health had a higher frequency of seeking preventive dental care (Araújo et al., 2009; Camargo et al., 2009; Gilbert et al., 2003; Matos&Lima-Costa, 2006; Okunseri et al., 2008b; Pavi et al., 2010; Thomson et al., 2010; Woolfolk et al. 1999; Wu et al., 2011). In addition, poor SROH was associated significantly with unfavorable oral health behaviors (Ekbäck et al., 2009; Kim et al., 2010; Locker et al., 2009; Okunseri et al., 2008b; Wu et al., 2011).

Associations between self-perceptions of general health status and SROH have been reported in several studies (Atchison & Gift, 1997; Benyamini et al, 2004; Okunseri et al., 2008a, b).

Psychosocial factors (e.g., self-esteem, mastery, personal control, life satisfaction, stress, sense of cohesion, depression, resilience, social support) were found to be related to SROH (Benyamini et al.,2004; Finlayson et al., 2010; Locker, 2009; Martins et al.,2011; Peker & Bermek, 2011; Sanders & Spencer, 2005; Wu et al., 2011).

SROH was also associated significantly with oral functional problems and concerns (Ekbäck et al., 2009; Gilbert et al., 1998; Kim et al., 2010; Locker et al., 2009; Ugarte et al., 2007).

2. Method

2.1 Data source and sample

This study used the household interview data which were collected during my PhD thesis. The survey was conducted by a market research company (Mayak) on a representative quota sample of 1200 Istanbul adults aged 18 years and over (response rate 88 %). This cross-sectional survey was undertaken in November and December 2003. The present study sample was restricted to 979 adults who answered the question on the SROH. Data were collected through personal interviews and carried out in the participants' homes by eight trained professional interviewers. A detailed description of the sampling, design and procedures of the survey has been reported elsewhere (Peker&Bermek,2011). The Ethics Committee of the Faculty of Medicine, the University of Istanbul approved the study protocol.

2.2 Measures
The dependent and independent variables which were used in this study are summarized below.

2.2.1 Dependent variable
SROH was assessed by using a single item question "How would you rate your oral health?" with possible ordinal responses: excellent, very good, good, fair and poor (Dolan et al., 1998). The answers were later dichotomized for analysis purposes, with participants who rated their oral health as excellent, very good, or good categorized as good and those who rated their oral health as fair or poor categorized as bad.

2.2.2 Independent variables
Independent variables were examined across for domains: (1) exogenous variables (age, gender); (2) personal characteristics of primary determinants of oral health (predisposing socio-demographic and health beliefs factors - education, marital status, oral health LOC beliefs, perceived general health status; enabling characteristics - socio-economic status, having dental insurance; need factors - perceived dental treatment need, self-reported number of teeth, self-reported dental pain and dental problem, and   (3)   oral health behaviors (frequency of tooth brushing and dental attendance pattern).
Perceived dental treatment need was measured by the response to the question "Do you perceive any need for dental treatment at the moment?" The response was either yes or no.
A sum score of reported oral problems was computed from questions on broken tooth, position of teeth, swollen gums, bad breaths, and ulcers in the mouth, bleeding gums, colour of the teeth and gum abscess. This score was dichotomized as no reported oral problems vs. reported at least one oral problem. Self-reported number of teeth was based on response to the item "How many of your own teeth do you have?", which was dichotomized as less than 20 teeth vs. 20 or more teeth. Dental pain was assessed by asking whether the person had a toothache in the last 6 months. The response was either yes or no. Self- perceived health status was measured using a single-item self-rating of health (Benyamini et al., 2004; Borrell & Baquero, 2011; Okunseri et al., 2008b). Self-rated health (SRH) was based on responses to a single item ("How do you consider your health in general?"), which was dichotomized as Good (excellent/good/fair) vs. Bad (poor/very poor). The measure of self-reported oral health behaviors included two questions: tooth brushing frequency (≥ twice a day, ≤ once a day); and   dental attendance pattern (symptom–oriented / regular dental check–up at least once a year). Age was coded in three age categories: (18–30, 31–45, and 46 + years). Educational level was categorized into three groups according to years of completed schooling: primary (0–5 years), secondary (6–11 years), and higher (more than 11

years). Socio–economic status (SES) was measured by using the VERI Socio-Economic Status Index (Tüzün, 2000). It is a social stratification model developed by the Veri Research Company in Turkey, made up of an equal-weight combination of values based on average educational level and working status of the household members, life facilitating property ownership, area of residence and house ownership. SES was categorized into three groups according to VERI Socio-Economic Status Index score: low (4-9), middle (11-14), and high (15-20). Marital status was recorded as married and not married (never married, separated, widowed or divorced). Health insurance status was coded as uninsured and insured. The Multidimensional Oral Health LOC Scale, a validated measure using 26 items assessed on a 4-point scale ranging 'strongly disagree' to 'strongly agree' was used to measure beliefs about adults' control over oral health (Peker & Bermek, 2011). This scale consists of four subscales, namely the Internal, External-Dentist, External-Chance, and External-Socialization agents. These subscales indicate the degree to which a person believes that his/her oral health outcomes are controlled by himself/herself, by chance, by the dentist's recommendation and advice, by the dentist's preventive dental care, or by socialization agents (e.g., family member, friends, colleagues, relatives etc.). Subscale scores are calculated by adding the scores of all the items within a particular subscale, and dividing the sum by the number of items. Higher scores reflect stronger endorsement of the subscales. Cronbach's alpha of the scale in this sample was 0.71.

2.3 Data analysis

The data were analyzed by using SPSS version 11.5 for Windows (SPSS, Inc, Chicago, IL, USA). A combination of descriptive, bivariate and multivariate statistical methods was used for this analysis. Chi square test was used for categorical variables, and the independent sample t-test was use for continuous variables. Finally, a binary logistic regression analysis with stepwise backward elimination (likelihood ratio) was applied to determine the relationship between the dependent variable and independent variables. The variables that had shown statistical significance at the 5% level in the bivariate analysis with at least one the outcomes studied were entered into the model for logistic regression analysis. Estimates of model fit (Omnibus test) and odds ratios (ORs) with their corresponding 95 percent confidence intervals (CIs) were computed. In all statistical analyses, the significance level was set to $p < 0.05$. Age, education, and oral health LOC beliefs scores were entered as continuous variables in the model. Nagelkerke R2 was used to describe the proportion of the total variance explained by the multivariate models.

3. Results

The sample consisted of 492 men and 487 women and the mean (SD) age was 36.52 (13.58) years; 68% had formal school education equal to or less than 8 years, 57% had a moderate SES, 57% were married, and 40 % had no health insurance. Overall, 65% of the study sample reported having bad oral health, while 71% rated general health as good. 18% reported having had regular dental checkups, 35% brushed twice a day or more. 29% of adults reported having dental pain during the past six months, 36% had dental problems, and 27% reported no need for dental treatment. 67% reported that they had less than 20 teeth.

Internal consistency reliability, as measured by Crohnbach's alpha, was 0.71 for the Multidimensional Oral Health LOC Scale, and 0.82 for the Internal subscale, 0.79 for the

External/Dentist subscale, 0.71 for the External/Chance subscale, and 0.72 for the External/Socialization agents subscale. The mean item subscale scores   were 3.49 (SD=0.43, range = 1.82 - 4) for Internal, 2.77 (SD =0.57, range = 1-4) for External /Dentist, 1.97 (SD =0.57, range = 0.86 – 4) for External / Chance, and 2.70 (SD = 0.79, range = 0.50 – 4) for External/Socialization agents

Independent variables		Bad SROH n (%)	Good SROH n (%)	P value
Gender	Female	297 (46.8)	190 (55.1)	0.014
	Male	337 (53.2)	155 (44.9)	
Age	18–30 years	328 (51.7)	72 (20.9)	<0.001
	31–45 years	210 (33.1)	131 (38)	
	46 + years	96 (15.1)	142 (41.2)	
Education	Primary or less	418 (65.9)	244 (70.7)	0.022
	Secondary	153 (24.1)	58 (16.8)	
	Higher	63 (9.9)	43 (12.5)	
Dental attendance	Regular	97 (15.3)	79 (22.9)	0.003
	Symptoms-oriented	537 (84.7)	266 (77.1)	
Toothbrushing	≥ twice a day	208 (33.7)	127 (38.5)	0.143
	≤ once a day	409 (66.3)	203 (61.5)	

Table 1. Exogenous and behavioral characteristics of the studied sample according to SROH (n=979)

The frequencies of the independent variables were assessed in this study in relation to SROH are shown in Table 1 and Table 2. Health insurance (P<0.001), gender (P=0.014), age (P<0.001), education (P=0.022), marital status (P<0.001), dental attendance pattern (P=0.003), Internal (P<0.001), Dentist (P<0.001), and Chance (P=0.006) oral health LOC beliefs, the self-reported number of teeth (P<0.001), dental pain (P<0.001), and SRH (P= 0.003)   were significantly associated with the SROH. SROH was not associated with SES (P=0.287), the frequency of tooth brushing (P=0.143), having dental problems (P=0.227), perceived need for dental treatment (P=0.160), and Socialization agents LOC beliefs (P=0.602).

Stepwise binary logistic regression analyses were performed to examine the association the independent variables with good SROH. In the final model, only four variables were found to be associated with good SROH. This model indicated a good fit (Ombinus test: chi-square = 445.200, p<0.0001) and with correct classification of 76.8 percent of the adults. The final model explained 52.4 % of the variance in good SROH (Nagelkerke's R2 = 0.524). As seen in Table 3, having good SROH was associated significantly with increasing age (P<0.001; odds ratio [OR]=2.03; 95% confidence interval [CI]= 1.64 -2.53) regular dental attendance (P=0.013; odds ratio [OR]=0.75; 95% confidence interval [CI]= 0.59 -0.94), higher Dentist LOC beliefs (P<0.001; odds ratio [OR]=2.05, 95% confidence interval [CI]= 1.52-2.76), and lower Chance LOC beliefs (P=0.001; odds ratio [OR]=0.62, 95% confidence interval [CI]= 0.47-0.83).

Independent variables		Bad SROH n (%)	Good SROH n (%)	P value
SES	Low	154 (24.3)	96 (27.8)	0.287
	Moderate	371 (58.5)	184 (53.3)	
	High	109 (17.2)	65 (18.8)	
Health Insurance	No	280 (44.2)	109 (31.6)	<0.001
	Yes	354 (55.8)	236 (68.4)	
SRH	Bad	537 (84.7)	266 (77.1)	0.003
	Good	97 (15.3)	79 (22.9)	
Marital status	Married	315 (49.7)	241 (69.9)	<0.001
	Non –married	319 (50.3)	104 (30.1)	
Dental pain	Yes	486 (76.7)	206 (59.7)	<0.001
	No	148 (23.3)	139 (40.3)	
Self-reported number of teeth	0-19	316 (49.8)	341 (98.8)	<0.001
	20-32	318 (50.2)	4 (1.2)	
Self-reported dental problems	No	416 (65.6)	213 (61.7)	0.227
	Yes	218 (34.4)	132 (38.3)	
Perceived dental treatment need	No	177 (27.9)	82 (23.8)	0.160
	Yes	457 (72.1)	263 (76.2)	
Internal LOC beliefs (Mean ± SD)		3.44 (0.42)	3.57 (0.42)	<0.001
Dentist LOC beliefs (Mean ± SD)		2.67 (0.54)	2.93 (0.60)	<0.001
Chance LOC beliefs (Mean ± SD)		2.01 (0.54)	1.90 (0.60)	0.006
Socialization agents LOC beliefs (Mean ± SD)		2.71 (0.77)	2.68 (0.83)	0.602

SD, standard deviation

Table 2. Predisposing, enabling and need characteristics of the studied sample according to SROH (n=979)

Independent variables	OR (95 % CI)	P-value
Age (years)	2.03 (1.64–2.53)	<0.001
Dental attendance (0= regular, 1= symptoms-oriented)	0.75 (0.59–0.94)	0.013
Dentist LOC Beliefs (range=1–4)	2.05 (1.52–2.76)	<0.001
Chance LOC Beliefs(range=0.86–4)	0.62 (0.47–0.83)	0.001

CI, confidence interval; OR, odds ratio

Table 3. Stepwise binary logistic regression for the association between good SROH and the independent variables

4. Discussion

This study is one of the first to examine a global rating of oral health among Istanbul adults aged 18 years and over using a a representative quota sample. SROH is subjective patient-centered measure of oral health which involve the individual in the decision making process and assessment of their oral health (Locker,1988; Pinelli & Loffredo,2007). Thus, the subjective evaluation of oral health conditions of adults affected by cultural beliefs and socio-demographic and behavioral factors is more important for designing effective oral health programs and services (Andersen & Davidson, 2007; Butani et al., 2008; Gilbert et al., 1998; Kaplan & Baron-Epel, 2003; Kim et al., 2010; Matthias et al., 1995; Pattussi et.al, 2010).

The focus of this study analysis centers around the relation of a comprehensive set of exogenous variables, personal characteristics of primary determinants of oral health (predisposing socio-demographic and health beliefs factors, enabling characteristics, need factors) and oral health behavioral characteristics.

Bivariate analysis showed that being female, having regular dental attendance, having health insurance, bad SRH, older age, being married, and having lower natural teeth were strongly associated with good SROH.

In contrast to previous studies (Gift et al., 1998; Kim et al., 2010; Okunseri et al., 2008b; Reisine & Bailit,1980), we found that older adults were more likely to rate their oral health better than younger adults. Consistent with previous studies (Patussi et al., 2010; Reisine & Bailit, 1980), we found that males tended to rate their oral health worse than females. There are some variations in the referents which were used for the SROH according to socio-demographic characteristics, with age being the main source of variation (Locker et al., 2009). Age and sex differences in perceived oral health could be attributed to differences in oral health related expectations (Ekbäck et al., 2009; Carr et al., 2001).

Istanbul adults with lower education level were more likely to report good SROH. It is known that the use of specific referents for the self-assessment health may vary by education (Krause & Jay, 1994). This finding was inconsistent with previous studies suggesting that less educated adults were more likely to rate their oral health as fair / poor (Atchison & Gift, 1997; Finlayson et al., 2010; Gift et al., 1998; Matthias et al., 1995). This discrepancy can be explained by the fact that Turkish adults with lower education level have lower levels of health literacy (Ozdemir et al., 2010). Recent studies suggest that health literacy is associated with educational attainment in self-rated health and in regular dental attendance pattern among older adults (Bennett et al., 2009). In addition, oral health literacy-related outcomes are risk indicators for poor self-reported oral health among rural-dwelling Indigenous Australians (Parker & Jamieson, 2010).

We found that adults who were married were more likely to report good SROH. Similar finding has been reported in a recent study conducted in Somali adults (Okunseri et al., 2008a).

Associations between SROH and socio-economic position markers (e.g., education, occupation, household income, household wealth, subjective social status and childhood socio-economic position) have been reported in several studies (Borrell&Baquero, 2011; Finlayson et al., 2010; Locker, 2009; Pattussi et al., 2010; Wu et al., 2011). In contrast, in the present study, SES (measured by the VERI Socio-Economic Status Index) is not associated with SROH. This discrepancy may be due to using composite SES index instead of well-accepted indicators of SES.

Consistent with previous studies (Abelsen, 2008; Araújo et al., 2009; Camargo et al., 2009; Gilbert et al., 2003; Locker & Miller, 1994; Matos & Lima-Costa, 2006; Maupomé et al., 2004; Okunseri et al., 2008b; Pavi et al., 2010; Petersen et al., 2000; Thomson et al., 2010; Woolfolk et al., 1999; Wu et al., 2011), we found that good SROH was strongly associated with regular dental attendance. It is known that an important part of maintaining good oral health is the use of appropriate dental services (Petersen & Yamamoto, 2005).

A recent qualitative study showed that adults rating their oral health as "excellent" were more likely to refer to health behaviors such as brushing and flossing twice a day and regular preventive dental visits (Locker et al., 2009). In previous studies, tooth brushing frequency was found to be related to SROH among both Korean adults aged 45-64 years (Kim et al., 2010) and Hmong adults living in the United States (Okunseri et al., 2008b). In contrast, in the present study and other ones (Martins et al., 2011), the frequency of tooth brushing is not associated with self-perception.

Dental insurance is associated with SROH consistent with previous studies (Coulter et al., 2004; Okunseri et al., 2008b). In our country, the national health insurance system was introduced in 2008 and covers oral health care. Recent study showed that if enrollees' out-of-pocket costs were increased for dental care, there was a decreasing likelihood of their reporting excellent oral health (Coulter et al., 2004).

We found that dental pain was associated with poor SROH consistent with previous studies (Atchison & Gift, 1997; Locker et. al, 2010; Martins et al., 2010) . We found that SROH was not associated with perceived treatment need and having oral problems. However, these results were different from previous studies and reported that the perceived need was greater among individuals who perceived that their oral health was poor/very poor (Kim et al., 2009; Martins, 2009, 2010; Matos & Lima-Costa, 2006). SROH was associated with self–reported oral functional or psychological limitations (Atchison & Gift, 1997; Gift et al., 1998; Kim et al., 2009; Martins et al., 2009, 2010, 2011; Ojofeitimi et al, 2007; Seremidi et al., 2009). Adults who rated their oral health as "poor" were more likely to report having a current oral problem and perceived treatment needs (Locker et al., 2009). Self-perceived need for treatment was usually measured by asking people about the existence of any dental problems or by using constructed variables that combined the need for treatment with the existence of signs and symptoms of diseases, because functional and psychological impacts of the oral disease seem to be as important, if not more, as the clinical indicators while estimating the dental needs (Seremidi et al., 2009). In this study, self-perceived need for treatment was measured by asking whether or not the respondent had a need for dental treatment. Oral functional limitation related to oral health problems was not measured.

We found an inverse association between SROH and the number of self-reported natural teeth. This finding is inconsistent with previous studies showing that having higher natural teeth is strongly associated with good SROH (Jones et al., 2001; Okunseri et al., 2008 a,b; Ugarte et al., 2007). This may be explained by the fact the adults assessed their oral health positively when they could chew everything and were free from a long history of pain and other problems associated with the natural dentition (Kim et al., 2010; Locker et. al, 2005; Matos & Lima-Costa, 2006; Martins et al., 2010, 2009). The decision to use the numbers of self-reported natural teeth as subjective oral health outcome in this study was made for a number of reasons. In this study, the association was further analyzed by creating two categories of remaining teeth (1–19 and 20–32 teeth), because these criteria for the number of teeth are widely used in research from several different age groups and in different countries (Axelsson & Helgadottir, 1995; Pitiphat et al, 2002; Ueno et al., 2010; Unell et al., 1997). Studies show that the number of natural teeth estimated by questionnaires is in good agreement with clinical examinations (Pitiphat et al, 2002; Unell et al., 1997) and patients' reported number of remaining teeth provide reasonably valid data on the actual number of teeth within a population group (Ueno et al., 2010). Furthermore, self-reported data would be used for measuring oral health conditions in populations at lower cost, less resource involvement and within shorter timeframes (Jones et al., 2001). Due to the limited budget and the deadline for the completion of the study, performing a clinical examination was not feasible in this study.

We found an inverse relationship between SROH and SRH. Although many studies suggest that the individuals who reported good/excellent oral health are more likely to report good/excellent general health (Atchison & Gift, 1997; Benyamini et al., 2004; Okunseri et al., 2008a,b), we found an inverse relationship between SROH and SRH. This result is consistent with previous studies suggesting that there is a deficit in perceptions of oral health relative to general health at all stages of adulthood and spanning the socio-economic spectrum (Sanders & Slade, 2006). Oral health and general health appear to be mostly unrelated in healthy population, because oral health and general health have different determinants (Kieffer & Hoogstraten, 2008).

In addition to material and behavioral factors, psychosocial factors may mediate the link between individual socio-economic status and health (Finlayson et al., 2010, Locker, 2009; Poortinga et al, 2008). Thus, many studies have examined the association between psychosocial factors (e.g.self-esteem, life satisfaction, stress, self-confidence, self-liking, self-competence, perfectionism, sense of cohesion, depression, resilience, social support) and oral health in adults (Benyamini et al., 2004; Finlayson et al., 2010; Locker, 2009; Martins et al., 2011; Wu et al., 2011). There are a few studies that have examined the relationship between personal control and SROH (Finlayson et al., 2010, Sanders & Spencer, 2005). In this study, the Multidimensional Oral Health LOC Scale was used to measure beliefs about adults' control over oral health (Peker & Bermek., 2011). The relationship between the SROH and LOC beliefs has been investigated only in a few studies (Kent et al., 1984; Peker & Bermek, 2011). Consistent with these studies, we also found that adults with high Dentist LOC and low Chance LOC were more likely to report good SROH. The findings of a recent study in Istanbul adults (Peker& Bermek, 2011) support the results of prior studies that health beliefs may mediate the link between individual socio-economic status and health (Broadbent et al., 2006; Butani et al., 2008, , Kiyak,1993; Poortinga et al., 2008). It is known that oral health beliefs influence adult's oral health behavior and self-ratings of oral health (Broadbent et al., 2006; Butani et al., 2008, , Kiyak,1993). Numerous studies showed that LOC beliefs were strongly associated with general and oral health behaviors (Bailey et al., 1981; Borkowska et al., 1998; Grotz et al., 2011; Mangelsdorff & Brush, 1978; Norman et al., 1998; Peker & Bermek, 2011, Steptoe & Wardle, 2001). Individuals who have strong beliefs in Internal control and in the control of Powerful others and weak beliefs in Chance control are likely to develop advantageous health behavior (Grotz et al., 2011; Norman et al., 1998; Peker & Bermek, 2011, , Steptoe & Wardle, 2001). An understanding of the role of oral health beliefs on self-ratings oral health may be useful in the design of oral health promotion programs and it provides clear guidance to assist oral health professionals to promote favorable oral health behaviors in their patients (Butani et al., 2008; Gilbert et al., 1998; Holt et al.,2003; Lee etal., 1993; Nakazono et al., 1997; Peker & Bermek, 2011).

The results of multivariate analyses showed that good SROH was strongly associated with regular dental attendance, older age, a higher Dentist LOC beliefs and a lower Chance LOC beliefs. The final model explained 52.4 % of the variance in good SROH (Nagelkerke's R2 = 0.524). Two components of the Multidimensional Oral Health LOC Scale were predictors of good SROH among Istanbul adults. This is in contrast to a previous study that suggests that oral health beliefs represent a distinct dimension which may not be critical to a study of perceived oral health (Atchison &Gif, 1997).

4.1 Limitations of the study and implications for future research

There are several limitations to this study that should be considered in the interpretation of the results. This study did not include clinical measures and examinations by dentists, and therefore the results pertain only to the associations found between self-reports of oral health. Thus, future studies are needed to evaluate the relationships between the clinical measures and self-reported oral health measures in adult population. Future study is needed to assess the validity and reproducibility of self-reported oral health (Pinelli & de Castro Monteiro Loffredo, 2007). Data were collected via self-report questionnaires, which might have introduced a "social desirability" bias. The cross-sectional design did not explain causation and changes over time in SROH. However, it does suggest future research questions on the development of the model of SROH in adults. Longitudinal studies would increase the knowledge on determinants of SROH further. Due to the cross-sectional nature of the data, the time sequence between some covariates and oral health was not well defined. There may be unmeasured factors such as cultural attitudes toward oral health and dental care, oral health outcomes, clinical status, psychological factors, and institutional barriers that could contribute to the differences in SROH among populations. We used the composite SES index to measure the socio-economic status of respondents. Some studies of SES and health have suggested that income is the best SES predictor of the SRH and SROH (Locker, 2009; Nummela et al., Sanders et al., 2006, von dem Knesebeck et al., 2003). Thus, future studies are needed to examine the association between income and SROH.

Further qualitative studies are needed to investigate the referents and meanings that underlie SROH and to examine the relationship between SROH and SRH among adults.

To measure the clinical, functional and psychosocial outcomes of oral disorders, future studies should be focused on the relation of SROH to the clinical measures and comprehensive subjective oral health measures. In addition, future studies using a combined measure of perceived need of any dental care may provide more detailed information about the relationship among SROH, self-perceived need for treatment and oral functional limitation (Seremidi et al., 2009).

5. Conclusions

This study is one of the first to examine a global rating of oral health among Istanbul adults aged 18 years and over using a a representative quota sample. Almost half of the study sample rated their oral health as bad. Older age, regular dental visit, a higher Dentist LOC beliefs and a lower Chance LOC beliefs are significantly associated with good SROH. Oral health programs and services should not only target treatments for dental disease, but should also include component that determine the subjective evaluation of oral health conditions of adults affected by cultural health beliefs, socio-demographic and behavioral factors. There is no oral health policy emphasizing prevention-oriented dental care and regular dental visit in Turkey. The results of this study could provide helpful information for oral health professionals to develop national oral health policy. Taking into account the oral health LOC beliefs that reinforce a good SROH may help the oral health professionals and dental health educators to develop health promotion programs. Age – specific oral health education and promotion programs is a good starting point for increasing oral health awareness and knowledge about the associations between oral and general health as well as improving regular dental attendance of Istanbul adults.

6. Acknowledgement

The data used in this paper were derived from my doctoral dissertation; I would like to thank my dissertation committee of Gülçin Bermek, Mustafa Şenocak and Nesrin Hisli Şahin for their advice and comments. I thank Mr. Necdet Süt and Dr. Ömer Uysal for their help with the statistical analysis and to Mr. Taner Gönç for his help processing and collecting data. This study was financially supported by the Istanbul University Research Foundation (Grant no. T-217 / 06032003).

7. References

Abelsen, B. (2008). What a difference a place makes: Dental attendance and self-rated oral health among adults in three counties in Norway. *Health & Place*, Vol.14, No.4, pp.829–840, ISSN 1353-8292

Akarslan, Z.Z.; Sadik, B.; Sadik, E.& Erten, H. (2008). Dietary habits and oral health related behaviors in relation to DMFT indexes of a group of young adult patients attending a dental school. *Medicina Oral Patologia Oral y Cirugia,* Vol.13, No.12, pp. E800-E807, ISSN:1698-4447

Andersen, R. M. (1995) Revisiting the behavioral model and access to medical care: Does it matter? *Journal of Health and Social Behavior*, Vol. 36, No.1,pp. 1-10, ISSN 0022-1465

Andersen, R.M.& Davidson, P.L.(1997). Ethnicity, aging, and oral health outcomes: A conceptual framework. *Advances in Dental Research*, Vol.11, No.2, pp.203–209. ISSN:0895-9374

Araújo, C.S.; Lima Rda, C.; Peres, M.A.& Barros, A.J.(2009). Use of dental services and associated factors: a population-based study in southern Brazil. *Cadernos de saúde pública*, Vol. 25, No.5, pp.1063-1072, ISSN 0102-311X

Arnljot, H.A.; Barnes, D.E.; Cohen, L.K.; Hunter, P.B.V.& Ship I.I.(1985). *Oral health care systems: an international collaborative study*, Quintessence Publishing Company Ltd, ISBN 9781850970019, London, England.

Arslan, A.; Orhan, K.; Canpolat, C.; Delilbasi, C.& Dural, S. (2009). Impact of xerostomia on oral complaints in a group of elderly Turkish removable denture wearers. *Archives of Gerontology and Geriatrics*, Vol.49, No.2, pp.263-267, ISSN 0167-4943

Atchison, K.A. & Andersen, R.M. (2000). Demonstrating Successful Aging Using the International Collaborative Study for Oral Health Outcomes. *Journal of Public Health Dentistry*, Vol.60, No.4, pp: 282-288, ISSN 0022-4006

Atchison, K.A.& Gift, H.C. (1997). Perceived oral health in a diverse sample. *Advances in Dental Research*, Vol.11, No.2, pp.:272-280, ISSN 0895-9374

Axelsson, G& Helgadottir, S. (1995). Comparison of oral health data from self-administered questionnaire and clinical examination. *Community Dentistry and Oral Epidemiology,* Vol. 23, No.6, pp. 365–368, ISSN 0301-5661

Bailey, C.; Dey, F.; Reynolds, K.; Rutter, G.; Teoh, T. & Peck, C. (1981). What are the variables related to dental compliance? *Australian Dental Journal,* Vol. 26, No.1, pp. 46–48, ISSN 0045-0421

Baker, S.R. (2009). Applying Andersen's behavioural model to oral health: what are the contextual factors shaping perceived oral health outcomes? *Community Dentistry and Oral Epidemiology,* Vol.37, No.6, pp.485-494, ISSN 0301-5661

Baran, I.& Nalcaci, R . (2011). Self-reported problems before and after prosthodontic treatments according to newly created Turkish version of oral health impact profile. *Archives of Gerontology and Geriatrics,* Vol.53,No.2, pp.e99-e105, ISSN 0167-4943

Bennett, I.M.; Chen, J.; Soroui, J.S. & White, S.(2009). The contribution of health literacy to disparities in self-rated health status and preventive health behaviors in older adults. *Annals of Family Medicine,* Vol.7, No.3, pp.204-211, ISSN 1544-1709

Benyamini,Y.; Leventhal, H.& Leventhal, E.A.(2004). Self-rated oral health as an independent predictor of self- rated general health, self-esteem and life satisfaction. *Social science & medicine,* Vol.59, No.5, pp.1109–1116, ISSN 0277-9536

Borkowska, E.D.; Watts, T.L.P.& Weinman, J. (1998). The relationship of health beliefs and psychological mood to patient adherence to oral hygiene behaviour. *Journal of Clinical Periodontology,* Vol. 25, No.3, pp. 187-193, ISSN 0303-6979

Borrell, L.N. & Baquero, M.C. (2011). Self-rated general and oral health in New York City adults: assessing the effect of individual and neighborhood social factors. *Community Dentistry and Oral Epidemiology,* Vol.39, No.4, pp.361-371, ISSN 0301-5661

Broadbent, J.M.; Thomson, W.M. & Poulton, R. (2006). Oral health beliefs in adolescence and oral health in young adulthood. *Journal of Dental Research,* Vol. 85, No.4,pp.339-343, ISSN 0022-0345

Butani, Y.; Weintraub, J.A. & Barker, J.C. (2008). Oral health-related cultural beliefs for four racial/ethnic groups: assessment of the literature. *BioMed Central Oral Health,* Vol. 8, Available from http://www.biomedcentral.com/1472-6831/8/26

Caglayan, F.; Altun, O.; Miloglu, O.; Kaya, M.D.& Yilmaz, A.B.(2009). Correlation between oral health-related quality of life (OHQoL) and oral disorders in a Turkish patient population. *Medicina Oral Patologia Oral y Cirugia,* Vol.14, No.11, pp. e573-578, ISSN:1698-4447

Camargo, M.B.; Dumith, S.C. & Barros, A.J. (2009). Regular use of dental care services by adults: patterns of utilization and types of services. *Cadernos de saúde pública,*Vol.25, No.9, pp. 1894-1906, ISSN 0102-311X

Carr, A.J.; Gibson, B. & Robinson, P.G. (2001). Measuring quality of life: Is quality of life defined by expectations or experience? *British Medical Journal,* Vol.322, No. 7296, pp. 1240-1243, ISSN 0959-8138

Chen, M.;Andersen, R.M.; Barmes, D.E.; Leclercq, M.H.& Lyttle, C.S. (1997). *Comparing oral healthcare systems,* World Health. Organization, *ISBN* 92-4-156188-2,Geneva,Switzerland.

Coulter, I.; Yamamoto, J.M.; Marcus, M.; Freed, J.; Der-Martirosian, C.; Guzman-Becerra, N.; Brown, L.J. & Guay, A. (2004). Self-reported oral health of enrollees in capitated and fee-for-service dental benefit plans. *The Journal of the American Dental Association*, Vol .135, No.11, pp. 1606-1615, ISSN 0002-8177

Dahl, K.E.; Wang, N.J.; Skau, I.& Ohrn, K.(2011). Oral health-related quality of life and associated factors in Norwegian adults. *Acta Odontologica Scandinavica*, Vol.69, No.4,pp.208-214, ISSN 0001-6357

Dolan, T.A.; Peek, C.W.; Stuckm, A.E. & Beck, J.C. (1998). Three – year changes in global oral health rating by elderly dentate adults. *Community Dentistry and Oral Epidemiology*, Vol. 26, No. 1, pp. 62–69, ISSN 0301-5661

Ekbäck, G.; Astrøm, A.N.; Klock, K.; Ordell, S. & Unell, L. (2009). Variation in subjective oral health indicators of 65-year-olds in Norway and Sweden. *Acta Odontologica Scandinavica*, Vol. 67, No. 4., pp. 222-232, ISSN 0001-6357

Finlayson, T.L.; Williams, D.R.; Siefert, K.; Jackson, J.S.& Nowjack-Raymer, R.(2010). Oral Health Disparities and Psychosocial Correlates of Self-Rated Oral Health in the National Survey of American Life. *American Journal of Public Health*, Vol.100, No.1,pp. 246–255, ISSN 0090-0036

Geckili, O.; Bilhan, H. & Bilgin, T. (2011). Impact of mandibular two-implant retained overdentures on life quality in a group of elderly Turkish edentulous patients. *Archives of Gerontology and Geriatrics*, Vol.53, No.2,pp.233-236, ISSN 0167-4943

Gift, H.C.; Atchison, K.A. & Drury, T.F. (1998). Perceptions of the natural dentition in the context of multiple variables. *Journal of Dental Research*, Vol.77, No. 7, pp.1529-1538, ISSN 0022-0345

Gilbert, G. H., Shelton, B. J., Scott Chavers, L., & Bradford, E. H. (2003). The paradox of dental need in a population-based study of dental adults. *Medical Care*,Vol. 41, No.1, pp. 119-134, ISSN 0025-7079

Gilbert, G.H.(2005). Racial and socioeconomic disparities in health from population-based research to practice-based research: the example of oral health. *Journal of Dental Education*, Vol.69,No.9,pp.1003-1014,ISSN 0022-0337

Gilbert, G.H.; Duncan, R.P.; Heft, M.W.; Dolan, T.A.& Vogel, W.B. (1998). Multidimensionality of Oral Health in Dentate Adults. *Medical Care*, Vol.36., No.7, pp.988-1001, ISSN 0025-7079

Gökalp, S.; Doğan, B.G.; Tekçiçek, M.; Berberoğlu, A. & Ünlüer, Ş. (2010). National survey of oral health status of children and adults in Turkey. *Community Dental Health*, Vol.27, No.1, pp. 12–17, ISSN 0256-539X

Grotz, M.; Hapke, U.; Lampert, T. & Baumeister, H. (2011). Health locus of control and health behaviour: results from a nationally representative survey. *Psychology, Health & Medicine*, Vol.16, No. 2, pp.129-140, ISSN 1354-8506

Holt, C.L.; Clark, E.M.; Kreuter, M.W. & Scharff, D.P. (2000). Does locus of control moderate the effects of tailored health education materials? *Health Education Research*, Vol. 15, No.4, pp. 393–403, ISSN 0268-1153

Jones, J.A.; Kressin, N.R.; Spiro A, 3rd.; Randall, C.W.; Miller, D.R.; Hayes, C.; Kazis, L. & Garcia, R.I. (2001). Self-reported and clinical oral health in users of VA health care. The journals of gerontology. Series A, *Biological Sciences and Medical Sciences*,Vol. 56, No.1,pp. M55-M62. ISSN:1079-5006

Kaplan, G. & Baron-Epel, O. (2003). What lies behind the subjective evaluation of health status? *Social Science & Medicine*, Vol .56, No.8, pp. 1669-1676, ISSN 0277-9536

Kargul, B. & Bakkal, M. (2010). Systems for the previsions of oral health care in the Black Sea countries Part 6: Turkey. *Journal of Oral Health and Dental Management,* Vol.9, No.3, pp. 115-121, ISSN 1583-5588

Kent, G.G.; Matthews, R.G. & White, F.H. (1984) Locus of control and oral health. *The Journal of the American Dental Association,*Vol. 109, No.1, pp. 67–69, ISSN 0002-8177

Kieffer, J.M.& Hoogstraten, J. (2008).Linking oral health, general health, and quality of life. *European Journal of Oral Sciences,* Vol.116, No.5, pp.445-450, ISSN 0909-8836.

Kim, H.Y.; Patton,L.L.& Park, Y.D. (2010). Assessment of predictors of global self-ratings of oral health among Korean adults aged 18-95 years. *Journal of Public Health Dentistry,*Vol.70,No.3,pp. 241–244, ISSN 0022-4006

Kiyak, H,A. (1993). Age and culture: influences on oral health behaviour. *International Dental Journal,* Vol. 43, No. 1, pp.9-16,ISSN 0020-6539

Krause, N.M. & Jay, G.M. (1994). What do global self-rated health items measure? *Medical Care,* Vol. 32, No.9, pp.930-942, ISSN 0025-7079

Lee, K.L.; Schwarz, E. & Mak, K.Y. (1993) Improving oral health through understanding the meaning of health and disease in a Chinese culture. *International Dental Journal ,* Vol. 43, No.1, pp.2-8, ISSN 0020-6539

Locker, D. & Gibson, B. (2005). Discrepancies between self-ratings of and satisfaction with oral health in two older adults populations. *Community Dentistry and Oral Epidemiology,* Vol. 33, No.4,pp.280–288, ISSN 0301-5661

Locker, D. (1988). Measuring oral health: a conceptual framework. *Community Dental Health,* Vol.5,No.1,pp.3-18,ISSN 0265-539X .

Locker, D. (1996). Applications of self-reported assessments of oral health outcomes. *Journal of Dental Education,* Vol.60, No.6, pp. 494–500, ISSN 0022-0337

Locker, D. (2009). Self-esteem and socioeconomic disparities in self-perceived oral health. *Journal of Public Health Dentistry,* Vol.69, No.1, pp.1-8, ISSN 0022-4006 .

Locker, D.& Miller, Y. (1994). Subjectively reported oral health status in an adult population. *Community Dentistry and Oral Epidemiology,* Vol. 22,No.6, pp.425–430,ISSN 0301-5661

Locker, D.; Maggirias, J. & Wexler, E. (2009). What frames of reference underlie self-ratings of oral health? *Journal of Public Health Dentistry,* Vol.69,No.2,pp.78-89,ISSN 0022-4006

Locker, D.; Wexler, E. & Jokovic, A. (2005). What do older adults' global self-ratings of oral health measure? *Journal of Public Health Dentistry,* Vol.65,No.3,pp.146–152, ISSN 0022-4006

Lundegren, N.; Axtelius, B.; Akerman, S.; Perera, I. &, Ekanayake, L. (2011) Self perceived oral health, oral treatment need and the use of oral health care of the adult population in Skåne, Sweden. *Swedish Dental Journal,* Vol.35, No. 2, pp. 89-98, ISSN 0347-9994

Mangelsdorff, A.D. & Brush, W.A. (1978) Locus of control as a predictor of dental care requirements. *The Journal of Preventive Dentistry,* Vol. 5, No.5, pp. 29–30, ISSN 0096-2732

Martins, A.B.; Dos Santos, C.M.; Hilgert, J.B.; de Marchi, R.J.; Hugo, F.N.& Pereira Padilha, D.M.(2011). Resilience and self-perceived oral health: a hierarchical approach. *Journal of the American Geriatrics Society,* Vol.59,No.4,pp.725-731,ISSN 002-8614.

Martins, A.M.; Barreto, S.M. & Pordeus, I.A. (2009) Objective and subjective factors related to self-rated oral health among the elderly. *Cadernos de Saúde Pública*, Vol.25, No 2, pp. 421-435, ISSN 0102-311X

Martins, A.M; Barreto, S.M.; Silveira, M.F.; Santa-Rosa, T.T.& Pereira, R,D. (2010). Self-perceived oral health among Brazilian elderly individuals. *Revista de Saúde Pública*,Vol.44,No.5,pp.912-922,ISSN 0034-8910

Matos, D.L.& Lima-Costa, M.F. (2006).Self-rated oral health among Brazilian adults and older adults in Southeast Brazil: results from the SB-Brasil Project, 2003. *Cadernos de Saúde Pública*,Vol.22,No.8,pp.1699-1707,ISSN 0102-311X

Matthias, R.E.; Atchison, K.A; Lubben, J.E.; De Jong, F. & Schweitzer, S.O. (1995). Factors affecting self-ratings of oral health. *Journal of Public Health Dentistry*, Vol. 55, No.4, pp. 197-204, ISSN 0022-4006

Maupomé, G.; Peters, D. & White, B.A. (2004). Use of clinical services compared with patients' perceptions of and satisfaction with oral health status. *Journal of Public Health Dentistry*,Vol. 64, No.2, pp.88–95, ISSN 0022-4006

Nakazono, T.T.; Davidson, P.L. & Andersen, R.M. (1997). Oral health beliefs in diverse populations. *Advances in Dental Research*, Vol.11, No. 2, pp. 235-244, ISSN 0895-9374

Namal, N.; Can, G.; Vehid, S.; Koksal, S.& Kaypmaz, A. (2008). Dental health status and risk factors for dental caries in adults in Istanbul, Turkey. *Eastern Mediterranean Health Journal*, Vol.14, No.1,pp.110-118, ISSN1020-3397

Norman, P.; Bennet, P.; Smith, C. & Murphy, S. (1998). Health Locus of Control and Health Behaviour. *Journal of Health Psychology*, Vol. 3, No. 2, pp.171- 180, ISSN 1359-1053

Nummela, O.P.; Sulander, T.T., Heinonen, H.S. & Uutela, A.K. (2007). Self-rated health and indicators of SES among the ageing in three types of communities. *Scandinavian Journal of Public Health*, Vol.35, No.1, pp. 39-47, ISSN 1403-4948

Ojofeitimi, E.O.; Adedigba, M.A.; Ogunbodede, E.O.; Fajemilehin, B.R. & Adegbehingbe, B.O. (2007). Oral health and the elderly in Nigeria: a case for oral health promotion. *Gerodontology*, Vol. 24, No.4, pp.231-234, ISSN 0734-0664

Okunseri, C.; Hodges, J.S. & Born, D.O. (2008a). Self-reported oral health perceptions of Somali adults in Minnesota: a pilot study. *International Journal of Dental Hygiene*,Vol.6,No.2,pp.114-118,ISSN 1601-5029

Okunseri, C.; Yang, M.; Gonzalez, C.; LeMay, W.& Iacopino, A.M. (2008b). Hmong adults self-rated oral health: a pilot study. *Journal of Immigrant and Minority Health* , Vol.10,No.1,pp.81-88,ISSN 1557-1912

Ostberg, A.L.& Hall-Lord, M.L.(2011). Oral health-related quality of life in older Swedish people with pain problems. *Scandinavian Journal of Caring Sciences*, Vol.25, No.3,pp.510-516, ISSN 0283-9318.

Ozdemir, H.; Alper, Z.; Uncu, Y. &, Bilgel, N. (2010). Health literacy among adults: a study from Turkey. *Health Education Research*, Vol.25, No.3, pp.464-477, ISSN 0268-1153

Oztürk, L.K.; Furuncuoğlu, H.; Atala, M.H.; Uluköylü, O.; Akyüz, S.& Yarat A. (2008). Association between dental-oral health in young adults and salivary glutathione, lipid peroxidation and sialic acid levels and carbonic anhydrase activity. *Brazilian Journal of Medical and Biological Research*, Vol. 41, No.11,pp.956-959, ISSN 0100-879X

Parker, E.J. & Jamieson, L.M. (2010). Associations between indigenous Australian oral health literacy and self-reported oral health outcomes. *BioMed Central Oral Health*, Vol. 10, Available from http://www.biomedcentral.com/1472-6831/10/3

Pattussi, M.P.; Peres, K.G.; Boing, A.F.; Peres, M.A.& da Costa, J.S.(2010). Self-rated oral health and associated factors in Brazilian elders. *Community Dentistry and Oral Epidemiology*,Vol.38,No.4,pp.348-359, ISSN 0301-5661

Pavi, E.; Karampli, E.; Zavras, D.; Dardavesis, T. & Kyriopoulos, J. (2010). Social determinants of dental health services utilisation of Greek adults. *Community Dentistry and Oral Epidemiology*, Vol. 27, No. 3, pp.145-150, ISSN 0301-5661

Peek, C.W.; Gilbert, G.H.; Duncan, R.P.; Heft, M.W. & Henretta, J.C. (1999). Patterns of change in self-reported oral health among dentate adults. *Medical Care*, Vol. 37, No.12, pp.1237–1248, ISSN 0025-7079

Peker, K. & Bermek, G.(2011). Oral health: locus of control, health behavior, self-rated oral health and socio-demographic factors in Istanbul adults. *Acta Odontologica Scandinavica*, Vol.69, No.1,pp.54-64, ISSN 0001-6357

Petersen, P.E. & Yamamoto, T. (2005). Improving the oral health of older people: the approach of the WHO Global Oral Health Programme. *Community Dentistry and Oral Epidemiology*; Vol.33, No.2, pp.81-92, ISSN 0301-5661

Petersen, P.E.; Aleksejuniene, J.; Christensen, L.B.; Eriksen, H.M. & Kalo, I. (2000). Oral health behavior and attitudes of adults in Lithuania. *Acta Odontologica Scandinavica*, Vol. 58, No. 6, pp. 243-248, ISSN 0001-6357

Pinelli, C. & de Castro Monteiro Loffredo,L. (2007). Reproducibility and validity of self-perceived oral health conditions. *Clinical Oral Investigations*, Vol.11,No.4,pp.431-437,ISSN 1432-6981

Pitiphat, W.; Garcia, R.; Douglass, C. & Joshipura, K. (2002). Validation of self-reported oral health measures. *Journal of Public Health Dentistry*, Vol. 62, No. 2, pp. 122–128, ISSN 0022-4006

Poortinga, W.; Dunstan, F.D. & Fone, D.L. (2008). Health locus of control beliefs and socio-economic differences in self-rated health. *Preventive Medicine*, Vol.46, No. 4, pp. 374-380, ISSN 0091-7435

Reisine, S.T. & Bailit, H.L. (1980). Clinical oral health status and adult perceptions of oral health. *Social Science and Medicine*, Vol.14A, No.6, pp. 597-605, ISSN 0160-7979

Sanders, A.E. & Slade, G.D. (2006). Deficits in perceptions of oral health relative to general health in populations. *Journal of Public Health Dentistry*, Vol. 66, No. 4, pp. 255-62, ISSN 0022-4006

Sanders, A.E.& Spencer, A.J.(2005). Why do poor adults rate their oral health poorly? *Australian Dental Journal*, Vol.50,No.3,pp.161-167, ISSN 0045-0421

Sanders, A.E.; Slade, G.D.; Turrell, G.; John Spencer, A. & Marcenes, W. (2006). The shape of the socioeconomic-oral health gradient: implications for theoretical explanations. *Community Dentistry and Oral Epidemiology*, Vol.34, No. 4, pp. 310-319, ISSN 0301-5661

Seremidi, K.; Koletsi-Kounari, H. & Kandilorou, H.(2009). Self-reported and clinically-diagnosed dental needs: determining the factors that affect subjective assessment. *Oral Health & Preventive Dentistry*, Vol.7, No. 2, pp. 183-190, ISSN 1602-1622

Steptoe, A. & Wardle, J. (2001). Locus of control and health behaviour revisited: a multivariate analysis of young adults from 18 countries. *British Journal of Psychology*, Vol. 92, No.4 , pp. 659-672, ISSN 0007-1269

Thomson, W.M.; Williams, S.M.; Broadbent, J.M.; Poulton, R. & Locker, D. (2010). Long-term dental visiting patterns and adult oral health. *Journal of Dental Research*, Vol. 89, No. 3, pp. 307-311, ISSN 0022-0345

Tüzün, S. (2000). Kentsel Türkiye Hane ve Bireyleri İçin Bir Tabakalaşma Modeli Olarak Veri Sosyo-ekonomik Statü İndeksi (VERİ S.E.S.İ.). İçinde: *Mübeccel Kıray İçin Yazılar*, Atacan F, Ercan F, Kurtuluş H & Türkay M, (Eds.), pp. 371-385, Bağlam Yayıncılık, ISBN 9756947446, Istanbul, Türkiye

Ueno, M.; Zaitsu, T.; Shinada, K.; Ohara, S. & Kawaguchi, Y. (2010). Validity of the self-reported number of natural teeth in Japanese adults. *Journal of Investigative and Clinical Dentistry*, VOl.1,No.2,pp. 79–84, ISSN 2041-1626

Ugarte, J.; Abe, Y., Fukuda, H.; Honda, S.; Takamura, N.; Kobuke, Y.; Ye, Z.; Aoyagi, K.; Mendoza, O. & Shinsho, F. (2007). Self-perceived oral health status and influencing factors of the elderly residents of a peri-urban area of La Paz, Bolivia. *International Dental Journal*, Vol. 57, No. 1, pp. 19-26, ISSN 0020-6539

Unell, L.; Soderfeldt, B.; Halling, A.; Paulander, J. & Birkhed, D. (1997). Oral disease, impairment, and illness: congruence between clinical and questionnaire findings. *Acta Odontologica Scandinavica*, Vol. 55, No.2, pp. 127–132, ISSN 0001-6357

Unlüer, S.; Gökalp, S. & Doğan, B.G. (2007). Oral health status of the elderly in a residential home in Turkey. *Gerodontology*, Vol. 24, No.1, pp.22-29, ISSN:0734-0664

von dem Knesebeck, O.; Lüschen, G.; Cockerham, W.C. & Siegrist, J. (2003). Socioeconomic status and health among the aged in the United States and Germany: a comparative cross-sectional study. *Social Science and Medicine* , Vol. 57, No. 9, pp. 1643-1652, ISSN 0160-7979

Woolfolk, M. W., Lang, W. P., Borgnakke, W.S., Taylor, G. W., & Nyquist, L. W. (1999). Determining dental checkup frequency. *Journal of the American Dental Association*, Vol. 130, No.5, pp. 715-723, ISSN 0002-8177

Wu, B.; Plassman, B.L.; Liang, J.; Remle, R.C.; Bai, L.&Crout, R.J.(2011). Differences in self-reported oral health among community-dwelling black, Hispanic, and white elders. *Journal of Aging and Health*, Vol. 23, No.2, pp.267-288,ISSN 0898-2643

12

Krill Enzymes (Krillase®) an Important Factor to Improve Oral Hygiene

Kristian Hellgren
Specialistkliniken, Helsingborg
Sweden

1. Introduction

Prevention of gingivitis is largely governed by limiting the development of oral dental plaque and biofilm formation. It is also broadly acknowledged that accumulation of microorganisms are of pivotal importance in the initiation and progression of gingivitis and associated oral diseases (Socransky, Haffajee, 2005). We propose that krill enzymes (Krillase®) as they disintegrate cell surface structures and diminish bacterial adhesion to be a novel and innovative method for prevention of gingivitis.

Krillase® is isolated from the digestive tract of Antarctic krill (*Euphausia superba*), a shrimp like animal constituting an enormous biomass in the Antarctic convergence. The harsch ecological situation in the Antarctica implies that krill has an exceptionally effective digestive apparatus containing a co-operative multi-enzyme system involving both endo- and exopeptidases. Moreover, these enzymes have much lower activation energies than those of mammalian enzymes ensuring fast and highly efficient breakdown of diverse biological substrates (Hellgren et al, 1999).

The objective for the development of Krillase® has been to maintain the natural composition of krill enzymes intact throughout the purification process. Krillase® is defined as a mixture of acidic endopeptidases (trypsin- and chymotrypsin-like enzymes) and exopeptidases (carboxypeptidase A and B).

The final product (chewing gum) is well characterized with respect to stability, enzyme activity, uniformity and biocompability. Data from toxicology, pharmacology, pre- resp clinical studies give evidence for a broad safety profile.

Krill enzymes, due to their unique synergistic action, have been proven to exert both quantitative and qualitative effects on dental plaque/biofilm as well as on bacterial adherence to teeth surfaces. This leads to significant decrease in plaque accumulation and reduction in occurrence of gingivitis and caries pathogenesis (Hellgren, 2009).

In summary, Krillase® constitutes an important future alternative to a variety of other more toxic chemicals presently marketed for oral use including bisguanid, triclosan, aminoalcohols.

2. Clinical studies

In our recent study the effect of Krillase® chewing gum on gingival inflammation and dental plaque formation was investigated (Hellgren, 2009). Ten healthy volunteers aged 21-

45 (average age 22.4 yrs) chewed Krillase for 10 minutes after each ?meal in conjunction with normal oral hygiene measures. The test chewing gums contained either 6.0 or 0.06U of Krillase ® versus placebo, and were chewed four times a day during a 10 day test period. In a double-blind cross-over design, each participant concluded three consecutive trial periods for each gum The severity of gingival bleeding was measured by probing gingival pockets at selected teeth including first molar and forward in each jaw, initially and after each test period. In parallel a plaque index was established.

A therapeutic dose of 0.06U Krillase in the chewing gum reduced the mean gingival bleeding index by 54% compared to baseline ($p < 0.05$) and significantly better ($p < 0.05$) than the placebo gums reduction of 21% compared to baseline. Also the Mean Simplified Debris Index which measures (Green, Vermillion, 1964) decreased by 60% from its initial status for the 0.06U Krillase® gum ($p < 0.05$) and 14% as compared to placebo gum. The high dose (Krillase®, 6.0U) did not improve the efficacy. There was no significant statistical difference between the Krillase® gums and placebo on the Simplified Debris Index. None of the subjects reported any adverse reactions or events during the entire trial period. The chewing gum was reported to be neutral in taste. This study verified that a process of pathogenic plaque formation is disturbed by Krillase®, possibly via disruption of oral biofim and affecting adhesive properties of the oral bacteria. This, results in a numerical decrease of plaque formation and a significant reduction of gingival bleeding compared to a placebo chewing gum.

Krillase® profile and mode of action is well adopted to improve gingival health. These clinical data clearly illustrate the superiority of Krillase® compared to placebo gums.

Placebo gums, however, also diminish the number of gingival bleeding sites, something that might be associated both to the mechanical effect of chewing gum as well as to the known placebo phenomenon like unconscious awareness of oral hygiene of study participants.

These findings are in adherence with previous in pre- and clinical studies demonstrating that Krillase® disintegrates bacterial surface adhesive proteins and hampers colonization of dental surfaces (Hahn Berg, 2003).

In another study (Hellgren, unpublished data) we demonstrated that a less voluminous plaque and bleeding were observed on teeth treated with Krillase® gum than placebo both in short (5 days) and long term (14 days) perspective.

The patients in this double-blind crossover study had initially healthy gingival condition provided by professional cleansing in dental office in conjunction with thorough oral hygiene instructions. Thereafter each patient was given chewing gum (Krillase® gum or placebo gum) to be chewed five times a day for 10 min after the meals. During the test period of 5 or 14 days, the patients were instructed to eat normally but to restrain from any other oral hygiene measures apart from the prescribed chewing gums. After the first test period the baseline is restored and the patient started with the test period 2. The same procedure is then repeated for the third test period. Plaque index (PLI), gingival bleeding (BOP) and photographs were performed after each the test period and compared with the baseline values (Löe, Sillnes, 1963; Löe et al 1965; Löe1967).

At the end of each test period (day 5 or 14) the teeth's were dyed with Diaplaque® (coloring plaque as red), clinical evaluations as well as photographing were performed.

In addition to the usual and somewhat subjective clinical evaluations performed by independent observers such as dentists or hygienists, we also included a quantitative imaged based assay in this study. Clinical evaluations are normally both time consuming and subjective, therefore further evaluations were performed by advanced computerized image analyses to objectively quantify the color differences in plaque formation and extension in the test photographs. To normalize all photographs before analysis a reference mm/gray scale in every photograph was used as an internal standard. Based on the reference scale the photos are corrected both for the geometric and photometric distortions. Thus, the reference gray scale in the photos makes it possible to recreate the original color reflectance values in each pixel in spite of variations in color temperature of the illumination, photographic emulsion and other factors, which cannot be fully controlled. The resulting data gave an accurate account of plaque extension in each particular tooth. Both subjective observer based evaluations and objective computerized analyses of standardized clinical photographs confirmed that patients chewing Krillase® chewing gum clearly formed less plaque than when chewing placebo gums after in 5 as well as 14 days trials. Some results are shown in **Figures 1-2**.

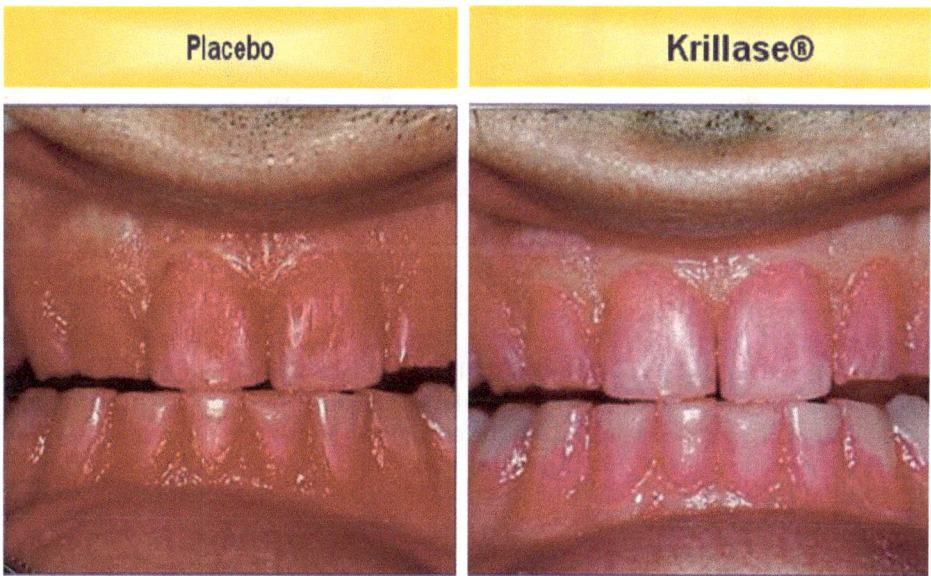

Fig. 1. Dental plaque extension after 14 days of treatment

Dental plaque development is closely associated with gingivitis and caries. Krillase® broad enzyme specificity in combination with its low autolysis warranted further studies on microbial adhesion in the oral cavity. SEM on *in vitro* plaque visualized that Krillase® significantly reduced the number of adhering microorganisms (Hahn Berg et al, 2001). These findings were further confirmed by elipsometry (Hahn Berg, 2003) data. The observed modifications of salivary and microbial proteins by Krillase® resulted in overall decrease of oral microflora abilities to attach. These findings are also supported by *in vivo* plaque study where Krillase® clearly detached microorganism from plaque accumulated on dentures (Hahn Berg, 2003).

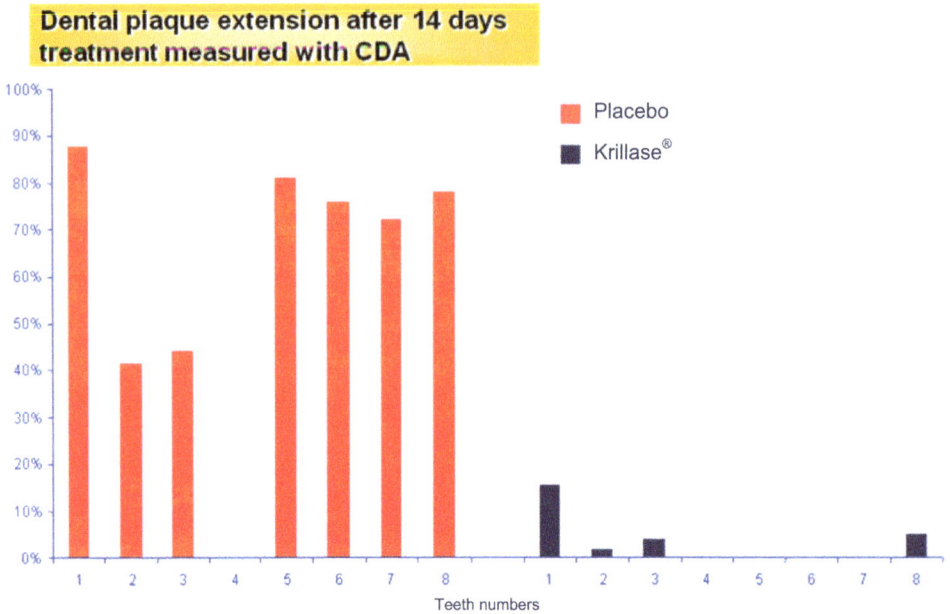

Fig. 2. Dental plaque extension after 14 days of treatment measured with CDA

Furthermore, our results also reveals that dental plaque exposed to carbohydrates in the presence of Krillase® looses most of its ability to produce acids causing the characteristic pH drop. The mechanism behind this phenomenon is unknown, but merits further and future investigations.

Another important observation is that krill enzymes besides counteracting bacterial adhesion does not alter the normal oral microflora, in contrast to the action of chlorhexidine or antibiotics. This is important since the current opinion is that oral ecosystem should not be altered by dental products. By disintegrating cell surface protein structures and in this way limiting bacterial adhesion, Krillase® treatment results in significant reduction of plaque accumulation and improves gingivits.

3. Discussion

Microorganisms continuously colonize oral surfaces forming initially dental plaque. The toxic products from plaque bacteria, like lactic acid from digested carbohydrates, induce local inflammation, gingivitis, periodontitis leading to caries and ultimately to tooth loss. Mechanical removal of plaque is still the most efficient way to prevent its accumulation and consequently development of dental diseases. A number of agents such as desinfectants/antiseptica (chlorhexidine, triclosan, herbal extracts), surfactants (sodium lauryl sulphate), sugar substitutes (xylitol) and enzymes (dextranases) are used for prevention against caries.

We have shown that Krillase® disruption of dental biofilm (pellicle) associated with diminished bacterial adherence to oral surfaces successfully prevents plaque formation and gingival inflammation. These findings are supported by a series of both *in vitro* data as well as clinical studies.

A therapeutic dose of 0.06U of Krillase® was sufficient as complement to normal oral hygiene. A dramatic reduction in number of gingival bleeding sites as well as the plaque index was noted when chewing Krillase® gums were compared to initial status. The higher dose does not seem to improve the efficacy, in line with our earlier *in vitro* observations pointing to a substrate-enzyme dependency.

Another study further corroborate these results where less plaque and bleeding were observed on teeth treated with Krillase® gum compared to a placebo gum both in short (five days) and longer term (14 days). Krillase® plaque retarding effect was documented in patients with baseline washout using professional cleaning and the refraining from any oral hygiene for 10-14 days.

These clinical findings confirm the previous observations demonstrating that Krillase® efficiently remove fimbriae from the cell surface of plaque bacteria as well as detach them from dentures worn by patients.

To conclude, we propose that regular chewing Krillase® gum represent a novel and valid strategy to prevent plaque formation and gingivitis consequently improving general oral hygiene. Being highly biocompatible and with no side effects, Krillase® constitutes a promising candidate for modern preventive oral care.

4. References

[1] Socransky SS, Haffajee AD, Periodontal microbiology ecology, *Periodontal 2005; 38: 135-187*

[2] Hellgren L, Karlstam B, Mohr V, Vincent J, Peptide hydrolases from Antarctic krill – an important new tool with a promising medical potential, *In Biotechnological applications of cold-adapted organisms, p 63-74; eds R Margesin, F Schinner, Springer Verl Berlin Heidelberg 1999*

[3] Hellgren K Assessment of Krillase® chewing gum for the reduction of gingivitis and dental plaque, *J Clin Dent 20:99-102, 2009*

[4] Hellgren K, Efficacy of Krillase® chewing gum on gingivitis and dental plaque formation, *Unpublished data*

[5] Greene JC, Vermillion JR, The simplified oral hygiene index, *J Amer Dent Assoc 68: 7-13, 1964*

[6] Löe H, Silness J, Periodontal disease in pregnancy: I. Prevalence and severity, *Acta Odontologica Scand 21: 533-551, 1963*

[7] Löe H, Theilade E, Jensen SB, Experimental gingivitis in man, *J Periodont 36: 177-187, 1965*

[8] Löe H, Oral hygiene in the prevention of caries and periodontal disease, *Int Dent J 50: 129-139, 2000*

[9] Löe H, The gingival index, the plaque index and the retention index systems, *J Periodontol 38: 610-616, 1967*

[10] Hahn Berg C, Kalfas S, Malmsten M, Arnebrant T, Proteolytic degradation of oral biofilms *in vitro* and *in vivo*: potential of proteases originating from *Euphausia superba* for plaque control, *Eur J Oral Sci 109: 316-324, 2001*

[11] Hahn-Berg CI, Properties of interfacial proteinaceous films with emphasis on oral systems, *PhD thesis, Inst Surface Chem, Stockholm and Dept Food Technol, Lund University, Lund, 2003*

13

Towards Oral Health Promotion

José Roberto de Magalhães Bastos et al.*

University of São Paulo/ Faculty of Dentistry at Bauru

Brazil

1. Introduction

What is the concept of health? What is oral health? What is the concept of health and oral health promotion? Is there a prescription to follow for any individual or a population? Can this universal prescription be refined to serve both developed and developing countries as well as populations with social deprivation characteristics? Many other questions could be raised before the discussion of oral health promotion or health promotion, yet the fact is that oral health is an important part of general health (1). Previous studies have thoroughly documented the association between oral health and other health conditions as well as also oral health's relation to quality of life (2, 3). However, health promotion cannot be targeted to only health sector efforts; intersectorial actions are necessary to make oral health more affordable. Therefore, it is not possible to improve oral health without assembling the evolution of the concept of health promotion.

2. Oral health

Would it be possible to conduct oral health promotion on a regular basis? In the first place, the concept of health and oral health should be clear to as many professionals as possible. The internationally accepted definition of the World Health Organization is a good start for clarification, because in the preamble of its constitution, it describes health as "a state of complete physical, mental and social well-being and not merely the absence of disease and infirmity" (4).

The primary concern must be professionals' idea of health as more than the absence of disease, and to do so, it is necessary for professionals to understand what would be classified as a disease or as infirmity. Although this chapter does not aim to delve deeply into the philosophy of health, illness and disease, it can help readers to understand disease overall as a disturbance in the balance of the health-disease process.

The complete state of physical, mental and social well-being would be too hard to explain in full to a person; nevertheless, this must be considered a target to health promotion practitioners. Consider this issue as a gradient of health wherein these three dimensions

*Magali de Lourdes Caldana[1], Luis Marcelo Aranha Camargo[2], Ariadnes Nobrega Oliveira[1], Ricardo Pianta Rodrigues da Silva[3], Angela Xavier[1], Fábio Silva de Carvalho[1] and Roosevelt da Silva Bastos[1]

[1]*University of São Paulo/Faculty of Dentistry at Bauru, Brazil*
[2]*University of São Paulo/ Biomedical Sciences Institute, Brazil*
[3]*São Lucas University, Brazil*

(physical, mental and social) cause the person to be healthier or unhealthier, depending on their condition (Fig. 1).

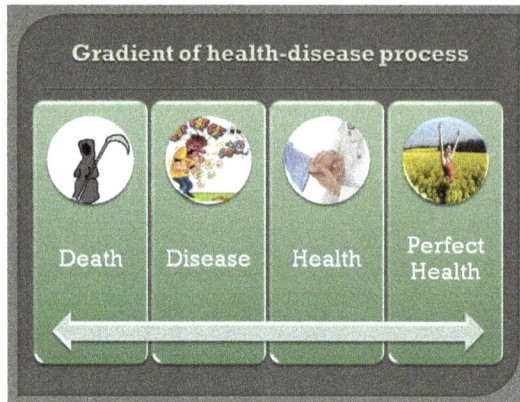

Fig. 1. Gradient of health-disease process

Oral health is another important concept to be clarified. Through time, many definitions have been presented with the aim to establish a state of acceptable oral health. Chaves (5) (1986) describes oral health as a harmonious state with normality patterns and a sound mouth. Yewe-Dyer (6) (1993) conceptualizes oral health as a mouth state with associated support structures where the possible diseases are controlled, the future diseases are inhibited and the occlusion is enough to chew food and the teeth present a healthy social appearance. These authors normally emphasize the absence of problems in the oral tissues such as teeth, gums and oral mucosa, but as Chaves (5) (1986) emphasizes, health is a personal state and it is impossible to exist in part, that is, as an entity of an isolated organ or system. Nevertheless, for practical reasons, this chapter handles the partial concept, as the partial concept is commonly used in oral health and dental health, with the aim of identifying partial objectives in public policies. Still, the concept of health as a whole cannot be far from a professional's understanding in any health specialty.

3. Reminding history and the development of concepts

The term "health promotion" first appeared in 1920 in Winslow at the end of the First World War with the strengthening of workers' organizations. The Winslow community was organized and prepared to develop policies that ensured the implementation of education programs to improve the health of the community's population (7).

After the end of World War II in 1945, the United Nations (UN) was founded and the scope of one of the UN's main discussions was the additional creation of a global health organization. The nations worldwide organized themselves in order to maintain peace and to establish criteria for the maintenance of harmony between countries. This was an important milestone for humanity to unite the nations in the post-war environment around the entity that governs not only the crucial issues of that time (such as the concept of living in peace with others) but also trade relations and health (4).

In 1946, Sigerist defined as the essential tasks of medicine as health promotion, prevention of disease and accident and curative care. He said that health is promoted by providing decent living conditions, good working conditions, education, culture, physical forms of leisure and rest. He called for coordinated efforts of politicians, trade unions and employers, educators and medical professionals. He felt that the lattermost people, as health experts, should set the standard for health settings and pursue them (8).

On July 22, 1946, Sigerist lead the World Health Conference in New York, which catalyzed the establishment of the World Health Organization (WHO). The United Nations inaugurated the WHO's activities in 1948, and the World Health Organization (WHO) opened its doors in the preamble of launching its charter and gave a definition if health that also provides its contributors with a goal they must reach (4).

The preamble of the WHO's constitution presents basic principles for happiness and harmonious relationships and the source of security for all people. It also discusses the actions that nations should take to provide to their populations with the rights of every human being without distinction of race, religion, political beliefs, and economic or social conditions. In this regard, governments technically possess responsibility related to health care services and therefore must achieve good results through policies in social and health areas.

The definition of health (4) as a *state of complete physical, mental and social and not merely the absence of disease or infirmity* was a great step for humanity. This definition provides a basis for all professionals around the world to follow, and it includes well-being as a major objective. This definition also adds the physical term undertaking somatic issues, the psychological health to be considered, and finally the social aspect of health. Living in harmony with society becomes a prerequisite of obtaining health. Furthermore, this definition does not stagnate and stops at a definitive point; instead, it continues by explaining that health is not simply the exclusion of suffering from the hardships of a disease. This definition has received some criticism, because it uses abstract terms such as state of complete well-being, and it sometimes characterizes health from the perspective of a particular individual and his relationship with his own physique, his mind and his social relations. As such, it does not highlight the importance of the health of a community. However, this definition brings together the concept of quality of life, as it shows different dimensions of an individual's health in terms of his or her physical, mental and social aspects.

In 1974, the Canadian Minister of Health and Welfare announced "A new perspective on the health of Canadians" that was so important it became known as the "Lalonde Report", immortalizing the name of this authority (9). In this document, for the first time, the term "health promotion "became part of an official government publication. The report begins its preface of the document with the following sentence:

Good health is the bedrock on which social progress is built. A nation of healthy people can do those things that make life worthwhile, and as the level of health increases so does the potential for happiness.

Motivated by the need to contain costs of the ministry, Marc Lalonde based his concerns upon the important concept of social determinants in health. He presented the process of his health-disease model in four parts: the environment (natural and social), lifestyle (behaviors that affect health), human biology (genetics and human function) and the organization of health services. Although this report was an advanced concept for its time, it was strongly behaviorist and based on individual decisions, thus highly preventivist. One of the criticisms launched at this report points out that the people who are affected by health problems are possibly to be blamed for living with their iniquities (10).

In Alma-Ata, the International Conference on Primary Health Care took place and was attended by 134 delegations and 67 international organizations. The Declaration of Alma-Ata first of all reaffirmed strongly the WHO's definition of health by stressing that health should be considered a fundamental human right. The declaration also said that other sectors, social or economic, should concentrate their efforts into the health sector to achieve the "greatest social objective" (11).

The Declaration of Alma-Ata defined and granted international recognition to the concept of primary health care, so Health for All by the Year 2000 should have used it as a strategy to make their mission a reality. The meeting ended by calling attention to the urgent need for government involvement, especially in developing countries, so that international action actually coincided with the commitment of governments, WHO, UNICEF (UN Children's Fund), non-governmental organizations, other international agencies, all workers in the area and the entire world community. WHO's goal is to create a commitment to primary health care and to channel increased technical and financial support to the detriment of investments in armaments and military equipment so that in the year 2000, the world population would reach an acceptable levels of health (11).

After eight years, the First World Conference on Health Promotion gathered thirty-five nations in 1986 to the Canadian capital. Its participants then disclosed the Ottawa Charter as a result of their discussions. New Health Promotion has established itself as a landmark. This event served to create the health sector's strategy for people throughout the world. Fundamental conditions and resources were cited as prerequisites for improving health, such as peace, education, food, income, stable ecosystem, sustainable resources, social justice and equity. Since the founding of the charter, several strategies have been listed and recommended for implementation throughout the world and are listed as follows (12).

1. **Develop healthy public policies based on health promotion.** In relation to equity in health, it was recommended that politicians should become aware that any of their decisions, not only their decisions in the specific area of health, could lead to better or worse living conditions for the population, so health promotion goes beyond good attendance, care and service.

2. **Supplant supportive environments into societies.** The environment's impact on the well being of people is undeniable. Thus, the protection of natural resources and the search for a suitable environment for the unfolding of life, whether in the area of technology, labor, energy production or urbanization should be observed continuously as to constitute positive factors for the communities.

3. **Community action should strengthen due to the importance of health to the population's engagement for decision-making strategies and their implementation.** The requirement in this goal is the public's access to information, learning opportunities and financial support for health issues. This is the concept of empowerment put into practice.

4. **The development of personal skills.** The individual might be prepared for the various stages of their existence that they will face throughout life. The risk of chronic disease incidence and disease's external causes should be addressed in a timely manner. We should not forget the necessary participation of educational, professional, commercial and voluntary institutions and even the government.

5. **Institutions should reorient health services.** Specifically, health services were advised to redirect their "compass" of attention so that it was not focused solely on clinical and emergency services. Professionals should also combine their experiences to give one

another a comprehensive approach that enables them to understand and respect the cultural peculiarities of each community that they assist. Finally, the Ottawa Charter ends with the commitments that its participants had made to a strong alliance with public health, It urges the international community to commit to public health, as well: "The Conference is firmly convinced that if people in all walks of life, nongovernmental and voluntary organizations, governments, the World Health Organization and all other bodies concerned join forces in introducing strategies for health promotion, in line with the moral and social values that form the basis of this charter, Health For All by the year 2000 will become a reality."

The Second International Conference on Health Promotion, held in Australia in 1988, reaffirmed, with the spirit of Alma-Ata by the Declaration of Adelaide (13), the five key points of the Ottawa Charter above. Additionally, it added four more:

1. **Support women's health.** Public policies that focus on this area address equal rights in the division of labor, performance of delivery according to the preferences and needs of women and the mechanisms that support working women, such as maternity leave.
2. **Food and nutrition**. The eradication of hunger and malnutrition must comprise a fundamental part of public policies for health. This eradication includes ample food in hospitals, schools, shelters and workplaces.
3. **Tobacco and alcohol**. This goal includes the implementation of any public policies aimed at reducing the production, distribution, marketing and consumption of these products.
4. **Creating healthy environments**. This conference encouraged the addition of ecology to public health in order to achieve socioeconomic development and sustainability in human use of the planet.

According to the Adelaide Declaration, health is both a fundamental right and a sound social investment. In order for improvements to occur, which will increase levels of citizens' health, investments from the government and private sectors are desperately needed in healthy public policies.

Many conferences ran around the world with health promotion at the center of their attention so that they could develop new concepts and continue the engagement of nations worldwide to achieve health for all (Sundsvall (14), Sweden, 1991; Jakarta (15), Indonesia, 1997; Mexico City (16), Mexico, 2000).

Bangkok, Thailand, hosted the Sixth International Conference on Health Promotion in 2005 (17). The Bangkok Charter reaffirmed and analyzed concepts and strategies reported by the previous conferences. This meeting discussed the current condition of the social determinants of health, which the Bangkok conference found to be very different from the time they were disclosed by the Ottawa Charter:

- Increasing inequality within countries and between countries;
- New patterns of consumption and communication, global procedures and marketing;
- Changes in the environment that affect all parts of the world; and
- The growing process of urbanization.

New challenges were raised, among them the fact that women and men are affected unequally, and increased vulnerability caused inequalities in the health of children, excluded groups, disabled and indigenous peoples (WHO, 2005).

Strategies to promote a globalized health strategy while respecting the autonomy of nations with their particular cultural characteristics were discussed in an attempt to control positively the determinants of health.

The commitments to "Health for All" were confirmed by the health ministers present:
1.   Make health promotion a central concern in the global development agenda;
2.   Make health promotion a core responsibility for government as a whole;
3.   Make health promotion a major focus of communities and civil society;
4.   Make health promotion a requirement of good corporate practice.

Given the non-materialization of shares based on the resolutions set out in previous conferences, the Bangkok Charter has completed its appeal to member countries to apply the theory in the practice of health promotion, public policies. Partnerships should be implemented for this purpose.

In 2009, the Nairobe conference for health promotion took place (18) with the aim to address health and development. The globalized world allowed financial crisis to interfere with the national economies in general, so the health systems were also affected. Global warming and climate instability was another source of concern, and the conference gave special attention to lower income countries as well as security threats.

Health promotion appears in the field of public health as a paradigm of transformative actions that aim to improve living conditions. With that change, it became necessary to conceive of health in a positive vision, seeking an expanded awareness that is integrated, complex, intersectional and pertinent to the environment, current modes of production and various lifestyles (19, 20).

Similarly, the conceptual framework of health promotion highlights the influence of the social health of individuals and populations. Scientific studies contribute to addressing the challenges related to health and quality of life that, combined with social components, are essential for individuals and communities to achieve a high health level profile (21, 22).

The current juncture is marked by social inequalities. In response, contemporary health promotion emphasizes the importance of social determinants in search of models of care that go beyond the medical curative effect. Thus, the present state of public health raises discussions about the new design for health managers, health professionals and society (23).

The discussion of health promotion has ventured into different settings, representing a change in the direction of health actions. This discussion is searching for a way to attempt social transformation, given the fact that promoting health today means to fight poverty naturalization so that social issues are recognized for what they are, which is social inequality (7, 20, 24).

It is noteworthy that relative social deprivation (more than the absolute) is associated with poorer health. In practice, this theory means that populations with high economic disparities will also feature high disparities in health states. Health promotion must be integrated equally on all social levels in order to address consistently the model of social determinants of health (25).

The commitment of the actions proposed by the Ottawa Charter aims to break with the fragmentation of the current health care model, imposing practices that can overcome the culture of medicalization and at the same time ally to the production of health through strategies that promote changes in lifestyle and promote the autonomy of individuals and social groups (23). Thus, health promotion requires intersectoral cooperation and joint actions, such as legislation, tax system and fiscal measures, education, housing, social services, primary health care, employment, leisure, transport and urban planning, among other segments. To achieve effective health promotion, however, these joints should not be geared to the demands of the international market, but targeted to the needs of the population in question (23).

It is important to think of health promotion as an important tool that catalyzes new modes of care and health management that improve the quality of life. It can also catalyze other realities that may make it possible to achieve equity in health (23).

Meanwhile, health determinants have begun to be the focus of attention with the aim of improving life and reducing disparities between countries and amongst the localities within countries.

4. Approaching the community

The selection of a criterion is important to the oral health promotion of any population. This criterion is influenced by philosophical, political and professional matters. Obviously, the biological events that arise from a disease have been apparent since Louis Pasteur and Robert Koch demonstrated the importance of microbiology for the treatment and prevention of any infectious disease. Additionally, epidemiological research has shown many other influences may concur to the incidence of different problems relating to the environment and the health state of a person or a population and the social determinants of health (26) (Fig. 2).

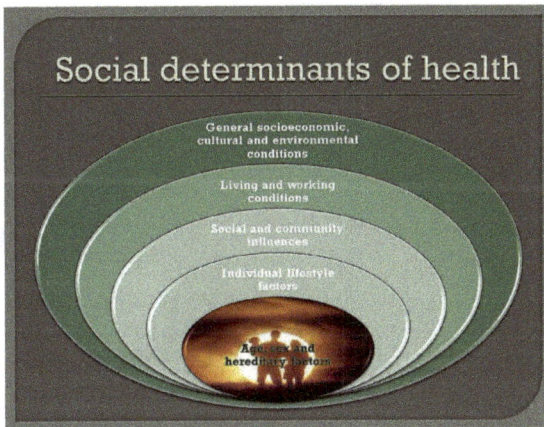

Fig. 2. Social determinants of health

The social determinants of health may be well exemplified in the upstream and downstream tale (27). As man lies beside a stream and hears a scream from downstream. The man recognizes a person drowning, and as fast as he can, he rescues the person when he hears another scream. Again, he rushes downstream and rescues another person, but the screams never end. As fast as possible between the rescues, he calls for medical help and many health professionals and swimmers came together to provide specialized assistance with ambulances, nurses and doctors, They all face a significant increase in the number of new cases of drowned people, sometimes with important cardiac complications. Suddenly, while the assistants were only helping the people who were already drowning in the water, somebody asks some important questions. "Why is a person who does not know to swim in the water downstream? Why is the number of people in this crazy situation so high and why don't out efforts stop the new cases downstream?" Finally, they ask the most important question, "What is pushing these people into the water upstream?" (Fig. 3).

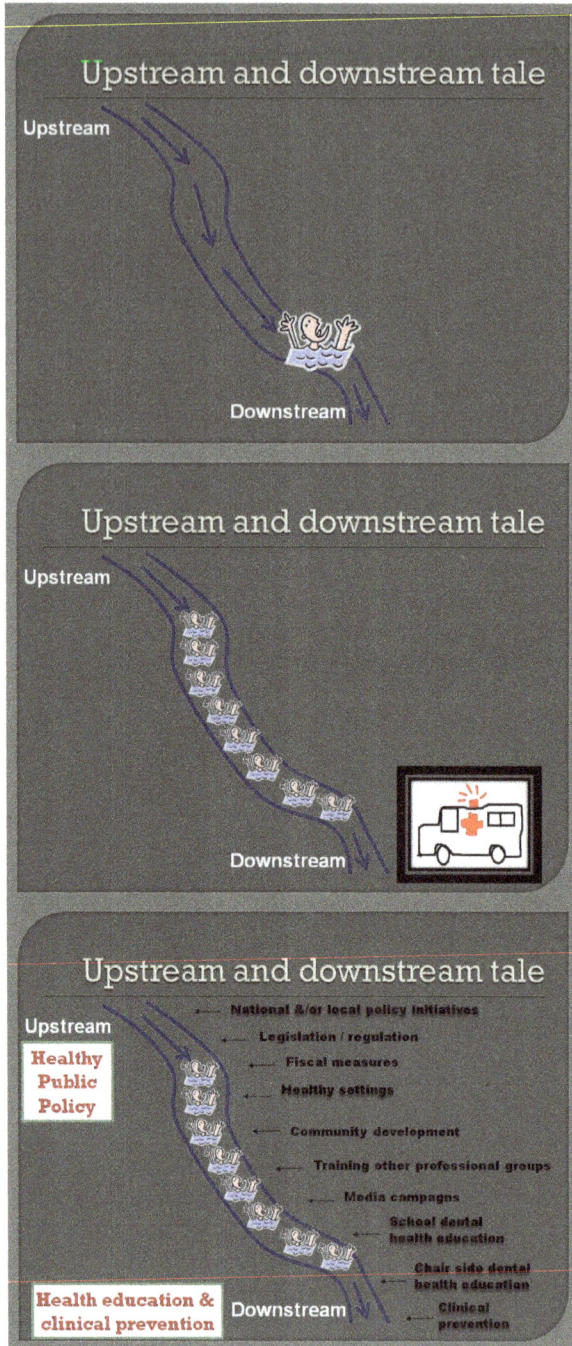

Fig. 3. Upstream and downstream tale

The drowning in this tale illustrates the diseases, such as dental caries and periodontal diseases. Social determinants of health, which are well represented by Dahlgren and Whitehead (26), would be representative of what is pushing people into the water. The assistance downstream to the "victims" is very important to the relief of actual health problems that are presently affecting people's lives, such as pain, infection and other consequences that destroy the organism and the quality of life. Unfortunately, the health policy planning is often forgotten. If there are no policy plans in action, new cases of drowning (disease) will continuously appear and perhaps increase, and the needs of diseased patients will highly increase as time goes by. A saying in Brazil likens this situation "to dry ice". This is the reason why upstream action is so important. The upstream actions are necessary to guide the whole population to be away from the "stream" toward a healthy life with a better range of choices offered by and for the whole community.

A disparity in the distribution of chronicled diseases, such as dental caries, happens between countries, across countries and amongst localities. What would be the appropriate approach to prevent health problems of a specific population?

Dental caries is still the most important disease that public health dentistry must combat. After the industrial revolution at the end of the eighteenth century, the spread consume of sugar cane throughout the globe caused a terrifying increase in the incidence of this disease (28-31). Preventive measures started to be effective within the early years of the twentieth century through the fluorosis studies, as they discovered the effect of fluorides and preventive effects on dental caries (32-35). The move to fluoridate the public water supply made possible a significant decrease in the prevalence of dental caries in young populations throughout the nineteenth century. The topical fluoridated products that are applied directly to the teeth professionally or at home made possible another remarkable decline in the prevalence of dental caries, first in the industrialized world. This technology later spread to developing countries. However, the decline, even within the industrialized world, was not evenly spread across the population, and the polarization of dental caries started to become a concern for researchers. Regular methods to prevent dental caries made possible a significant decrease in the prevalence of the disease and seems to have stopped near DMFT 1.00 in patients at twelve years old in many populations (36).

Epidemiological basic data are the baseline for establishing the criterion needed to balance the approach beyond a specific community in a strategy for the whole population, including high-risk groups, in a developed or developing community. The balance must attempt to answer a simple question. Will the population in focus benefit the most from a small decrease in the oral disease risk in a great number of people or a great decrease in the risk for a small population?

The British epidemiologist Geoffrey Rose (37-39) defined the first three possibilities for preventive measures regarding chronic diseases such as dental caries.

The high-risk strategy gathers preventive efforts to modify the risk distribution of a community (Fig. 4). While the strategy's attention focuses on a small group of the population, the rest of this population does not benefit (40) (Table 1).

Dental caries is a disease that affects all communities and has generalized causes with intrinsic social influence. Dental biofilm, fermentable carbohydrates, oral hygiene and fluoride exposure are directly associated with the incidence of dental caries and the whole community is exposed to all of these risk factors. These characteristics make dental caries a chronic disease that can be managed by the population approach. Obviously, such characteristics call for an intersectorial decision regarding social, economic, industrial, political and other sectors with the intention of a massive upstream action, that is, a population strategy (Fig. 5).

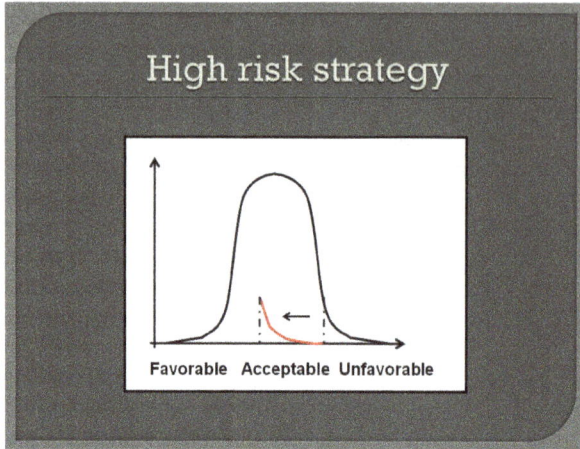

Fig. 4. High-risk strategy graphic

Advantages	Disadvantages
Appropriate intervention to the individual	Over prevention of a person
No intervention for those who are not exposed to a special risk	Palliative and temporary success
Ethically appropriate for the organization of dental services	Inappropriate behavioral strategy
Selectivity improves the risk-benefit ratio and therefore there are more cost-effective resources	Limited by poor prediction
	Reliability problems and costs
	Contribution to the overall control of the disease may be disappointing and small

Adapted from: Baelum, Sheiham and Burt, 2011(41).

Table 1. Advantages and disadvantages of the high-risk preventive approach

While the defenders of the high-risk approach attempt only the right arm of distribution, the population strategy intends to move all distribution to the left, carrying together the high-risk group, represented by the right arm of distribution (fig. 5).

Baelum, Sheiham and Burt (41) (2011) consider three main advantages to the population approach. First, they consider a radical approach. The social determinants of health would be addressed when the biological determinants of disease are targeted, such as the fermentable carbohydrates and the dental biofilm related to dental caries. Second, they propose a powerful approach. Public health education may focus on common risk factors for different diseases. For example, when parents control their child's sugar consumption through a better daily diet and control sweet snacks between meals, they may decrease the dental caries in their child as well as their child's likelihood of becoming obese and contracting other related health problems, such as diabetes and cardiovascular disease. Thirdly, they stress that the population preventive approach is appropriate. Any chronicle disease is associated with social problems of a society and this approach protects the "victims" from being blamed.

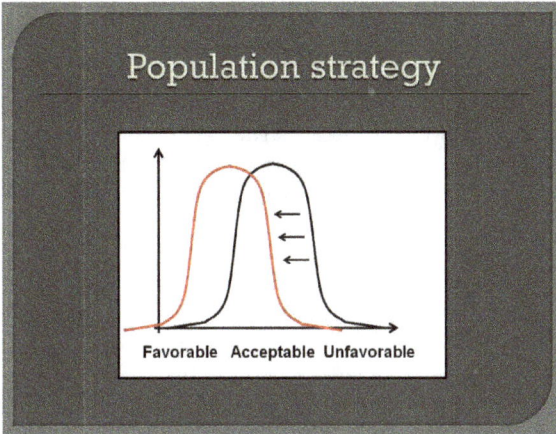

Fig. 5. Population strategy graphic

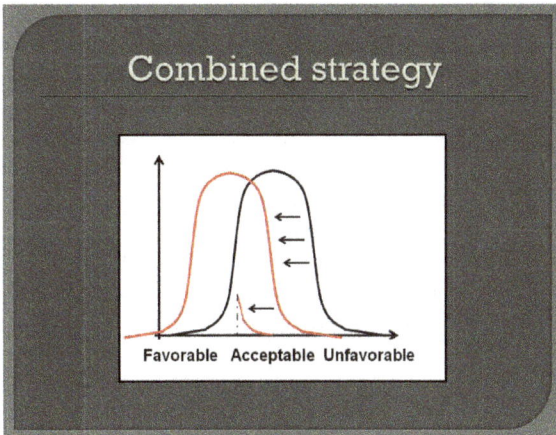

Fig. 6. Combined strategy graphic

Some disadvantages might arise during the population approach. The first one is a limitation in the acceptability of the preventive measures regarding the desire of people for visible, imminent and probable results according to the eye of a layman. Reliability is the second limitation; this topic is related to economic, political and other barriers. It is simple; the sugar industry is not interested in investing money in or otherwise endorsing educational lessons regarding carbohydrate consumption. The third limitation is the primary financial costs of this approach and the unknown benefits of educational and preventive measures.

Therefore, blending the population approach with some components of the high risk strategy seems to be the most acceptable way to implement preventive measures in a community so that the community can avoid the access inequality of the population approach and avoid the victim blaming related to the high risk approach (40). It is been named the combined strategy (Fig. 6).

5. Project USP in Rondônia: An example

The project USP in Rondônia emerged in 2002 with the aim of health promotion for a population devoid of attention in this regard. The Faculty of the Dentistry of Bauru offers two grade degrees, Dentistry and Speech, Language Pathology and Audiology Sciences. Students from both grading courses participate in activities in the far state of Rondônia regarding dentistry and speech pathology, prevention activities, health promotion, health assistance and rehabilitation.

Twice a year, expedition teams provide health services to the population in an area bounded by the urban and rural areas of a municipality within the State of Rondônia, Monte Negro and the adjacent rural riverine population. A large percentage of this population lives far from the centers of reference and thus remains oblivious to the basic conditions of sanitation, education and basic health programs (primary, secondary and tertiary). Therefore, the project "USP in Rondônia" researches local realities in order to boost the actions already undertaken in the municipality and thus provide better quality of life for this underprivileged population(41).

The state of Rondônia was created by complementary law No. 41, December 22th 1981, which rose from the federal territory with the same name, whose dismembered territory consisted of areas from the states of Amazonas and Mato Grosso, previously called Guaporé Territory. The geographic surface of Rondônia is 243,044 km2, representing 7.11% of the North Region and 2.98% of the entire area of Brazil. Its colonization is directly linked to economic cycles occurring in that region, such as the cycles of gold and rubber.

The municipality of Monte Negro originated from Boa Vista and was transformed into a city by law No. 378 on February 13th, 1992, with designation of Monte Negro, named because of an accidental relief of its territory. Its population totals 14,091 inhabitants according to the demographic census (2010), and 52.57% of this population is male and 47.43% female. Of this total population, 6,701 people live in rural areas and 7,390 in the urban area. It has 1,931.37 km² and a population density of 7.30 inhabitants per Km². Its Human Development Index (HDI) is 0.685 and the average per capita income in 2000 was R$ 170.88 (around US$ 100.00). It derives its main economy from logging/wood processing, followed by local trade, agriculture (mainly coffee, corn, rice) and cattle feeding (Fig. 7).

The rural riverine communities attended are Calama, Rio Preto and Demarcação, which are all localized in the northern region of Rondônia. Calama is a district of Porto Velho with 3,400 inhabitants and has two schools for children. The basis of its local economy is fishing and planting cassava, i.e., subsistence agriculture. The community of Rio Preto is distant three hours from Calama by river, and it is located on the bank of the Madeira River. It is composed of about 25 families who live in tracts that are subdivided where families live based on subsistence agriculture, animal husbandry (chicken, pigs) and fishing. The community does not present any kind of commerce or local health clinic. If community members wish to purchase food, medicine or assistance of any kind, they must travel by boat to the District of Calama. The community of Demarcação is also on the banks of the Madeira River and comprises about 300 people. They acquire their electricity from a generator and the community has a good organizational structure. The basis of the local economy is fishing and subsistence agriculture. There is a spot healer who is highly respected by the community, and he is aware of many herbs that can treat diseases.

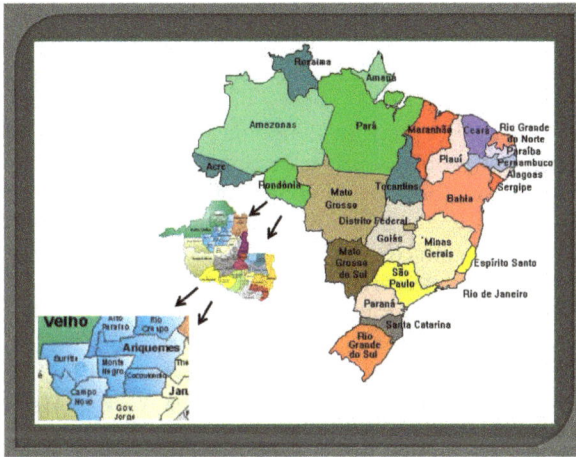

Fig. 7. Monte Negro, state of Rondônia, Brazilian Amazon

Situational diagnosis of Monte Negro:
- Dearth of and poor access to information;
- Population with low levels of education;
- Inadequate oral health and speech therapy;
- Lack of knowledge of teachers and educators;
- Lack of information for the community's health workers and health agents;
- A large percentage of the population lacks basic sanitation; and
- They all experience difficulties in accessing health care, especially the people living in rural areas.

Situational diagnosis of the rural riverine population:
- Low levels of education and no notion of citizenship;
- Lack of expectation for the improvement of living conditions;
- Lack of even the minimum conditions of sanitation;
- Lack of access to basic services;
- Lack of access to health care;
- Lack of means to prevent dental caries and speech problems;
- Difficulty accessing medicines; and
- Need for training of professionals in the field of education and health.

In addition, the diagnosis included a lack of basic hygiene, sanitation, general health and basic dental and speech notions. This revealed the need for a population strategy with educational activities that involve the local teachers and community workers and health professionals so that they can become multipliers of knowledge and information throughout the year, aiming to improve the standard of health for their entire community.

Among the rural riverine populations that benefited from this project highlight are the communities of the Lower Rio Madeira (Tabajara), Calama, Rio Preto, Demarcação, Santa Luzia D'Oeste and Nova Brasilândia D'Oeste.

During the first expedition, i.e., from 2002 until 2011, a total of 13,499 patients were attended to for a total of 37,976 procedures. This work of health promotion benefits the entire population of the city, rural and coastal populations, as well as promoted the welfare activities also carried out in educational activities with not only the patients who attended, but also their family members, teachers, educators and health professionals, making them all multipliers of information to continue with the work of health education during the months' interexpeditions.

The actions taken by the project "USP in Rondônia" have direct and indirect impacts on quality of life and health of people of urban, rural and rural riverine communities, where improvements are found top be increasing through the implementation of education-prevention activities and assistance in the field of dentistry, speech and language therapy and audiology to patients. Such activities are undertaken with patients treated in clinical and educational activities in kindergartens, schools and PETI (Program for the Elimination of Child Labour) and health education activities with schoolteachers, educators and Community Health Agents.

Over the course of almost ten years of design, we observed a high number of welfare activities in which people benefited greatly from further work in Health Education with influential people in the community enabling information to reach thousands of others, because they acted as a chain of multipliers for health in this municipality.

Dentistry, Speech, Language Pathology and Audiology attended 13,499 patients for a total of 37,976 procedures. It is noteworthy that the procedures installed 172 total dentures and 64 partial dentures in addition to 110 hearing aids.

Training courses about health education for teachers and for the Community Health Agents are a result of the locals' participation and community involvement with the project, which aims to increase the benefit provided. Some individuals' gain in professional knowledge might spread to the entire community, depending on their roles in the community.

Age	dft (SD)	DMFT (SD)	DT (SD)	MT (SD)	FT (SD)	Caries Free (%)	SiC Index	Care Index (%)
5	3.15 (3.12)	-	2.67 (3.06)	0.00 (0.00)	0.48 (1.15)	34.42	6.65	23.30
12	-	3.41 (2.69)	2.53 (2.24)	0.25 (0.64)	0.63 (1.45)	14,81	6,70	21,72
15-19	-	5.98 (4.19)	3.27 (2.87)	1.09 (1.59)	1.62 (2.66)	8,16	10,61	29,40
35-44	-	16.00 (7.30)	2.21 (2.33)	9.79 (8.65)	4.00 (4.16)	0,00	24,38	25,00
65-74	-	25.96 (9.82)	0.89 (1.60)	24.71 (10.74)	0.36 (1.15)	1,78	32,00	1,41

Table 2. Dental caries profile by component (decayed teeth [DT(SD)], missing teeth [MT(SD)] and filling teeth [FT(SD)]) of Monte Negro population, Rondônia state, in 2008

The improvement of general health, oral health, speech, language, audiology and behaviors for healthier daily habits can be observed over the intervening years. The tables 2 and 3 shows the results of the epidemiological surveys conducted in the rural riverine population and in the municipality of Monte Negro during the years 2005/2006(42) and 2008(43).

To review the aspects of speech, language pathology and audiology science, the project team conducted an epidemiological survey of hearing disorders in the urban population between 2005 and 2007 and found the prevalence of disabling hearing loss in the town to be3.81%, with 3.43% at moderate loss and 0.38% at severe loss. This prevalence might be considered low compared to the prevalence in Canoas in southern of Brazil, which was 6.8% (44). Note that the results found in the North of Brazil (Monte Negro) are within the range of data found in studies supported by the World Health Organization (45), which range from the lowest incidence (2.1%) in Oman and the highest incidence (7.8%) in North Vietnam. It is noteworthy that the survey of Monte Negro made adjustments for hearing aids, which benefited 52 patients with hearing impaired analog devices, donated by the company Phonak, at a total of 110 devices. These patients are still professionally followed.

Age		DMFT (SD)		p (Test t)
Monte Negro	Rural Riverine	Monte Negro	Rural Riverine	
5	4-5	3.15* (3.12)	4.31* (3.42)	0.03
	12	3.41 (2.69)	2.65 (3.01)	0.07
15-19	18	5.98 (4.19)	5.42 (5.33)	0.24
	35-44	16.00 (7.30)	17.73 (8.61)	0.10
	65-74	25.96 (9.82)	21.56 (11.95)	0.05

* dft data

Table 3. Comparison of the dental caries profile of Monte Negro (2008) and rural riverine populations (2005-2006)

The sustainability of the Project "USP in Rondônia" has always been a concern since its beginning. Since 2005, it has invested in training courses for teachers and community health professionals. The Course in Health Education Project believes that this type action is of fundamental importance, because these professionals have the function to multiply information for this population, providing autonomy and independence.

Investments, acquisitions of new equipment, means of divulgation within and outside the academic community and the motivation of the teamwork involved provides higher credibility and support to the entire population for this project. The assessments are made on each shipment of activities undertaken and the results obtained for both the team's work and for the population served, so new actions are planned constantly according to the observed changes in the pattern of the population's health.

6. Final considerations

"Health promotion is the process of enabling people to increase control over, and to improve, their health. To reach a state of complete physical, mental and social well-being, an individual or group must be able to identify and to realize aspirations, to satisfy needs, and to change or cope with the environment. Health is, therefore, seen as a resource for everyday life, not the objective of living. Health is a positive concept emphasizing social and personal resources, as well as physical capacities. Therefore, health promotion is not just the responsibility of the health sector, but goes beyond healthy life-styles to well-being". This part of the Ottawa Charter (1986) is still in context.

The individual health counseling toward changing personal behavior will not last if there is no frequency in sessions. A community in need of health promotion must be accessed by two main aspects, a common risk factor and the population approach, as "Project USP in Rondônia" has been doing since 2002.

7. References

[1] Watt RG. Strategies and approaches in oral disease prevention and health promotion. Bull World Health Organ. 2005;83(9):711-8.

[2] Kumar S, Goyal A, Tadakamadla J, Tibdewal H, Duraiswamy P, Kulkarni S. Oral health related quality of life among children with parents and those with no parents. Community Dent Health. 2011;28(3):227-31.

[3] Saintrain MV, de Souza EH. Impact of tooth loss on the quality of life. Gerodontology. 2011.

[4] WHO. Constitution of World Health Organization. New York: World Health Organization; 1946.

[5] Chaves M. Odontologia Social. São Paulo: Artes Médicas; 1986. 448 p.

[6] Yewe-Dyer M. The definition of oral health. Br Dent J. 1993;174(7):224-5.

[7] Sícoli JL, Nascimento PR. Promoção de saúde: concepções, princípios e operacionalização. Interface: Comunicação, Saúde, Educação. 2003;7(12):101-22.

[8] Nunes ED. Henry Ernest Sigerist: pioneiro da história social da medicina e da sociologia médica. Educ Med Salud. 1992;26(1):70-81.

[9] Lalonde M. A new perspective on the health of Canadians. Ottawa: Ministry of Supply and Services of Canada; 1981.

[10] Heidmann ITSB, Almeida MCP, Boehs AE, Wosny AM, Monticelli M. Promoção de saúde: trajetória histórica de suas concepções. Texto Contexto Enfermagem. 2006;15(2):352-8.

[11] WHO, UNICEF. Declaration of Alma Ata. International Conference on Primary Health Care. Alma Ata: World Health Organization; 1978.

[12] WHO. 1st Global Conference on Health Promotion: Ottawa 1986. Geneve: WHO; 1986.

[13] WHO. 2nd Global Conference on Health Promotion: Adelaide 1988. Geneve: WHO; 1988.

[14] WHO. 3rd Global Conference on Health Promotion: Sundsvall 1991. Geneve: WHO; 1991.

[15] WHO. 4th Global Conference on Health Promotion: Jakarta 1997. Geneve: WHO; 1997.

[16] WHO. 5th Global Conference on Health Promotion: Mexico 2000. Geneve: WHO; 2000.

[17] WHO. 6th Global Conference on Health Promotion: Bangkok 2005. Geneve: WHO; 2005.

[18] WHO. 7th Global Conference on Health Promotion, Nairobi 2009. Geneve: WHO; 2009.

[19] Lefèvre F, Lefèvre AMC. Promoção de saúde: a negação da negação. Rio de Janeiro: Vieira & Lent; 2004.

[20] Westphal MP. Promoção da saúde e prevenção de doenças. In: Campos GWS, Minayo MCS, Akerman M, Júnior MD, Carvalho YA, editors. Tratado de saúde coletiva. Rio de Janeiro: FIOCRUZ; 2006.

[21] Buss PM. Promoção de saúde e qualidade de vida. Ciênc Saúde Coletiva. 2000;5(1):163-77.

[22] Menossi MJ, Oliveira MM, Coimbra VCC, Palha PF, Almeida MCP. interdisciplinaridade: um instrumento para a construção de um modelo assistencial fundamentado na promoção da saúde. Rev Enferm UERJ. 2005;13:252-6.

[23] Silva JG, Gurgel AA, Frota MA, Vieira LJES, Valdés MTM. Promoção da saúde: possibilidades de superação das desigualdades sociais. Rev Enferm. 2008;16(3):421-5.

[24] Czesrenia D, Freitas CM. Promoção de saúde: conceitos, reflexões , tendências. Rio de Janeiro: FIOCRUZ; 2003.

[25] Marcondes WB. A convergência de referências na promoção da saúde. Saúde e Sociedade. 2004;13(1):5-13.

[26] Dahlgren G, Whitehead M. Policies and strategies to promote social equity in health. Stockholm: Institute for Future Studies; 1991.

[27] Watt RG. From victim blaming to upstream action: tackling the social determinants of oral health inequalities. Community Dent Oral Epidemiol. 2007;35(1):1-11.

[28] Woodward M, Walker AR. Sugar consumption and dental caries: evidence from 90 countries. Br Dent J. 1994;176(8):297-302.

[29] Helöe LA, Haugejorden O. "The rise and fall" of dental caries: some global aspects of dental caries epidemiology. Community Dent Oral Epidemiol. 1981;9(6):294-9.

[30] Dijs F. [Sugar and the birth of dentistry]. Ned Tijdschr Tandheelkd. 2004;111(6):243-5.

[31] Moore WJ. The role of sugar in the aetiology of dental caries. 1. Sugar and the antiquity of dental caries. J Dent. 1983;11(3):189-90.

[32] Newbrum E. Cariology. Baltimore: Williams & Wilkins; 1983.

[33] Jiménez-Farfán MD, Hernández-Guerrero JC, Juárez-López LA, Jacinto-Alemán LF, de la Fuente-Hernández J. Fluoride consumption and its impact on oral health. Int J Environ Res Public Health. 2011;8(1):148-60.

[34] Tenuta LM, Cury JA. Fluoride: its role in dentistry. Braz Oral Res. 2010;24 Suppl 1:9-17.

[35] McGrady MG, Ellwood RP, Pretty IA. Why fluoride? Dent Update. 2010;37(9):595-8, 601-2.

[36] Marthaler TM. Changes in dental caries 1953-2003. Caries Res. 2004;38(3):173-81.

[37] Rose G. Sick individuals and sick populations. Int J Epidemiol. 1985;14(1):32-8.

[38] Rose G. Sick individuals and sick populations. 1985. Bull World Health Organ. 2001;79(10):990-6.

[39] Rose G. Sick individuals and sick populations. Int J Epidemiol. 2001;30(3):427-32; discussion 33-4.

[40] Rose G. High-risk and population strategies of prevention: ethical considerations. Ann Med. 1989;21(6):409-13.

[41] Baelum V, Sheiham A, Burt B. Controle da cárie em populações. In: Fejerskov O, Kidd E, Nyvad B, Baelum V, editors. Cárie dentária: a doença e seu tratamento clínico. São Paulo.: Santos; 2011. p. 616.

[42] Silva RH, Castro RF, Cunha DC, Almeida CT, Bastos JR, Camargo LM. [Dental caries in a riverine community in Rondônia State, Amazon Region, Brazil, 2005-2006]. Cad Saude Publica. 2008;24(10):2347-53.

[43] Bastos RS, Silva RP, Maia-Junior AF, Carvalho FS, Merlini S, Caldana ML, et al. Dental caries profile in Monte Negro, Amazonian state of Rondônia, Brazil, in 2008. J Appl Oral Sci. 2010;18(5):437-41.

[44] Béria JU, Raymann BC, Gigante LP, Figueiredo AC, Jotz G, Roithman R, et al. Hearing impairment and socioeconomic factors: a population-based survey of an urban locality in southern Brazil. Rev Panam Salud Publica. 2007;21(6):381-7.

[45] WHO. Ear and hearing disorders survey. Protocol for a population-based survey of prevalence and causes of deafness and hearing impairment and other ear diseases. Prevention of Blindness and Deafness (PBD). Geneva: WHO; 1999.

14

HIV/AIDS and Oral Health in Socially Disadvantaged Communities

Febronia Kokulengya Kahabuka[1] and Flora Masumbuo Fabian[2]
[1]*Muhimbili University of Health and Allied Sciences, School of Dentistry,*
[2]*International Medical and Technological University*
Tanzania

1. Introduction

The chapter begins with a brief overview of HIV/AIDS. Different oral manifestations of HIV/AIDS are reported with the fact that the oral lesions parallel the decline in the number of CD4 cells and an increase in viral load. The chapter also presents a trend of occurrence of oral manifestations before ARV and during ARV era. Moreover, the impact of HIV/AIDS on oral health of the people living with HIV/AIDS (PLWHA) in socially disadvantaged communities particularly in those living in Sub Saharan Africa where majority of HIV positive individuals reside is discussed. In addition, a need for a balanced diet by PLWHA is specified and a narration of functional impairment due to HIV/AIDS related oral conditions which often render these people unable to eat properly is presented. Knowledge of Oral manifestations of HIV/AIDS among dental practitioners, medical practitioners and people living with HIV/AIDS as well as the influence of this knowledge to the care for PLWHA is explored. A brief description of the care expectations of PLWHA from the medical and dental personnel is sighted. Eventually, recommendations for possible interventions are provided.

2. Overview of HIV/AIDS

Human immunodeficiency virus (HIV) is a lentivirus, a member of the retrovirus family that causes Acquired Immunodeficiency Syndrome or AIDS (Douek et al., 2009), an infectious disease in humans, in which progressive failure of the immune system allows life-threatening opportunistic infections and various cancers to thrive. HIV infection in humans is considered pandemic by the World Health Organization (WHO). HIV has been shown to have infected about 0.6% of the world's population and since its discovery in 1981 to the year 2006 AIDS has killed more than 25 million people. In 2009, AIDS claimed an estimated 1.8 million lives, down from a global peak of 2.1 million in 2004. However, a peak of an estimated 2.6 million people were newly infected in 2009 (UNAIDS report 2010). A disproportionate number of AIDS deaths occur in Sub-Saharan Africa, retarding economic growth and exacerbating the burden of poverty (Greener, 2002). UNAIDS report that Sub-Saharan Africa remains by far the worst-affected region, with an estimated 22.5 million people currently living with HIV/AIDS (67% of the global total), 1.3 million deaths (72% of the global total) and 1.8 million new infections (69% of the global total). However, the number of new infections declined by 19% across the region between 2001 and 2009, and by more than 25% in 22 sub-Saharan African countries during this period (UNAIDS report 2010).

2.1 Types of HIV, virulence and mode of attack

Two types of HIV have been characterized: HIV-1 and HIV-2. HIV-1 is the virus that was initially discovered and termed both LAV and HTLV-III. It is more virulent, more infective and is the cause of the majority of HIV infections globally (Centers for Disease Control and Prevention 2001, Gilbert, et al., 2003). The lower infectivity of HIV-2 compared to HIV-1 implies that fewer of those exposed to HIV-2 will be infected per exposure. Because of its relatively poor capacity for transmission, HIV-2 is largely confined to West Africa (Reeves and Doms, 2002). The HIV is a frequently mutating retrovirus.

HIV infection has 3 stages; acute infection or primary infection stage, latency stage and AIDS. The acute infection lasts for several weeks and may include symptoms such as fever, lymphadenopathy that is swollen lymph nodes, pharyngitis presenting as sore throat, rash, muscle pain (myalgia), malaise and mouth and esophageal sore. During this stage most oral manifestations occur and these have been shown to be indicators for counseling and testing (Fabian et al., 2009). The latency stage is the second stage and it involves few or no symptoms and can last anywhere from two weeks to twenty years or more depending on the individual. AIDS, is the final stage of HIV infection, and is defined by low CD4+ T cell counts (fewer than 200 per microliter), presence of various opportunistic infections such as various parasitic, viral and microbial infections, cancers and other conditions. A small percentage of HIV-1 infected individuals retain high levels of CD4+ T-cells without being on antiretroviral therapy. However, most have detectable viral load and will eventually progress to AIDS without treatment, albeit more slowly than others. These individuals are classified as HIV controllers or long-term non-progressors (LTNP). People who maintain CD4+ T cell counts and also have low or clinically undetectable viral load without anti-retroviral treatment have also been given the name of elite controllers or elite suppressors (ES) (Blankson, 2010; Grabar et al., 2009).

2.2 Testing for HIV

The first and most common blood test for patients who are suspected of having HIV infection, is usually the enzyme-linked immunosorbent assay (ELISA) test for the presence of HIV antibody in their blood. HIV-1 testing consists of initial screening with the ELISA to detect antibodies to HIV-1. Specimens with a nonreactive result from the initial ELISA are considered HIV-negative. Specimens with a reactive ELISA result are retested in duplicate (Piatak, et al., 1993). If the result of either duplicate test is reactive, the specimen is reported as repeatedly reactive and undergoes confirmatory testing with a more specific supplemental test such as the Western blot or, less commonly, an immunofluorescence assay (IFA). Only specimens that are repeatedly reactive by ELISA and positive by IFA or reactive by Western blot are considered HIV-positive and indicative of HIV infection. Specimens that are repeatedly ELISA-reactive occasionally provide an indeterminate Western blot result, which may be either an incomplete antibody response to HIV in an infected person or nonspecific reactions in an uninfected person. The combination of the ELISA and Western blot tests is more than 99.9% accurate in detecting HIV infection within four to eight weeks following exposure. The polymerase chain reaction (PCR) test can be used to detect the presence of viral nucleic acids in the very small number of HIV patients who have false-negative results on the ELISA and Western blot tests. These tests are also used to detect viruses and bacteria other than HIV and AIDS. In socially disadvantaged communities however, these procedures of testing may not be feasible due to social constraints specifically poor social economic environments. This is where the oral manifestations become important indicators and most probably testing may depend only on ELISA test and CD_4 level counts.

3. Oral manifestations of HIV infection

Over 30 different oral manifestations of HIV disease have been reported since the beginning of the AIDS epidemic (Schiødt & Pindborg, 1987). Several groups of these oral manifestations are known. They may be; infections, neoplasms or other manifestations. Infections include fungal, viral or bacterial. Whereas, the most common neoplasms are Kaposi's Sarcoma and Non-Hodgkin's Lymphoma. The others category include non-specific or Aphthous-like ulcers, idiopathic thrombocytopenic purpura, mucosal melanin pigmentation and salivary gland diseases.

3.1 Fungal infections

Fungal infection or Oral Candidiasis (broadly known as thrush) is a relatively frequent problem for people who are HIV positive. People with candidiasis often notice changes in taste perception, which may make food undesirable. Oral candidiasis has been described to occur during the acute stage of HIV infection, (Dull et al., 1991) but it occurs most commonly with falling CD4+ T-cell count in the middle and late stages of HIV disease. Several reports indicate that most persons with HIV infection carry a single strain of Candida during clinically apparent candidiasis and when candidiasis is quiescent (Miyasaki et al., 1992). Oral Candidiasis may present in either of the following forms; pseudomembranous candidiasis, erythematous candidiasis, hyperplastic candidiasis, or angular cheilitis.

3.1.1 Pseudomembranous candidiasis

Pseudomembranous candidiasis is by far the most common form of oral candidiasis. Pseudomembranous candidiasis appears as a white "curd-like" material (Fig. 1) that when wiped off reveals an underlying erythematous mucosa (Shiboski et al., 2009). Removable plaques on the oral mucosa are caused by overgrowth of fungal hyphae mixed with desquamated epithelium and inflammatory cells. This type of candidiasis may involve any part of the mouth or pharynx. Generally, the clinical diagnosis is made on the basis of appearance.

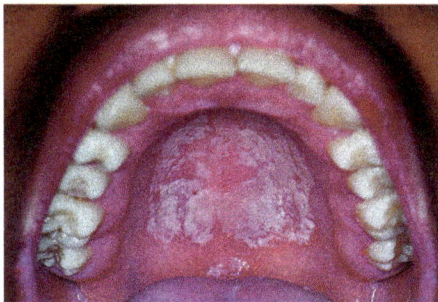

Fig. 1. Pseudomembranous candidiasis on the palate (a courtesy of F. Kahabuka)

3.1.2 Erythematous candidiasis

Erythematous candidiasis appears as flat, red patches of varying size (Fig. 2). It commonly occurs on the palate and the dorsal surface of the tongue (Shiboski et al., 2009). Erythematous candidiasis is frequently subtle in appearance and clinicians may easily overlook the lesions, which may persist for several weeks if untreated. Identification of fungal hyphae in the lesion is necessary to make a definitive diagnosis. Both Erythematous candidiasis and Pseudomembranous candidiasis can cause changes in taste perception and/or pain and a burning sensation.

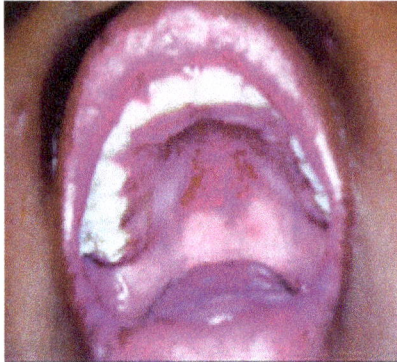

Fig. 2. Erythematous candidiasis on the palate (a courtesy of F. Kahabuka)

3.1.3 Hyperplastic candidiasis

This type of candidiasis is unusual in persons with HIV infection. The lesions appear white and hyperplastic. The white areas are due to hyperkeratosis and, unlike the plaques of pseudomembranous candidiasis, hyperplastic candidiasis cannot be removed by scraping. The lesions may be confused with hairy leukoplakia. Diagnosis of hyperplastic candidiasis is made from the histologic appearance of hyperkeratosis and the presence of hyphae in the lesion.

3.1.4 Angular cheilitis

Angula cheilitis appears as an erythema and/or fissuring either unilaterally or bilaterally at the corners of the mouth (Shiboski et al., 2009). It can appear alone or in conjunction with another form of intraoral candidiasis. This condition is easily mistaken for chapped lips.

3.2 Viral infections

Members of the human herpesvirus (HHV) and human papillomavirus (HPV) families are the most common causes of primary viral infections of the oral cavity. Nonetheless, many other viral infections can affect the oral cavity in humans, either as localized or systemic infections.

3.2.1 Herpes simplex

Oral herpes simplex is a viral condition associated with herpes simplex virus type 1 (HSV-1). It is characterized by the eruption of serum-filled vesicles, or blisters (sometimes referred to as "cold sores" or "fever blisters") on the face, lips, or mouth. Herpes simplex lesions may be large, painful, and more prone to secondary infection in HIV-positive individuals. These lesions can cause pain and decrease the ability to eat comfortably.

3.2.2 Herpes zoster

Oral herpes zoster generally causes skin lesions. Following a prodrome of pain, multiple vesicles appear on the facial skin, lips, and oral mucosa. Skin and oral lesions are frequently unilateral and follow the distribution of the maxillary and/or mandibular branches of the trigeminal nerve. The skin lesions form crusts and the oral lesions coalesce to form large ulcers. The ulcers frequently affect the gingiva, so tooth pain may be an early complaint. The reactivation of varicella zoster virus (VZV) causes herpes zoster (shingles). The disease occurs in the elderly and the immunosuppressed.

3.2.3 Human Papillomavirus (HPV) lesions

HPV-associated lesions frequently occur in the oral cavity, including the lip and sides of the tongue. HPV lesions in the oral cavity may appear as solitary exophytic, papillary or multiple nodules. They may be sessile or pedunculated and appear as multiple, smooth-surfaced raised masses resembling focal epithelial hyperplasia or as multiple, small papilliferous or cauliflower-like projections. Lesions caused by HPV are common on the skin and mucous membranes of persons with HIV disease. HPV lesions tend to be more serious and more difficult to treat in HIV-positive people. A few reports also suggest that these oral lesions may be more prevalent, or the number of lesions may be greater in people with HIV.

3.2.4 Cytomegalovirus

Oral ulcers caused by cytomegalovirus (CMV) have been reported (Jones et al., 1993). These ulcers can appear on any mucosal surface and may be confused with aphthous ulcers (Heinic et al., 1993), necrotizing ulcerative periodontitis (NUP), (Dodd et al., 1993), and lymphoma. Unlike aphthous ulcers, however, which usually have an erythematous margin, CMV ulcers appear necrotic with a white halo, (Langford et al., 1990). Diagnosis of CMV ulcers is made from a biopsy but immunohistochemistry may be helpful.

3.2.5 Hairy Leukoplakia and Epstein-Barr virus

Oral hairy leukoplakia (HL), which presents as a nonmovable, corrugated or "hairy" white lesion on the lateral margins of the tongue, occurs in all risk groups for HIV infections, although less commonly in children than in adults, (Nadal et al., 1992). HL occurs in about 20% of persons with asymptomatic HIV infection and becomes more common as the CD4+ T-cell count falls, (Feigal et al 1991). HL lesions vary in size and appearance and may be unilateral or bilateral. The surface is irregular and may have prominent folds or projections, sometimes markedly resembling hairs. Occasionally, however, some areas may be smooth and flat. Lesions occur most commonly on the lateral margins of the tongue and may spread to cover the entire dorsal surface. While this condition may resemble thrush, hairy leukoplakia lesions cannot be wiped off, unlike the lesions of thrush. Hairy leukoplakia is thought to be caused by the Epstein-Barr virus (Frezzini et al., 2006). It is also associated with infectious mononucleosis. Since this condition is rarely seen unless the CD4 cell count is low, it is less common in areas where combination anti-HIV therapy is readily available. A definitive diagnosis requires identification of Epstein-Barr virus infected epithelial cells.

3.3 Bacterial infections

The most common oral lesions associated with bacterial infection are periodontal diseases.

3.3.1 Periodontal disease

Periodontal disease is a fairly common problem in both asymptomatic and symptomatic HIV-infected patients, (Masouredis et al., 1992, Winkler et al., 1992). It can take two forms: the rapid and severe condition called necrotizing ulcerative periodontitis (NUP), (Glick et al., 1994) and its associated and possibly precursor condition called linear gingival erythema (LGE), (Grbic et al., 1995). The presenting clinical features of these diseases often differ from those in non-HIV-infected persons in that unlike for non-HIV-related periodontal disease LGE and NUP often occur in clean mouths where there is very little plaque or calculus to account for the gingivitis.

3.3.2 Linear Gingival Erythema

The gingival (gum) condition originally known as HIV-gingivitis, and now called linear gingival erythema (LGE), appear as a distinct band of erythema of the gingival margin that does not respond to removal of local factors. LGE may be painful may bleed and may progress to periodontal disease. Sometimes LGE may be mistaken for ordinary gingivitis which usually is not painful and does not lead to periodontal disease.

3.3.3 Necrotizing Ulcerative Periodontal disease

Necrotizing ulcerative periodontitis (NUP), which previously was called HIV-periodontitis, is a condition associated with rapid soft tissue and bone loss, including exposure of the bone; rapid deterioration of tooth attachment; and the premature loss of teeth. Periodontal disease may go unnoticed until the tissues supporting the teeth are so damaged as to cause the loss of a tooth.

3.4 Neoplasms

Several opportunistic tumors (cancers or neoplasms) are associated with HIV infection. Two of them namely; Kaposi's sarcoma (KS) and non-Hodgkin's Lymphoma (NHL) occur most frequently and may manifest in the oral cavity. Both of these conditions are seen when immune suppression is severe and an individual has an AIDS diagnosis (a CD4 cell count below 200 cells/mm^3).

3.4.1 Kaposi's Sarcoma

Kaposi's sarcoma (KS) is the most common neoplasm in people with HIV. KS may occur intraorally, either alone or in association with skin and disseminated lesions, (Ficarra et al 1988). Intraoral lesions have been reported at other sites and may be the first manifestation of late-stage HIV disease (AIDS).

KS can appear as a red, blue, or purplish lesion that do not blanch (whiten) with pressure. It may be flat or raised, solitary or multiple. Lesions' size ranges from small to extensive, often they enlarge rapidly and may become exophytic (grow outward). The most common oral site is the hard palate (Shiboski et al., 2009), but lesions may occur on any part of the oral mucosa, including the gingiva, soft palate, buccal mucosa and in the oropharynx, (Fig 3). Occasionally, yellowish mucosa surrounds the KS lesion. Oral KS lesions may enlarge, ulcerate, and become infected. Good oral hygiene is essential to minimize these complications. Biopsy and histologic examination are important in order to make a definitive diagnosis.

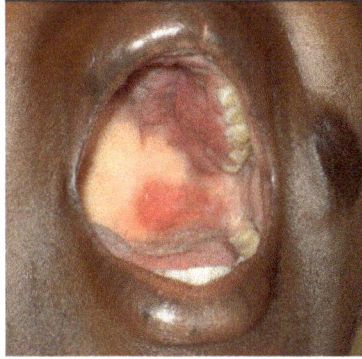

Fig. 3. Kaposi's sarcoma on the palate and skin (a courtesy of O. Hamza)

3.4.2 Non-Hodgkin's lymphoma

Diffuse, undifferentiated non-Hodgkin's lymphoma (NHL) is a frequent HIV-associated malignancy. NHL is the second most common tumor associated with HIV/AIDS (Frezzini et al., 2006), it can occur anywhere in the oral cavity. Most often NHL occurs as a soft, tumor-like mass (with or without involvement of underlying bone) that may enlarge rapidly. The lesion may present as firm, painless swelling that may be ulcerated but may also appear as necrotic or nonulcerated masses. Oral NHL may be confused with major aphthous ulcers and rarely as a pericoronitis associated with an erupting third molar. Histologic examination of biopsy specimens is required in order to make a definite diagnosis of NHL.

4. Other oral lesions associated with HIV disease

4.1 Oral ulceration

Oral ulcers resembling recurrent aphthous ulcers (RAUs) in HIV-infected persons are reported with increasing frequency. The cause of these ulcers is unknown. Proposed causes include stress and unidentified infectious agents. In HIV-infected patients, the ulcers are well circumscribed with erythematous margins. The ulcers of the minor RAU type may appear as solitary lesions of about 0.5 to 1.0 cm. The herpetiform type appears as clusters of small ulcers (1 to 2 mm), usually on the soft palate and oropharynx. The major RAU type appears as extremely large (2 to 4 cm) necrotic ulcers. The major RAUs are very painful and may persist for several weeks. The ulcers usually occur on nonkeratinized mucosa; this characteristic differentiates them from those caused by herpes simplex.

4.2 Aphthous stomatitis

Aphthous stomatitis (canker sores) is a common condition regardless of HIV status. In HIV-positive individuals the ulcers or sores may be slow to heal, and aphthous ulcers minor are more likely to become aphthous ulcers major.

4.3 Idiopathic Thrombocytopenic Purpura

Idiopathic thrombocytopenic purpura (ITP) has been reported to occur in HIV-infected patients. Oral lesions may be the first manifestation of this condition. They may present as petechiae, ecchymoses and hematoma anywhere on the oral mucosa. Spontaneous bleeding from the gingiva can occur, and patients may report finding blood in their mouths on waking up.

4.4 Salivary Gland Disease and Xerostomia

Bilateral parotid gland enlargement occurs in HIV infected individuals. Salivary gland disease associated with HIV infection (HIV-SGD) can present as xerostomia with or without salivary gland enlargement. Salivary gland enlargement in children and adults with HIV infection usually involves the parotid gland (Fig 4). The enlarged salivary glands are soft but not fluctuant. The enlarged parotid glands can be a source of annoyance and discomfort. HIV-infected patients may also experience dry mouth in association with taking certain medications (such as ddI, antidepressants, antihistamines, and antianxiety drugs) that can hinder salivary secretion.

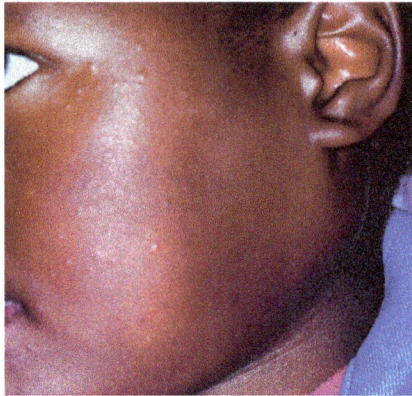

Fig. 4. Unilateral Parotid gland enlargement (a courtesy of F. Kahabuka)

4.5 Mucosal melanin pigmentation

Single and multiple oral mucosal melanotic macules have been reported to occur in HIV infected individuals. Some have been associated with zidovudine therapy. Their significance is not known and thus no treatment is indicated.

5. The relationship of HIV and oral health

Essentially, oral manifestations of HIV/AIDS are opportunistic diseases or manifestations of immune deficiency or derangement. They are not caused directly by HIV and in fact the same lesions occur in association with other immune deficiency disorders. Most oral health problems can be found in people who are either HIV positive or negative. But there are some differences worthy noting. Some conditions are found more often in PLWHA than the normal population. These include Oral candidiasis, Aphthous stomatitis (canker sores) and herpes simplex. Few oral health conditions are seen almost exclusively in people living with HIV/AIDS which include Oral Hairy Leukoplakia and opportunistic tumors, while some that are found in both populations are more problematic for people with HIV, especially those with advanced disease. Regarding dental caries, it is known that some medications used by people living with HIV/AIDS and even HIV itself may cause decreased salivary flow, or dry mouth, which is known to contribute to rampant caries. This type of caries frequently develops at the cervical region of the tooth, and the cervical area is more likely to decay at a faster rate. While periodontal diseases can occur in anyone regardless of his/her HIV status, one particularly severe form (necrotizing ulcerative periodontitis) and a related condition (linear gingival erythema) appear to be unique to those with compromised immune systems. Many of the earliest manifestations of the immune suppression associated with HIV infection occur in the mouth – particularly oral candidiasis, but also viral and sometimes severe bacterial infections, including tuberculosis. The presence of these lesions may be an early diagnostic indicator of immunodeficiency and HIV infection, may change the classification of the stage of HIV infection, and is a predictor of the progression of HIV disease (Lifson et al., 1994). The dental and oral health professions therefore have a key role in early diagnosis, and in the management of these distressing infections.

6. Trend of occurrence of oral manifestations before ARV and during ARV era

Oral manifestations of HIV infection are a fundamental component of disease progression with up to 90% of HIV-seropositive patients developing oral lesions through the course of their HIV-infection (Arendorf et al., 1998, Dios et al., 2000, Patton et al., 2000, Samaranayake et al., 2002). Occurrence of the oral lesions parallels the decline in the number of CD4 cells counts less than 200 cells/mm^3, and an increase in viral load greater than 3000 copies/mL, xerostomia, poor oral hygiene and smoking, (Aquirre et al., 1999, Tappuni & Fleming, 2001). Oral lesions are thus independent indicators of the HIV disease progression.

Following the introduction of highly active antiretroviral therapy (HAART), the oral manifestations of human immunodeficiency virus infection has changed drastically, (Aguirre et al., 1999, Domaneschi et al., 2011, Johnson 1999, Patton et al., 2000). HAART is effective in suppressing plasma-HIV viral load below a detectable level and elevating CD4 cell counts. One study noted a reduction of oral lesions from 47.6% pre-HAART to 37.5% during the HAART era (Patton et al., 2000). The study further reported a significant reduction in oral hairy leukoplakia and necrotizing ulcerative periodontitis, but on the other hand found no significant change in the incidence of oral candidiasis, oral ulcers and Kaposi's sarcoma. However, an increase was observed to occur in the HAART era of the salivary gland disease (Patton et al., 2000), and of oral warts (Greenspan et al., 2001, King et al., 2002).

Reports from few countries in the Sub Saharan Africa present a closely similar picture. In Tanzania Hamza et al., (2006) observed oral lesions in 39.5% of the patients whereas Fabian et al., (2009) reported at least one oral lesion in 45% of the PLWHA they examined while Mwangosi & Majenge, (2011) reported a prevalence of oral manifestations to be 23.5%. In Kenya Butt et al., (2001) reported over 80% prevalence of candidiasis of the hyperplastic, erythematous and pseudomembraneous types, 27.9% prevalence of lymphadenopathy and angular cheilitis, while oral Kaposi's sarcoma was seen in 13% of the patients. Six years later, Butt et al., (2007) encountered oral manifestations with highest prevalence in the oral cavity to include: angular cheilitis 32.4%, hyperplastic candidosis (labial mucosa) 15%, erythematous candidosis (gingival) 5%, Kaposis sarcoma (hard/soft palate) 2.9% and Parotid enlargement 2%. Shiboski (2002) in South Africa reported that oral candidiasis (OC) was the most common oral lesion among HIV-infected women, and that the preliminary findings suggest that HAART is associated with a decreasing OC incidence. A study by Rwenyonyi et al., (2011) among Ugandan children living with HIV/AIDS recorded one or more oral lesions in 73% of the children examined. Furthermore, they found cervical lymphadenopathy (60.8%), oral candidiasis (28.3%) and gingivitis (19.0%) to be the most common soft tissue oral lesions. They reported that the overall frequency distribution of soft tissue oral lesions was significantly lower in children on highly active antiretroviral therapy (HAART) as compared to their counterparts not on HAART.

7. Knowledge of oral manifestations of HIV/AIDS, infection control and dental care services to people living with HIV and AIDS

7.1 Knowledge of oral manifestations

Dental practitioners have satisfactory knowledge about HIV and AIDS as well as oral manifestations of HIV/AIDS. Dental students alike, especially in the last years of training have sufficient knowledge on HIV and AIDS. The attitude of dental practitioners and dental students towards HIV positive patients is good. Majority are willing to give dental treatment to HIV positive patients (Arjuna et al., 2011, Park et al., 2011, Turhan et al., 2010), though a few never treat HIV positive patients (McQuistan et al., 2010). In relation to HIV transmission, some dental students and even some dental personnel believe that HIV can be easily transmitted during clinical procedures. Some dentists, dental students and some dental school deans prefer that HIV/AIDS patients should be referred to specialized clinics (Ryalat et al., 2011, Vázquez-Mayoral et al., 2009). On the other hand, medical practitioners' knowledge of oral manifestations of HIV/AIDS is insufficient. Likewise people living with HIV/AIDS have limited awareness of oral manifestations of HIV/AIDS (Kahabuka et al., 2007). The limited knowledge and awareness may negatively impact oral health care delivery to the PLWA but may also limit utilization of dental care services even when they are available (Pereyra et al., 2011).

7.2 Knowledge on infection control measures

During provision of oral health care services, it is imperative to adhere to infection control to prevent transmission of diseases from patient to healthcare worker, healthcare worker to patient and patient to patient. Indeed, to be able to control cross infection of any blood borne diseases, the highest standards of infection control must be maintained in all clinical situations. This is essential in as far as controlling HIV spread is concern. Despite the importance of infection control in dental practice, a study by Uti et al., (2009) showed that while the level of knowledge of the dentists was generally acceptable, there was still partial compliance with recommended infection control procedures among Nigerian dentists as a result of inadequate supplies. Therefore, dental students and dental personnel must be provided with proper and current education on infection control as well as sufficient supplies in order to enhance positive attitude towards HIV positive patients. In the event a dental personnel or dental student finds himself/herself HIV positive appropriate action should be taken to protect patients and staff.

7.3 Dental care services to PLWHA

In socially disadvantaged communities, it is common to find people living with unmet dental care needs (Kikwilu et al., 2008). For people living with HIV/AIDS oral manifestations add to an already existing problem of unmet dental care needs. A number of factors contribute to this situation. Some of them are; high cost, unavailability of the services, lack of insurance and education, a shortage of dentists trained or willing to treat persons living with HIV/AIDS, patient fear and discomfort with dentists, stigma within health care systems, lack of awareness of the importance of regular dental care, and other competing priorities, (Mofidi & Gambrell, 2009, McQuistan et al., 2010). Like any health condition faced by HIV-positive people, early identification and treatment should be emphasized. In many cases, when PLWHA are attended by medical professionals for other ailments referral to a dentist should be made as soon as possible for management of oral lesions. The dental profession therefore, has an obligation to provide the required dental services to PLWHA.

8. Need for a balanced diet by people living with HIV/AIDS (PLWHA)

Food is the foundation of nutritional health. Nothing can replace food. It can be supplemented, adjusted, increased or decreased, but not entirely replaced. Food provides the building blocks of carbohydrates, proteins and fats (the macronutrients), as well as vitamins and minerals, (the micronutrients). The best way to make sure an individual gets all of these nutrients is by eating a wide variety of healthy foods every day (Centre for Disease Control 1987). Unfortunately during the acute stage, PLWHA develop oral manifestations most of which are painful conditions that may impair eating. Disturbances in eating hinders accomplishment of the PLWHA's need for a nutritionally balanced diet required much more than uninfected individuals because they need to naturally boost their immune system but also they need to deal with the weight loss. Moreover, AIDS is well known for causing severe weight loss known as wasting (WHO 2005). Whereas starving people tend to lose fat first, the weight lost during HIV infection tends to be in the form of lean tissue, such as muscle (WHO 2005). This type of wasting led to the term "slim" in some African countries during the early years of AIDS pandemic because AIDS sufferers lost a lot of lean tissue. In children, HIV is frequently linked to growth failure. One large European study found that children with HIV were on average around 7 kg (15 lbs) lighter and 7.5 cm (3 inches) shorter than uninfected children at ten years old (Kotler et al., 1989a). The double factors, that is inability to eat properly and the wasting caused by HIV infection make the PLWHA more vulnerable to nutritional insufficiency.

8.1 Weight loss and mortality

In a study done in Tanzania among people living with HIV/AIDS (Fabian et al., 2009) it was shown that the mean BMI in males was 21.01 ± 3.89 (SD) and in females the figure was 22.81 ± 3.85 (SD). In all, low BMI was significantly correlated with presence of oral candidiasis, angular cheilitis, lymph node enlargement, and oral ulcers. Moreover, candidiasis was associated with angular cheilitis and oral hairy leukoplakia, and dry mouth was related to lymph node enlargement and oral hairy leukoplakia. It is therefore assumed that people living with HIV/AIDS cannot eat well once they have oral lesions. The U.S. Centers for Disease Control and Prevention (CDC) recognized wasting as an AIDS-defining condition in 1987. The "wasting syndrome" is defined as a weight loss of at least 10% in the presence of diarrhea or chronic weakness and documented fever for at least 30 days that is not attributable to a concurrent condition other than HIV infection itself (Centre for Disease Control 1987). In practice, any involuntary weight loss of that magnitude is typically considered wasting.

A significant relationship between weight loss and mortality, disease progression, or both has been demonstrated in numerous prospective and retrospective studies both before the advent of effective antiretroviral therapy (ART) (Guenter, P. et al., 1993, Newell et al., 2003,

Wheeler et al., 1998 WHO 2005) and in the current era of treatment, in regions where such therapy is available, (Schwenk et al., 2000, Thiebaut et al., 2000). In addition to weight loss, depleted levels of body cell mass, which contains the metabolically active tissue, have been associated with increased risk of mortality in patients with HIV infection, (Guenter, P. et al., 1993). In socially disadvantaged communities, nutrition may become a major concern and probably the high mortality rate in Sub Saharan Africa may be contributed to, by poor nutrition.

Increased resting energy expenditure (REE) is a common finding in patients with HIV infection particularly in those with systemic secondary infections, (Heijligenberg et al., 1997, Shevitz et al., 1999). In addition, decreased energy intake has been found to be the primary contributor to wasting, particularly during periods of rapid weight loss rather than REE. Elevated REE may serve as a cofactor in accelerating weight loss and provides evidence of a failure to compensate for decreased energy intake. Studies using stable isotope techniques have demonstrated that total energy expenditure (TEE) is not significantly elevated in weight-stable patients with HIV infection, when compared with estimates of TEE in other studies of healthy adults (Heijligenberg et al., 1997). Patients losing weight have been found to have decreased levels of TEE, despite elevated rates of REE, reflecting a decrease in physical activity levels.

8.2 Treatment to reduce wasting

Intervention for wasting is important in the management of people living with HIV/AIDS. Treatment of secondary infections and other complications of HIV infection is an important factor in the management of wasting, as first evidenced by an increase in weight and body cell mass in patients with disseminated CMV infection treated with ganciclovir, (Kotler et al., 1989b). Opportunistic infections that interfere with swallowing such as candidiasis, herpes, or CMV esophagitis make the patients particularly susceptible to wasting. In addition to secondary infections, aphthous ulcers, chronic diarrhea, or malabsorption of any etiology; depression; and other contributors to anorexia should be treated.

8.3 Nutritional intervention to reduce wasting

Nutritional strategies to forestall or reverse wasting must work to maintain or increase energy intake. Patients with HIV infection can increase protein synthesis rates during periods of increased dietary intake, (Selberg et al 1995). However, nutritional supplementation alone is unlikely to fully restore weight or lean tissue in PLWHA. Dietary counseling is another important factor and when counseling is done by dietitians it can help individuals to identify target energy intake and food choices to suit individual tastes, practices, and tolerances. Issues such as the importance of maintaining energy intake should be emphasized, even during periods when eating is not pleasurable; and can give patients techniques for managing HIV- or medication-related symptoms such as anorexia, early satiety, nausea, vomiting, diarrhea, food intolerances, and oral or esophageal ulcers. Natural foods including homemade juices, fruits and naturally grown foods may be the most suitable types of foods during the periods when the HIV/AIDS complications are further complicated by oral and esophageal conditions.

Increases in net daily energy intake can be achieved with the use of oral supplements, despite some compensatory decrease in self-selected food consumption. Such supplements can be very useful in individuals for whom an inability or unwillingness to prepare or consume meals becomes an impediment to oral intake. A variety of liquid and solid oral supplements are available, including conventional preparations and specialized formulas for patients with specific intolerances such as fat malabsorption or lactose intolerance. Elemental formulas provide another option for individuals with malabsorptive disorders. Some studies suggest an increased benefit from special oral preparations containing specific amino acids and proprietary agents for PLWHA, (Clark et al., 2000, Pichard et al., 1998, Shabert et al., 1999). Until further data become available, the primary criteria for selection of a specific supplement should be tolerability and cost. However, use of food supplements in socially disadvantaged communities may not be practical because of unavailability.

As stated by the WHO (Petersen 2006) oral health professionals have a most important role to play in early detection of HIV/AIDS as part of their daily practice. It is needed to ensure that professionals do have the necessary skills but such skills may be obtained through systematic continuous education. In developing countries at some areas where oral health professionals are not available, specially trained primary health care workers may be instrumental in prevention of HIV/AIDS if they undertake examinations for detectable oral lesions.

9. Medical and dental service expectations of PLWHA

PLWHA have various expectations both from medical and dental personnel. For instance, Guenter, D. et al., (2010) reported that there are 3 forms of professional expert that PLWHA expect from their physicians, these included Medical/Clinical, Legal/Statutory and Moral/Ethical. With regard to the medical/ clinical expectations the PLWHA required HIV/AIDS specific knowledge and that the knowledge should be in a context of continuity over time and willingness to negotiate. The legal/statutory expectations included advocating on behalf of patients to gain access to the broader determinants of health determinants such as disability, housing, food and dietary supplements that PLWHA identified as necessary in effectively managing their illness. The PLWHA indicated that it was difficult to negotiate for moral authority of physicians. There is concern by the PLWHA that they are negatively judged, especially with regard to mode of transmission, drug use, sexuality and sexual practices. The PLWHA reported that they are open to constructive ethical and moral guidance regarding their health if they are treated in a nonjudgmental way by their physicians. Regarding expectations from dental personnel, a study done in Tanzania reported that PLWHA indicated a social need rather than a professional need (Shubi et al., 2006). The majority (95%) reported that they needed the Oral Health Professionals to have empathy, others (85%) indicated that they need the Oral Professionals to observe sterility and avoid discrimination while fewer (60%) indicated that they needed the professionals to set a separate special clinic for PLWHA or incorporate Oral Health services in the already existing special clinics for PLWHA.

10. Recommendations

Access to ARV remains low in socially disadvantaged communities. Oral manifestations affect quality of life through difficulties in food testing, chewing and swallowing. There is therefore need for immediate oral health care and referral, prevention and treatment of oral diseases. Oral health promotion is needed particularly among the socially disadvantaged communities especially in the developing countries. This can be accomplished through encouraging oral health professionals and public health professionals to work together to make oral health an integral component of optimum care management and introduction of surveillance of oral diseases associated with HIV/AIDS.

11. References

Aquirre, J.M., Echebarria, M.A., Ocina, E., Ribacoba, L. & Montejo, M. (1999). Reduction of HIV-associated oral lesions after highly active antiretroviral therapy. *Oral Surg Oral Med Oral Pathol Oral Radiol Endod.* 88(2):114-115.

Arendorf, T.M., Bredekamp, B., Cloete C.A., & Sauer, G. (1998). Oral Manifestations of HIV infection in 600 South African patients. *J Oral Pathol Med.* 27(4): 176-179.

Arjuna, N.B., Ellepola, A.N., Sundaram, D.B., Jayathilake, S., Joseph, B.K. & Sharma, P.N. (2011). Knowledge and attitudes about HIV/AIDS of dental students from Kuwait and Sri Lanka. *J Dent Educ.* 75(4):574-581.

Blankson, J.N. (2010). Control of HIV-1 replication in elite suppressors. *Discovery medicine 9* (46): 261–266. PMID 20350494.

Butt, F.M., Chindia, M.L., Vaghela, V.P., & Mandalia, K. (2001). Oral manifestations of HIV/AIDS in a Kenyan provincial hospital. *East Afr Med J.* 78(8):398-401.

Butt, F.M., Vaghela, V.P., & Chindia, M.L. (2007). Correlation of CD4 counts and CD4/CD8 ratio with HIV-infection associated oral manifestations. *East Afr Med J.* 84(8):383-8.

Centre for Disease Control. (1987). Revision of the CDC surveillance case definition for acquired immunodeficiency syndrome. Council of State and Territorial Epidemiologists; AIDS Program, *Center for Infectious Diseases.* MMWR Morb Mortal Wkly Rep. 36 Suppl 1:1S-15S.

Centers for Disease Control and Prevention. (2001). *Revised guidelines for HIV counseling, testing, and referral.* MMWR Recomm Rep. 50 (RR-19): 1–57. PMID 11718472.

Clark, R.H., Feleke, G., Din, M., Yasmin, T., Singh, G., Khan, F.A. & Rathmacher, J.A. (2000). Nutritional treatment for acquired immunodeficiency virus-associated wasting using beta-hydroxy beta-methylbutyrate, glutamine, and arginine: a randomized, double-blind, placebo-controlled study. *JPEN J Parenter Enteral Nutr.* 24(3):133-139.

Dios, P.D., Ocampo, A. & Miralles, C. (2000). Changing prevalence of human immunodeficiency virus-associated oral lesions. *Oral Surg Oral Med Oral Pathol Oral Radiol Endod.* 90(4):403-404.

Dodd, C.L., Winkler, J.R., Heinic, G.S., Daniels, T.E., Yee, K. & Greenspan, D. (1993). Cytomegalovirus infection presenting as acute periodontal infection in a patient infected with the human immunodeficiency virus. *J Clin Periodontal* 20:282-285.

Domaneschi, C., Massarente, D.B., de Freitas, R.S., de Sousa Marques, H.H., Paula, C.R., Migliari, D.A. & Antunes, J.L. (2011). Oral colonization by Candida species in AIDS pediatric patients. *Oral Dis.* 17(4):393-398. doi: 10.1111/j.1601-0825.2010.01765.x. Epub 2010 Nov 29.

Douek, D.C., Roederer, M. & Koup, R.A. (2009). Emerging concepts in the immunopathogenesis of AIDS. *Annu. Rev. Med.* 60: 471–84. doi:10.1146/annurev.med.60.041807.123549. PMC 2716400. PMID 18947296.

Dull, J.S., Sen, P., Raffanti, S., Middleton, J.R. (1991). Oral candidiasis as a marker of acute retroviral illness. *South Med J* 84:733-735, 739.

Fabian, F.M., Kahabuka, F.K., Petersen, P.E., Shubi, F.M. & Jürgensen, N. (2009). Oral manifestations among people living with HIV/AIDS in *Tanzania. Inter Dent J.* 59:187-191.

Feigal, D.W., Katz, M.H., Greenspan, D., Westenhouse, J., Winkelstein, W., Lang, W., Samuel, M., Buchbinder, S.P., Hessol, N.A., Lifson, A.R., Rutherford, G.W., Moss, A., Osmond, D., Shiboski, S., Greenspan, J.S. (1991). The prevalence of oral lesions in HTV-infected homosexual and bisexual men: Three San Francisco Epidemiologic Cohorts. *AIDS*. 5:519-525.

Ficarra, G., Berson, A.M., Silverman, S. Jr., Quivey, J.M., Lozada-Nur, F., Sooy, D.D., Migliorati, C.A. (1988). Kaposi's sarcoma of the oral cavity: a study of 134 patients with a review of the pathogenesis, epidemiology, clinical aspects, and treatment. *Oral Surg Oral Med Oral Pathol*. 66:543-550.

Frezzini, C., Leao, J.C., Cedro, M. & Porter, S. (2006). Aspects of HIV disease relevant to dentistry in the 21st century. *Dent Update*. 33(5):276-8, 281-2, 285-6.

Gilbert, P.B., McKeague, I.W., Eisen, G., Mullins, C., Guéye-Ndiaye., A., Mboup, S. & Kanki, P.J. (2003). Comparison of HIV-1 and HIV-2 infectivity from a prospective cohort study in Senegal. *Statistics in Medicine* 22 (4): 573–593. doi:10.1002/sim.1342. PMID 12590415

Glick, M., Muzyka, B.C., Salkin, L.M., Lurie, D. (1994). Necrotizing ulcerative periodontitis: a marker for immune deterioration and a predictor for the diagnosis of AIDS. *J Periodontol*. 65:393-397.

Grabar, S., Selinger-Leneman, H., Abgrall, S., Pialoux, G., Weiss, L. & Costagliola, D. (2009). Prevalence and comparative characteristics of long-term nonprogressors and HIV controller patients in the French Hospital Database on HIV. *AIDS*. 23 (9): 1163–1169. doi:10.1097/QAD.0b013e32832b44c8. PMID 19444075.

Grbic, J.T., Mitchell-Lewis, D.A., Fine, J.B., Phelan, J.A., Bucklan, R.S., Zambon, J.J., Lamster, I.B. (1995). The relationship of candidiasis to linear gingival erythema in HIV-injected homosexual men and parenteral drug users. *J Periodontol*. 66:30-37.

Greener, R. (2002). AIDS and macroeconomic impact. In *State of The Art: AIDS and Economics*. Forsythe, S.S. pp. 49–55 IAEN. ISBN 0960519610, 9780960519613

Greenspan, D., Canchola, A.J., MacPhail, L.A., Cheikh, B. & Greenspan, J.S. (2001). Effect of highly active antiretroviral therapy on frequency of oral warts. *Lancet*. 5;357(9266):1411-1412.

Guenter, P., Muurahainen, N., Simons, G., Kosok, A., Cohan, G.R., Rudenstein, R. & Turner, J.L. (1993). Relationships among nutritional status, disease progression, and survival in HIV infection. *J Acquir Immune Defic Syndr*. 6(10):1130-1138.

Guenter, D., Gillett, J., Cain, R. & Pawluch, D., Travers, R. (2010). What Do People Living With HIV/AIDS Expect From Their Physicians? Professional Expertise and the Doctor–Patient Relationship. *Journal of the International Association of Physicians in AIDS Care*. 9(6) 341-345.

Hamza, O.J.M., Matee, M.I.N., Simon, E.N.M., Kikwilu, E., Moshi, M.J., Mugusi, F., Mikx, F.H.M., Verweij, P.E. & van der Ven A.J.A.M. (2006). Oral manifestations of HIV infection in children and adults receiving highly active anti-retroviral therapy [HAART] in Dar es Salaam, Tanzania. *BMC Oral Health*. 18;6:12

Heijligenberg, R., Romijn, J.A., Westerterp, K.R., Jonkers, C.F., Prins, J.M. & Sauerwein, H.P. (1997). Total energy expenditure in human immunodeficiency virus-infected men and healthy controls. *Metabolism*. 46(11):1324-1326.

Heinic, G.S., Greenspan, D. & Greenspan, J.S. (1993). Oral CMV lesions and the HIV infected: early recognition can help prevent morbidity. *J Am Dent Assoc*. 124:99-105.

Jones, A.C., Freedman, P.D., Phelan, J.A., Baughman, R.A. & Kerpel, S.M. (1993). Cytomegalovirus infections of the oral cavity: a report of six cases and review of the literature. *Oral Surg Oral Med Oral Pathol.* 75:76-85.

Kahabuka, F., Fabian, F., Petersen, P.E. & Nguvumali, H. (2007). Awareness of HIV/AIDS and its oral manifestations among people living with HIV in Dar es Salaam, Tanzania. *Afri J of Aids Research.* 6: 91-95

Kikwilu, E.N., Masalu, J.R., Kahabuka, F.K., & Senkoro, A.R. (2008). Prevalence of oral pain and barriers to use of emergency oral care facilities among adult Tanzanians *BMC Oral Health.* 8: 28. Published online 2008 29. doi: 10.1186/1472-6831-8-28.

King, M.D., Reznik, D.A., O'Daniels, C.M., Larsen, N.M., Osterholt, D.M. & Blumberg, H.M. (2002). Human Papillomavirus-Associated Oral Warts among HIV-Seropositive Patients in the Era of Highly Active Antiretroviral Therapy: An Emerging Infection. *Clin Infect Dis.* 34:641-648.

Kotler, D.P., Tierney, A.R., Wang, J. & Pierson, R.N. Jr. (1989a). Magnitude of body-cell-mass depletion and the timing of death from wasting in AIDS. *Am J Clin Nutr.* 50(3):444-7

Kotler, D.P., Tierney, A.R., Altilio, D., Wang, J. & Pierson, R.N. (1989b). Body mass repletion during ganciclovir treatment of cytomegalovirus infections in patients with acquired immunodeficiency syndrome. *Arch Intern Med.* 149(4):901-5

Langford, A., Kunze, R., Timm, H., Ruf, B. & Reichet, P. (1990). Cytomegalovirus associated oral ulcerations in HIV-infected patients. *J Oral Pathol Med.* 19:71-76.

Lifson, A.R., Hilton, J.F., Westenhouse, J.L., Canchola, A.J., Samuel, M.C., Katz, M.H., Buchbinder, S.P., Hessol, N.A., Osmond, D.H., & Shiboski, S. (1994). Time from HIV seroconversion to oral candidiasis or hairy leukoplakia. among homosexual and bisexual men enrolled in three prospective cohorts. *AIDS.* 8:73-79.

Masouredis, C.M., Katz, M.H., Greenspan, D., Herrera, C., Hollander, H,. Greenspan, J.S. & Winkler, J.R. (1992). Prevalence of HIV-associated periodontitis and gingivitis in HIV-infected patients attending an AIDS clinic. *J Acquir Immune Defic Syndr.* 5:479-483.

McQuistan, M.R., Kuthy, R.A., Qian, F., Riniker-Pins, K.J., & Heller KE. (2010). Dentists'treatment of underserved populations following participation in community-based clinical rotations as dental students. *Journal of Public Health Dentistry.* 70:276-284.

Miyasaki, S.H., Hicks, J.B., Greenspan, D., Polacheck, I., MacPhail, L.A.., White, T.C., Agabian, N. & Greenspan, J.S., (1992). The identification and tracking of Candida albicans isolates from oral lesions in HIV-seropositive individuals. *J Acquir Immune Defic Syndr.* 5:1039-1046.

Mofidi, M. & Gambrell, A.M. (2009). Community-Based Dental Partnerships: Improving Access to Dental Care for Persons Living with HIV/AIDS. *Journal of Dental Education.* 73(11):1247-1259.

Mwangosi, I.E.A.T. & Majenge, J.M. (2011). Prevalence and awareness of oral manifestations among people living with HIV/AIDS attending counselling and treatment centres in Iringa Municipality, Tanzania. Tanzania *Journal of Health Research.*13: 205-213.

Nadal, D., de Roche, B., Buisson, M. & Seger RA (1992). Oral hairy leukoplakia in vertically and horizontally acquired HIV infection. *Arch Dis Child.* 67:1296-1297.

Newell, M.L., Borja, M.C. & Peckham, C. (2003). Height, Weight, and Growth in Children Born to Mothers With HIV-1 Infection in Europe. *Pediatrics* 111(1) e52-60.

Park, J.C., Choi, S.H., Kim, Y.T., Kim, S.J., Kang, H.J., Lee, J.H., Shin, S.C. & Cha, Y.J. (2011). Knowledge and attitudes of Korean dentists towards human immunodeficiency virus/acquired immune deficiency syndrome. *J Periodontal Implant Sci.* 41(1):3-9. Epub 2011 Feb 28.

Patton, L.L., McKaig, R., Strauss, R., Rogers, D. & Eron, J.J. Jr. (2000). Changing prevalence of oral manifestations of human immunodeficiency virus in the era of protease inhibitor therapy. *Oral Surg Oral Med Oral Pathol Oral Radiol Endod.* 89(3):299-304.

Pereyra, M., Metsch, L.R., Tomar, S., Valverde, E., Jeanty, Y., Messinger, S & Boza, H. (2011). Utilization of dental care services among low-income HIV-positive persons receiving primary care in South Florida. *AIDS Care.* 23(1):98-106.

Petersen, P.E. (2006). Policy for prevention of oral manifestations in HIV/AIDS - The approach of the WHO Global Oral Health Programme. *Adv Dent Res.* 19: 17-20

Piatak, M., Jr., Saag, M. S., Yang, L. C., Clark, S. J., Kappes, J. C., Luk, K. C., Hahn, B. H., Shaw, G. M. & Lifson, J.D. (1993). High levels of HIV-1 in plasma during all stages of infection determined by competitive PCR. *Science* 259 (5102): 1749–1754. doi:10.1126/science.8096089. PMID8096089.

Pichard, C., Sudre, P., Karsegard, V., Yerly, S., Slosman, D.O., Delley, V., Perrin, L. & Hirschel, B. (1998). A randomized double-blind controlled study of 6 months of oral nutritional supplementation with arginine and omega-3 fatty acids in HIV-infected patients. Swiss HIV Cohort Study. *AIDS.* 12(1):53-63.

Reeves, J.D. & Doms, R.W. (2002). Human Immunodeficiency Virus Type 2. *J. Gen. Virol.* 83 (Pt 6): 1253–1265. doi:10.1099/vir.0.18253-0. PMID12029140.

Rwenyonyi, C.M., Kutesa, A., Muwazi, L., Okullo, I., Kasangaki, A. & Kekitinwa A. (2011). Oral Manifestations in HIV/AIDSInfected Children. *European Journal of Dentistry* 5:291-298.

Ryalat, S.T., Sawair, F.A., Al Shayyab, M.H. & Amin, W.M. (2011). The knowledge and attitude about HIV/AIDS among Jordanian dental students: (Clinical versus pre clinical students) at the University of Jordan. *BMC Res Notes.* 15;4(1):191. [Epub ahead of print]

Samaranayake, L.P., Fidel, P.L., Naglik, J.R., Sweet, S.P., Teanpaisan, R., Coogan, M.M., Blignaut, E. & Wanzala, P. (2002). Fungal infections associated with HIV infection. *Oral Dis.* 8: 151-160.

Schiødt, M. & Pindborg, J.J. (1987). AIDS and the oral cavity. Epidemiology and clinical oral manifestations of human immune deficiency virus infection: a review. *Int J Oral Maxillofac Surg.* 16(1):1-14.

Schwenk, A., Beisenherz, A., Romer, K., Kremer, G., Salzberger, B. & Elia, M. (2000). Phase angle from bioelectrical impedance analysis remains an independent predictive marker in HIV-infected patients in the era of highly active antiretroviral treatment. *Am J Clin Nutr.* 72(2): 496 – 501

Selberg, O., Suttmann, U., Melzer, A., Deicher, H., Muller, M.J., Henkel, E. & McMillan, D.C. (1995). Effect of increased protein intake and nutritional status on whole-body protein metabolism of AIDS patients with weight loss. *Metabolism.* 44(9):1159-1165.

Shabert, J.K., Winslow, C., Lacey, J.M. & Wilmore, D.W. (1999). Glutamine-antioxidant supplementation increases body cell mass in AIDS patients with weight loss: a randomized, double-blind controlled trial. *Nutrition.* 15(11-12):860-864.

Shevitz, A.H., Knox, T.A., Spiegelman, D., Roubenoff, R., Gorbach, S.L. & Skolnik, P.R. (1999). Elevated resting energy expenditure among HIV-seropositive persons receiving highly active antiretroviral therapy. *AIDS*. 13(11):1351-1357.

Shiboski CH (2002). HIV-related oral disease epidemiology among women: year 2000 update. *Oral Dis*. 8 (Suppl) 2:44-48.

Shiboski, C.H., Patton, L.L., Webster-Cyriaque, J.Y., Greenspan, D., Traboulsi, R.S., Ghannoum, M., Juvericc, R., Phelan, J.A., Reznik, D., Greenspan, J.S., The Oral HIV/AIDS Research Alliance, Subcommittee of the AIDS Clinical Trial Group. (2009). The Oral HIV/AIDS Research Alliance: updated case definitions of oral disease endpoints. J Oral Pathol Med 38:481-488

Shubi, F., Kahabuka, F.K., Fabian, F. & Nguvumali, H. (2006). Caries status and opinions of people living with HIV/AIDS on oral health care providers' desired behaviour. *Tanz Dent J*. 13:56-63.

Tappuni, A.R. & Flemming, G.J. (2001). The effect of antiretroviral therapy on the prevalence of oral manifestations in HIV-infected patients: a UK study. *Oral Surg Oral Med Oral Pathol Oral Radiol Endod*. 92(6):623-628.

Thiebaut, R., Malvy, D., Marimoutou, C. & Davis, F. (2000). Anthropometric indices as predictors of survival in AIDS adults. Aquitaine Cohort, France, 1985-1997. Groupe d'Epidemiologie Clinique du Sida en Aquitaine (GECSA). *Eur J Epidemiol*. 16(7):633-639.

Turhan, O., Senol, Y., Baykul, T., Saba, R. & Yalçin, A.N. (2010). Knowledge, attitudes and behaviour of students from a medicine faculty, dentistry faculty, and medical technology Vocational Training School toward HIV/AIDS. *Int J Occup Med Environ Health*. 23(2):153-160.

UNAIDS report on the global AIDS epidemic 2010. Available at http://www.unaids.org/globalreport/documents/20101123_GlobalReport_full_en .pdf (Accessed 2011-09-01).

Uti, O.G., Agbelusi, G.A., Jeboda, S.O. & Ogunbodede, E. (2009). Infection control knowledge and practices related to HIV among Nigerian dentists. *J Infect Dev Ctries*. 3(8):604-610.

Vázquez-Mayoral, E.E., Sánchez-Pérez, L., Olguín-Barreto, Y. & Acosta-Gío, A.E. (2009). Dental school deans' and dentists' perceptions of infection control and HIV/AIDS patient care: a challenge for dental education in Mexico. *AIDS Patient Care STDS*. 23(7):557-562.

Wheeler, D.A.., Gibert, C.L., Launer, C.A., Muurahainen, N., Elion, R.A., Abrams, D.I. & Bartsch, G.E. (1998). Weight loss as a predictor of survival and disease progression in HIV infection. Terry Beirn Community Programs for Clinical Research on AIDS. *J Acquir Immune Defic Syndr Hum Retrovirol*. 18(1):80-85.

Winkler, J.R., Herrera, C., Westenhouse, J., Robinson, P., Hessol, N., Buchbinder, S., Greenspan, J.S. & Katz, M.H. (1992). Periodontal disease in HIV-infected and uninfected homosexual and bisexual men. *AIDS* 6:1041-1043.

World Health Oorganization (2005). Consultation on Nutrition and HIV/AIDS in Africa: Evidence, lessons and recommendations for action.

15

The Influence of Smoking on Dental and Periodontal Status

Jindra Smejkalova, Vimal Jacob, Lenka Hodacova,
Zdenek Fiala, Radovan Slezak and Sajith Vellappally
Charles University in Prague, Medical Faculty in Hradec Kralove
Czech Republic

1. Introduction

Tobacco is one of the major toxic agents in our civilization. It's use is considered as one of the most common cause of mortality and morbidity in both developed and developing countries in present times. Of 260 million deaths which occurred in the developing world between 1950 and 2000, it is estimated that 50 million were due to smoking. Globally, smoking related mortality is set to rise from 3 million annually (1995 estimate) to 10 million annually by 2030, with 70 % of these deaths occurring in developing countries (Fagerström, 2002). Since 1970, smoking prevalence among men has slightly decreased, but among women, teenagers and children, smoking has increased dramatically. Sixty percent of children are exposed to Environmental Tobacco Smoke (ETS) at their homes (Mackay & Amos, 2003).

Tobacco is one of the most important risk factor for oral diseases including oral cancer, oral mucosal lesions, periodontal diseases, wound healing failure, dental implants failure, gingival inflammation, acute necrotizing ulcerative gingivitis and apthous ulcers (Vellappally et al., 2007; Jacob et al., 2007). There is substantial evidence suggesting that the risk of oral diseases increase with frequent use of tobacco and that quitting smoking results in reduced risk (Winn, 2001).

1.1 Smoking and dental caries

Smoking and its relation to dental caries is a subject of many opinions. From early reports in literature and in accordance with common belief smoking was thought to actually help to reduce dental caries (Hart, 1899; Gibbs, 1952). Schmidt, in 1951, reported that the increase in tobacco smoking was followed by a decrease in caries rate. Smoking increases thiocyanate level in saliva. Thiocyanate, a normal constituent of saliva, was found to have caries inhibiting effect (Reibel, 2003; Johnson & Bain, 2000). On the other hand, studies showed that smoking is associated with lower salivary cystatin activity and output of cystatin C is also reduced during gingival inflammation. Cystatins are thought to contribute to maintaining oral health by inhibiting certain proteolytic enzymes (Lie et al., 2001). In addition, studies have confirmed by earlier results that there were no significant differences in salivary flow rates between smokers and non-smokers (Reibel, 2003). The decreased buffering effect of smoker's saliva and the higher number of lactobacilli and *S. mutans group* may indicate an increased susceptibility to caries (Schmidt, 1951; Kassirer, 1994). To date, several investigators have discovered a correlation between an increased smoking level and dental caries (Axelsson et al., 1998; Bruno-Ambrosius et al., 2005). For example, in 1952, Ludwick and Massler reported that individuals who smoked more than 15 cigarettes daily had significantly higher number of decayed, missing, and filled teeth. In 1971, Ainamo found that increased smoking results in significantly high number of decayed surfaces per dentition. In 1990, Zitterbart confirmed an association between smoking and the prevalence of dental caries in adult males. Smokers had a significantly higher DMFT (Decayed, Missing, and Filled Teeth) score, untreated decayed surfaces, and missing surfaces. More cigarettes consumed per day resulted in more missing tooth surfaces in a smoker's mouth (Zitterbart et al., 1990). Statistical analyses from a study in Sweden in 1991 showed that smoking, as a habit and an increased number of cigarettes smoked per day, are positively correlated with the increased number of decayed, missing and filled teeth and number of initially decayed proximal surfaces (Hirsch et al., 1991). Even though studies did not establish a causative relationship, the recent study done on American female population in 2006, showed a correlation between cigarette smoking and the presence of dental caries (Heng et al., 2006).

Most of the studies mentioned above have taken into consideration other contributing factors to dental caries development, such as age, tobacco habits other than smoking, oral hygiene habits, eating habits, preventive visits to dentist (dental recalls) and overall health standards. Therefore elucidating the exact strength of dental caries in relation to smoking is difficult to identify.

Association between smoking and dental caries is well documented in older age groups (Locker, 1992; Jette et al., 1993). Among the middle-age (Axelsson et al., 1998) or young adults (Sgan-Cohen et al., 2000) results are inconsistent. Non-smokers reported more frequent healthy oral health behavior than did daily smokers (Telivuo et al., 1995). Studies indicate that smokers not only had bad oral hygiene and less sophisticated outlook on health, but also had different eating habits, presumably consuming higher amount of sugar containing products like soft drinks and snacks (Axelsson et al., 1998; Hirsch et al., 1991). Daily smoking was associated with increased use of sugar in tea and coffee, and with more frequent alcohol consumption (Telivuo et al., 1995). It was also found that smokers have poorer brushing habits than non-smokers (Ainamo, 1971; Kelbauskas et al., 2005; Macgregor, 1985). Also current smokers were less likely to report regular preventive visits to dentists and were reluctant to use accessory dental aids such as dental floss (Locker, 1992).

In natural tobacco, sugar can be present in a level up to 20 %$_{wt}$. In addition, various caries promoting factors such as sugars and sweeteners are added intentionally during tobacco manufacturing process (Talhout et al., 2006). Sugars used as cigarette additive include glucose, fructose, invert sugar (glucose/fructose mixture) and sucrose. In addition, many tobacco additives contain high amount of sugars, for example fruit juices, honey, molasses extracts, cones, maple syrup and caramel. The added sugars are usually reported to serve as flavor/casing and humectants. However, sugars also promote tobacco smoking, because they generate acids that neutralize the harsh taste and throat impact of tobacco smoke. Moreover, the sweet taste and the agreeable smell of caramelized sugar flavors are appreciated in particular by starting adolescent smokers (Talhout et al., 2006).

All the findings above can be argued for increased dental caries in smokers. Though a direct etiological relation is still lacking between smoking and dental caries, the above-mentioned studies and findings point to the conjecture that smoking has some influence in high caries incidence. Further studies, clinical trials and experiments are needed to confirm the independent effect of smoking as one of the causes of dental caries.

1.2 Smoking and periodontitis

The manifestation and progression of periodontitis, a multifactorial disease with microbial dental plaque as the initiator, is influenced by a variety of determinants and factors. They include subject characteristics, social and behavioral factors, systemic factors, genetic factors, tooth-related factors, microbial composition of dental plaque and other emerging factors (Nunn, 2003). Cigarette smoking is a significant risk factor for periodontal disease (Tanner, 2005), demonstrated by an increased loss of attachment (Hymann & Reid, 2003; Amarasena et al., 2003; Razali et al., 2005), development and progression of periodontal inflammation (James et al., 1999; Genco, 1996) and increased gingival recession (Müller et al., 2002). It has been estimated that smoking accounts for half of all periodontal diseases. There is epidemiological evidence which shows that cigarette smoking is a stronger risk factor for the presence of periodontitis compared to the presence of certain suspected periodontal pathogens (Darby et al., 2005). The number of cigarettes smoked per day is a major risk determining factor, doubling the risk for those in the lowest consumption category and increasing it six fold in the subgroup smoking more than thirty cigarettes per day (Tomar & Asma, 2000; Winn, 2001). Former smokers have lower rates of periodontitis than present smokers (Alabandar et al., 2000; Calsina et al., 2002; Johnson & Hill, 2004; Krejci & Bissada, 1999; Spickerman et al., 2003; Van Winkelhoff et al., 2001). Longitudinal studies indicate that periodontal disease may progress faster in smokers in comparison to non-smokers (Beck et al., 1997; Winn, 2001). Further research on this topic is necessary to expand the spectrum of knowledge acquired till date and to apply it clinically.

The Community Periodontal Index of Treatment Needs (CPITN) was developed for the 'Joint Working Committee' of the World Health Organization (WHO) and Federation Dentaire Internationale (FDI) by Jukka Ainamo, David Barmes, George Beagrie, Terry Cutress, Jean Martin, and Jennifer Sandro-Infirri in 1982. The CPITN procedure is recommended for epidemiological surveys of periodontal health. It uses clinical parameters and criteria relevant to planning and prevention of periodontal diseases and it records the common treatable conditions namely periodontal pockets, gingival inflammation and dental calculus (Ainamo & Ainamo, 1994). The CPITN is not intended as a comprehensive assessment of total past and present periodontal disease experience and it does not record irreversible changes such as gingival recession or other deviations from periodontal health such as tooth mobility or loss of periodontal attachment (Peter, 1999). Association between cigarette smoking and various oral diseases such as leukoplakia and oral cancers has been well documented but the role of cigarette smoking in the causation of periodontitis, however has not been widely investigated in the Czech Republic. In this study, the CPITN index was used to evaluate the influence of cigarette smoking on periodontitis.

2. Aim of the study

The aim of the study was to evaluate the different approach of smokers and non-smokers to the oral health and to monitor the influence of smoking habits on the oral health, namely on the periodontium and the teeth.

3. Methods

A cross-sectional population-based study was conducted in Czech Republic on a representative sample of 1684 respondents within the age group of 30 to 69 years. The project was conducted in cooperation with the Department of Hygiene and Preventive Medicine of Charles University in Prague, Medical Faculty in Hradec Kralove and Department of Dentistry of University Hospital in Hradec Kralove.

The study consisted of two parts - self reported questionnaire inquiry and clinical examination of oral health status including examination of teeth, periodontium and oral mucosa. Clinical investigations were performed by the uniformly instructed dentists. To limit the select bias caused by the fact that hospitalized patients usually do not represent the common population the respondents were selected from the patients hospitalized in the University Hospital as well as from patients of three practicing dentists.

3.1 Questionnaire investigation

All participants of this study were requested to answer the questionnaire which included questions concerning their personal history, economic status, educational qualification, profession and other important etiological factors of oral health, which can play a role of so called „confounding factors", like general health status, frequency of dental visit, brushing habits and dental aids used. We were also interested (though very tentatively) in the eating habits, the suitable and non suitable food. We inquired into the consumption of food with the risk for oral health (confections, sweet drinks), as well as of the food with the protective effect (fruit, vegetable as a sources of natural antioxidants). Respondents could make their choice among the answers: „ regularly, daily, several times a week, several times a month, less frequently, never." Questions concerning alcohol consumption were also included in the questionnaire.

Detailed attention was given to smoking history. Regular smokers were defined as individuals who, at the time of examination, smoked at least one cigarette daily. Occasional smokers were individuals who smoked less than one cigarette per day. Former or ex-smokers were defined as individuals who smoked at least 1 cigarette per day for 6 consecutive months and those who did not smoke at least for the past 6 months from the time of the study. Finally, non-smoker was a person, who never smoked for the period longer than 6 months. We also took into account the number of cigarettes smoked each day or week and the number of years of smoking.

The last section of the questionnaire was focused on a subjective assessment of the oral health by the respondents themselves and on their information level about the smoking harmfulness. The questionnaire clarity and the time necessary for filling it up were traced in the pilot study.

3.2 Clinical investigation

Dental status and periodontal status were assessed by DMF (Decayed, Missing, and Filled Teeth) and CPITN (Community Periodontal Index of Treatment Needs) indices respectively, which at present are considered to be sufficiently valid for population studies.

The dentition was evaluated by recording the number of the decayed (D), missing (M) and filled (F) teeth, and number of decayed teeth with fillings (D+F) as well. The index DMF was then calculated as a sum of all these four quantities: DMF = D + M + F + (D + F). Thus, in the total sum each tooth was counted only once.

The periodontal status and treatment needs were evaluated by the help of CPITN index (Community Periodontal Index of Treatment Need) using the alternative of this index for individual use in adults where in the individual sextants, all teeth were examined with the exception of the third molars only. The CPI 0 means a healthy periodontium; CPI 1 indicates the gingival bleeding on gentle probing. The CPI 2 code is characterized by the presence of retention factors for plaque on the given tooth surface, most often by supragingival and/or subgingival calculus. Furthermore, CPI 3 coding indicated the presence of shallow pockets up to 4-5 mm, while CPI 4 indicated deep pockets 6 mm or more. In cases where there were two teeth only in some sextant, this was not taken into account (CPI X). Edentulous individuals were excluded from this study.

To judge the impact of some selected variables such as smoking and certain "confounding" factors on the oral health, or the periodontium we used the treatment needs category of the CPITN index, which is related to the health care needs of inflamed periodontium. The value TN 0 (no treatment needed) corresponds with the CPI 0 in the given sextant. Classification CPI 1 conforms with TN I (oral hygiene necessary), whereas CPI 2 and CPI 3 correspond with TN II (oral hygiene needed, clearing up the calculus and other retention factors for plaque). CPI 4 is equal to TN III, which indicates the need for complex treatment (oral hygiene adjustment, clear out, need of tooth extraction and its replacement, need for surgical treatment of periodontal pockets, fixation of rather unstable teeth and other therapeutic modalities).

3.3 Statistical analysis

The statistical evaluation was performed by using NCSS 2007 program. Descriptive statistics, χ^2 test and logistic regression were done. To compare quantitative data (e.g. the age), Kruskal – Wallis analysis of dispersion with subsequent multiple matching (ANOVA) has been used. To evaluate qualitative data (e.g. the level of education) the X^2 test of independence in the contingent tables or Fisher's exact test was used.

For calculating the odds ratio for the selected variables (such as smoking, health status, education, frequency of teeth brushing, taking part in preventive check ups, food consumption even after the evening teeth brushing) we employed the method of multiple logistic regression.

4. Results

4.1 Results of questionnaire part of the study

During the 3 years period of data collection, we investigated 1 684 respondents. Participants were chosen randomly, with age above 69 years and less than 30 years being the only exclusion criterion. Our sample consisted of 792 males and 922 females with mean age of 44.2 years. There were 489 current smokers (369 regular and 120 occasional ones), 261 former smokers and 934 non-smokers among them (table 1).

The level of respondents´ education in individual groups is illustrated in table 2. People with the basic education represented 28.3%, 7.9% were skilled with graduation exam, 41.6% passed the high school and 22.2% had the university education. Majority of the respondents with the basic education (44%) were found to be regular smokers. The highest number among university educated persons (28.2%) was identified as non-smokers. Quite surprisingly, we found relatively high prevalence of people with the high school education as regular and occasional smokers. These results are significantly different (p < 0.001).

Smoker:	Males		Females		Total	
	n	%	n	%	n	%
Regular	206	26.0	163	18.2	369	21.9
Occasional	63	8.0	57	6.4	120	7.1
Ex-smoker	161	20.3	100	11.2	261	15.5
Non-smoker	362	45.7	572	64.2	934	55.5
Total	792	100.0	922	100.0	1684	100.0

Table 1. Classification according to cigarette smoking and gender ($p < 0.001$; χ^2 test)

Education	Regular smoker	Occasional smoker	Ex-smoker	Non-smoker	Total
Basic	44.0	25.0	26.8	23.0	28.3
Vocational	9.8	11.7	10.3	6.0	7.9
High school	35.8	45.0	44.1	42.8	41.6
University graduation	10.4	18.3	18.8	28.2	22.2
Total	100.0	100.0	100.0	100.0	100.0

Table 2. Educational qualification of respondents in percentage ($p < 0,001$; χ^2 test)

Table 3 shows the average monthly income per head in the family of our respondents. In our study, 3.7% of investigated persons belonged to the lowest income group, 30.4% in the middle, and 47.3% in the higher income group. About 5% of respondents did not know the exact family income, and 13.7% of them refused to answer. The income differences between smokers and non-smokers were not statistically significant (p= 0,665). From these results we can only find not statistically lower frequency of people with the higher incomes in the group of smokers.

Income/moths/person	Regular smoker	Occasional smoker	Ex-smoker	Non-smoker	Total
Not willing to disclose	14.5	15.1	11.7	13.7	13.7
< 5000 CZK	4.7	4.2	3.5	3.3	3.7
5000 – 10000 CZK	30.7	23.5	28.8	31.6	30.4
> 10000 CZK	44.1	51.3	52.1	46.8	47.3
Do not know	6.0	5.9	3.9	4.6	4.9
Total	100.0	100.0	100.0	100.0	100.0

Table 3. Characteristics according to the income, it means the net monthly earnings per person in the family ($p = 0,665$; χ^2 test)

As for the attitude towards oral health, we can conclude that the participation in the preventive check-ups by dentist was far from being optimal (table 4). In Czech Republic, the dental health care system provides its citizens the opportunity to participate in dental prevention programs two times yearly and this check ups are free of charge, paid from health insurance. From the results of our study we can see that prevention twice a year was performed by 64.8% respondents only, whereas 22.8% visited the dentist once a year. Nevertheless, the attitude of non-smokers and smokers towards preventive dental check-ups were different; whereby non-smokers visited their dentists more often than smokers and former smokers. Among regular smokers, 6.3% visited the dentist once in two years, 7.9% respondents took part in check-ups less frequently; and 8.7% never attended preventive check-ups. These findings were found to be statistically significantly different (p < 0.001).

Preventive check-ups	Regular smoker	Occasional smoker	Ex-smoker	Non-smoker	Total
2 times a year	52.3	63.0	62.8	70.6	64.8
Once a year	24.8	26.1	23.0	21.6	22.8
Once in 2 years	6.3	2.5	5.0	3.1	4.1
Less frequently	7.9	6.7	6.1	2.9	4.8
Never	8.7	1.7	3.1	1.8	3.5
Total	100.0	100.0	100.0	100.0	100.0

Table 4. Percentage of respondents participating in preventive dental check-ups (p < 0,001; χ^2 test)

We also found a different approach of smokers and non-smokers to the oral hygiene (table 5). Most of the investigated persons (87.6%) brushed their teeth twice or even three times a day. The majority of them were non-smokers, former or occasional smokers. Almost 90% of respondents from these groups brushed their teeth 2 – 3 times a day. The regular smokers did so in 78.2% only. More than 15% of regular smokers brushed their teeth once a day only and another 6.5% of them even less often. Results are statistically significant (p < 0.001).

	Regular smoker	Occasional smoker	Ex-smoker	Non-smoker	Total
3 times a day or more	7.3	7.6	5.8	14.7	11.2
2 times a day	70.9	83.1	83.8	75.6	76.4
Once daily	15.2	7.6	7.7	8.8	9.9
Less frequently	6.5	1.7	2.7	1.0	2.5
Total	100.0	100.0	100.0	100.0	100.0

Table 5. Tooth brushing frequency (%); p < 0.001; χ^2 test

Almost all the probands (98.3 %) used the tooth brush and tooth paste. Dental floss and interdental brushes were used by non-smokers and former smokers (p =0,001). Regular use of mouth wash were being performed regularly (12.7%) or occasionally (48.9 %) mainly by non-smokers and former smokers (p < 0.015).

Table 6 illustrates the eating habits of our respondents. We enquired about the consumption of risky foods (confectionary, sweet drinks) as well as protective ones (fruit, vegetable as a source of natural antioxidants). In this table we also included the questions concerning alcohol consumption.

Statistical evaluation revealed the consumption of sweets to be generally high. Nearly 14% of our respondents consumed confectioneries regularly or on a daily basis (13.8%), or at least several times a week (35.1 %). There was a statistically significant difference between smokers and non-smokers. The regular and former smokers consumed much less sweets than occasional smokers and non-smokers (p < 0.001). Also the consumption of sweetened drinks was rather high, 18.7% of respondents consumed sweetened drinks daily and more than one quarter of investigated persons (27.1%) had such drinks several times a week. The consumption of sweetened drinks was more popular among smokers compared to non-smokers (p < 0.001).

In case of a healthy diet consumed by the respondents such as the use of fruits and vegetables, the trend was just opposite. Fruits and vegetables were consumed regularly by 53% of respondents, significantly more often by the non-smokers and former smokers (p < 0.001).

The regular daily consummation of beer and wine was agreed by 7.5% of respondents. The regular smokers were leading this ladder (p < 0.001). 1.4% of investigated persons agreed to have consumed spirits on a regular daily basis. The regular smokers represented a marked majority, statistically significant (p < 0.001).

	Regular smoker	Occasional smoker	Ex-smoker	Non-smoker	Total
Sweets p < 0.001; χ^2 test					
Regular daily	13.2	15.3	12.6	14.2	13.8
Sweet drinks (soft drinks, coca-cola, juices) p < 0.001; χ^2 test					
Regular daily	27.0	23.5	16.5	15.4	18.7
Fruits and vegetables p < 0.001; χ^2 test					
Regular daily	38.0	47.5	54.9	58.9	52.9
Beer and vine p < 0.001; χ^2 test					
Regular daily	11.9	6.8	10.7	5.1	7.5
Distilled liquors p < 0.001; χ^2 test					
Regular daily	2.8	2.6	2.0	0.4	1.4

Table 6. Eating habits of respondents (in percentages)

An important difference between smokers and non-smokers was also found in the consumption of food and sweetened drinks after the evening teeth brushing (table 7), which was more frequent in smokers with comparison to non-smokers.

„After having brushed teeth in the evening:	Regular smoker	Occasional smoker	Ex-smoker	Non-smoker	Total
I never **eat or drink any sweet drinks or beer or milk"**					
Yes, that is true.	34,7	48,3	52,6	61,6	53,4
I usually do not eat or drink sweet drinks"					
Yes, that is true.	48,9	46,6	38,2	33,2	38,3
I still eat some food and drink sweet drinks"					
Yes, that is true.	16,4	5,2	9,2	5,3	8,3

Table 7. Food and sweet drinks consumption after the evening teeth brushing (%); χ^2 test

The last part of the questionnaire was aimed to the subjective assessment of oral cavity status by respondents themselves, on assessment of the quality of life in connection with the oral health, and finally on the knowledge of respondents regarding the harmfulness of smoking. Table 8 shows that half of respondents (53.6%) evaluated appearances of their own dentition as good, 44% were unsatisfied and 2.2% were not interested in evaluation. When taking into account the history of smoking we can see that non-smokers were satisfied with their dental health more often (57.9%) when compared with those with the smoking history. The lowest degree of satisfaction was found among the regular smokers. These findings were statistically markedly significant (p < 0.001). The status of teeth, gingivae and oral mucosa were considered to be in good condition by 49.6% of the investigated individuals. One quarter of total number considered this status as bad and 25.4% were not able to answer this question. When answering this question the non-smokers considered their oral health status being good more often than regular or even former smokers (p < 0.001). Regular and former smokers thought that their oral health is poorer when compared with the rest of population (p< 0.001).

Level of respondents' knowledge regarding the harmful effects of smoking is illustrated in table 9. According to our opinion these results were rather favorable. Nearly all the members of our study (95.6%) knew that smoking harms the health. Nevertheless, smokers showed statistically much poorer knowledge when compared with the non-smokers (p < 0.001). The awareness concerning negative influence of smoking on oral cavity was found to be low. Positive answer was obtained from 90.5%, but smokers response was markedly less frequent (78.9%) when compared to non-smokers or former smokers (p < 0.001). For the question whether they were informed about the negative effects of smoking on one's health by their dentist, the positive response rate was only 49%, mainly answered by regular smokers. On the contrary, the non-smokers were not informed (p < 0.001), which means that the health education was performed rather selectively, most often targeted on the smokers.

Questions:	Regular smoker	Occasional smoker	Ex-smoker	Non-smoker	Total
"Are you satisfied with the appearance of your teeth?" p < 0. 001; χ^2 test					
- satisfied	44,0	58,5	50,0	57,9	53,6
- non-satisfied	52,7	41,5	48,4	39,8	44,1
- I am not interested in it	3,3	0,0	1,6	2,3	2,2
"How do you assess the health status of your teeth, gingivae and oral mucosa?" p < 0. 001; χ^2 test					
- good	36,2	53,8	42,0	56,6	49,6
- bad	32,9	22,7	28,4	21,2	25,0
- I don't know	31,0	23,5	29,6	22,2	25,4
"In comparison with the others, do you think your oral health is": p< 0. 001; χ^2 test					
- better	19,7	17,9	24,8	34,0	28,3
- the same	52,6	65,8	50,0	50,8	52,2
- worse	27,7	16,2	25,2	15,2	19,6

Table 8. Subjective assessment of oral health by respondents (%)

Questions:	Regular smoker	Occasional smoker	Ex-smoker	Non-smoker	Total
"Do you think smoking is harmful for your health? " p < 0. 001; χ^2 test					
- yes	89,4	95,8	98,5	97,2	95,6
"Do you think smoking has bad influence on your oral health?" p < 0. 001; χ^2 test					
- yes	78,9	85,0	95,8	94,3	90,5
"Were you informed about the negative effect of smoking on your health by your dentist?" p < 0. 001; χ^2 test					
- yes	59,6	52,5	52,9	42,6	48,6

Table 9. Knowledge of respondents about the health consequences of smoking (%)

4.2 Results of clinical part of the study
4.2.1 Influence of smoking on DMF index

The assessment of a dental status showed that smokers had a significantly higher DMF index when compared to non-smokers (17.2 vs. 16; p = 0.001) (table 10), which had been caused mainly due to a higher number of decayed teeth (D) (1.06 vs. 0.7; p = 0.003), missing teeth (M) (5.65 vs. 4.53; p < 0.001) and decayed teeth with fillings (D+F) (1.46 vs. 1.03; p = 0.04).

Variables	Number of decayed teeth (D)		Number of missed teeth (M)		Number of filled teeth (F)		Number of decayed teeth with fillings (D+F)		DMF index	
	Mean ± s.d.	p-value	Mean ± s.d.	p-value	Mean ± s.d.	p-value	Mean ± sd.	p-value	Mean ± s.d.	p-value
Smoking:										
- smokers	1,06 ± 1,94	0,003 (**)	5,65 ± 6,82	<0,001 (***)	9,18 ±5,52	0,008 (**)	1,46 ± 2,56	0,046 (*)	17,23 ± 7,35	0,001 (**)
- non-smokers	0,70 ± 1,50		4,53 ± 5,93		9,84 ± 5,26		1,03 ± 1,76		16,05 ± 7,06	
Age:										
- younger 50	0,83 ±1,75	0,21 (NS)	2,88 ± 3,79	<0,001 (***)	9,58 ± 5,10	0,11 (NS)	1,20 ± 1,98	0,842 (NS)	14,41 ± 6,52	<0,001 (***)
- 50 or older	0,91 ±1,66		9,06 ± 8,01		9,57 ± 5,89		1,27 ± 2,48		20,70 ± 6,62	
Sex:										
- males	1,01 ±1,91	0,008 (*)	5,14 ± 6,67	0,508 (NS)	9,24 ± 5,29	0,028 (*)	1,28 ± 2,20	0,649 (NS)	16,56 ± 7,37	0,879 (NS)
- females	0,73 ±1,52		4,89 ± 6,03		9,83 ± 5,45		1,17 ± 2,14		16,57 ± 7,05	
Education:										
Basic	1,17 ± 2,32		6,75 ± 7,30		9,35 ± 5,66		1,37 ± 2,39		18,60 ± 7,26	
Vocational	1,14 ± 1,80	<0,001 (***)	4,62 ± 5,64	<0,001 (***)	9,21 ± 5,05	0,020 (*)	1,25 ±1,76	0,301 (NS)	16,10 ± 6,71	<0,001 (***)
High school	0,65 ± 1,25		4,65 ± 6,18		10,00 ± 5,32		1,14 ± 2,15		16,36 ± 6,93	
University	0,74 ± 1,35		3,56 ± 4,88		9,11 ± 5,23		1,20 ± 2,02		14,51 ± 7,16	
Preventive check-ups:										
Two times a year	0,66 ± 1,28		4,52 ± 5,61		10,10 ± 5,42		1,10 ± 2,11		16,33 ± 7,02	
Once a year	0,91 ± 1,56		4,79 ± 6,10		9,13 ± 5,13		1,37 ± 2,12		16,12 ± 7,16	
Once in 2 years	1,34 ± 1,68	<0,001 (***)	6,93 ± 8,16	<0,001 (***)	7,60 ± 4,59	<0,001 (***)	1,44 ± 2,31	0,003 (**)	17,00 ± 7,82	<0,001 (***)
Less frequently	1,54 ± 2,23		7,48 ± 8,54		8,78 ± 5,14		1,59 ± 1,93		19,38 ± 7,52	
Never	2,90 ± 4,80		9,46 ±10,05		5,09 ± 4,59		1,89 ± 3,21		19,19 ± 8,32	
Tooth brushing frequency:										
3 times or more	0,62 ± 1,32		5,70 ± 7,40		8,81 ± 5,43		0,86 ± 1,15		15,92 ± 7,26	<0,001 (***)
2 times/day	0,79 ± 1,49	<0,001	4,56 ± 5,77	<0,001	9,81 ± 5,33	<0,001	1,24 ± 2,22	0,677	16,31 ± 7,08	

Variables	Number of decayed teeth (D)		Number of missed teeth (M)		Number of filled teeth (F)		Number of decayed teeth with fillings (D+F)		DMF index	
	Mean ± s.d.	p-value	Mean ± s.d.	p-value	Mean ± s.d.	p-value	Mean ± sd.	p-value	Mean ± s.d.	p-value
Once daily	1,33 ± 2,06	(***)	6,50 ± 7,82	(***)	9,14 ± 5,44	(***)	1,28 ± 2,10	(NS)	18,28 ± 7,52	
Less frequently	2,32 ± 4,61		9,31 ± 8,35		6,30 ± 5,45		2,15 ± 3,62		19,57 ± 7,81	
Eating after evening tooth brushing:										
- Yes	1,85 ± 2,93	<0,001	7,33 ± 7,86	<0,001	8,07 ± 5,45	<0,001	1,60 ± 2,69	0,540	18,82 ± 7,68	<0,001
- No	0,77 ± 1,54	(***)	4,68 ± 6,00	(***)	9,76 ± 5,33	(***)	1,19 ± 2,10	(NS)	16,30 ± 7,09	(***)

Table 10. The impact of some variables on the DMF index value
s.d. = standard deviation

On the contrary, the mean number of teeth with fillings (F) was significantly higher in non-smokers than smokers (9.84 vs. 9.18; $p = 0,008$), which most probably corresponds with better participation of non-smokers in the follow-ups.

Smoking is one of many confounding factors which deteriorate the status of dentition and oral health in general. From the other variables of our study (table 10), the most influential predictors of dental status or DMF value are as follows: the age (linear relation), the level of education achieved (non-linear relation), taking part in preventive dental check-ups (non-linear relation), tooth brushing frequency (non-linear relation), and consumption of food/beverages after evening tooth brushing. Among the respondents in higher age group, there was a higher number of missing teeth (M). In our sample, the average number of missing teeth in respondents younger than 50 years reached 2.88, while in the age group of 50-69, it was 9.06 ($p < 0.001$). The number of missing teeth was higher in respondents with a lower educational status, lower frequency of preventive dental visits (less than once a year), lower frequency of tooth brushing (less than twice a day) and among those who consumed food/beverages after the evening tooth brushing. The number of decayed teeth was also higher in patients with a lower education, among those who brushed their teeth less than twice daily, among those who visited dentist less frequently and among those who consumed food/beverages after the evening tooth brushing. The same factors influenced significantly the number of filled teeth; nevertheless in this case it was a non-linear relation.

4.2.2 Influence of smoking on the periodontium

Negative influence of smoking on the periodontium was even more conclusive (table 11). While the non-smokers recorded higher prevalence of CPI 0 (healthy periodontium) in all sextants, the smokers had in all sextants a higher prevalence of CPI 3, or resp. CPI 4 (shallow or deep gingival pockets). Lower levels of CPI 1 (gingiva bleeding on probing) among smokers were undoubtedly caused by vasoconstriction effect of nicotine on the vessels of gingival plexus and an increasing keratinization of gingival epithelium.

Smoking is of course only one of the factors that affect the periodontal status. A wide range of demographic factors, such as age, educational level and socioeconomic factors, have been identified as associated with chronic inflammatory diseases (Gamonal et al., 1998). In table 12 we present the percentage of respondents with the highest CPI findings according to the level of age, sex, education, participation in preventive dental check-ups, tooth brushing frequency and smoking history. According to the results of χ^2 test of independence in contingency tables, all these variables had a statistically significant influence on CPI (p< 0.001).

	CPITN 0	CPITN 1	CPITN 2	CPITN 3	CPITN 4
1st sextant (p=0.076; χ^2 test)					
Smokers	5.6	27.2	13.9	34.5	7.3
Non-smokers	9.1	33.7	13.8	29.5	6.8
2nd sextant (p=0.016; χ^2 test)					
Smokers	17.4	31.7	24.0	15.0	5.2
Non-smokers	25.3	37.3	19.3	10.4	3.7
3rd sextant (p=0.021; χ^2 test)					
Smokers	7.0	23.7	16.4	32.8	9.8
Non-smokers	11.5	31.3	17.2	25.6	6.8
4th sextant (p=0.043; χ^2 test)					
Smokers	5.6	30.0	14.3	30.3	11.5
Non-smokers	10.2	35.2	14.1	27.2	6.5
5th sextant (p=0.007; χ^2 test)					
Smokers	4.2	14.3	58.9	15.7	3.5
Non-smokers	8.6	18.8	59.0	8.1	3.1
6th sextant (p=0.011; χ^2 test)					
Smokers	5.9	27,9	15,3	30,0	11,5
Non-smokers	10.2	37,1	14,4	24,5	6,8

Table 11. CPITN score (%) of smokers and non-smokers in each sextant

The primary aim of our survey was to assess the influence of smoking on oral health. Using the method of multivariable logistic regression we determined the odds ratio (OR) for eight selected variables on mean number of decayed teeth (D) and on periodontitis with TN III score. The reference value was set as number of D = 0 (e.g. absence of decayed teeth) and absence of CPI 4 (e.g. no deep gingival pockets were found). As a reference level for each of selected variable (odds = 1) the best particular value was considered, which means non-smoker, younger age, women, university educated respondent who brushes his/her teeth twice a day or even more often and those who participates in the dental preventive follow-ups twice a year.

	CPI 0	CPI 1	CPI 2	CPI 3	CPI 4
Smoking (χ^2 test; p < 0,001)					
Regular	1,1	9,2	27,4	36,9	25,4
Occasional	1,7	16,1	33,1	34,7	14,4
Ex-smoker	1,2	11,0	30,3	42,1	15,4
Non-smoker	1,8	18,6	30,7	35,2	13,7
Age (χ^2 test; p < 0,001)					
30-49 years	2.1	19.4	32.1	35.2	11.2
50-69 years	0.4	6.8	22.1	43.2	27.4
Sex (χ^2 test; p < 0,001)					
Males	1.3	12.4	26.1	41.7	18.4
Females	1.7	18.0	31.3	33.9	15.1
Education (χ^2 test; p < 0,001)					
Basic school	0,6	9,1	27,4	38,8	24,1
Vocational	0,8	17,6	26,7	39,7	15,3
High School	2,2	15,8	32,2	36,6	13,2
University	1,9	20,9	30,7	32,9	13,6
Participation on preventive check-ups (χ^2 test; p < 0,001)					
2 times a year	2,0	18,1	33,4	33,6	13,0
Once a year	0,5	11,1	26,0	42,7	19,6
Once in 2 years	0,0	10,4	23,9	40,3	25,4
Less frequently	3,9	5,3	22,4	36,8	31,6
Never	0,0	5,7	11,3	49,1	34,0
Tooth brushing frequency (χ^2 test; p < 0,001)					
3 times a day	2,3	25,4	32,2	25,4	14,7
2 times a day	1,5	15,0	31,3	38,1	14,1
Once daily	1,2	8,0	21,0	40,1	29,6
Less frequently	2,6	5,1	17,9	28,2	46,2

Table 12. Percentage of respondents with highest CPI in relation to selected variables

Our results in table 13 showed that incidence of decayed teeth is enhanced mainly by the consumption of food/beverages after evening tooth brushing (OR=1.68; p=0.011) and low participation in preventive check-ups (OR=1.77; p= 0.0013). Smoking increased the risk of decayed teeth as well (OR=1.23), but the result was not significant (p=0.061). Nevertheless, our findings confirmed the fact that there exists a dose and effect relationship with smoking. Though not statistically significant in our study, the number of dental caries occurrence increased in individuals who smoked more than 10 cigarettes per day.

Different results were found when assessing the influence of smoking on periodontium (table 14). The risk for periodontitis with TN III score (which means the findings of CPI 4) was statistically increased with age (OR=2.63; p<0.001), low tooth brushing frequency (OR=2.18; p<0.001), and low participation in dental prevention check-ups (OR=1.8; p=0.007). Smoking increased the risk as well (OR=1.33), but the result was not significant (p=0.065). Nevertheless, the risk markedly increases with the number of cigarettes smoked. Smoking 11 or more cigarettes a day increased the risk of periodontitis (CPITN III), which emphasizes the need for a complex dental care (OR=1.98, p=0.0043). Smoking of 10 or less cigarettes per day increases the risk of periodontitis (CPITN III grade) as well, but in this case, not significantly (OR = 1.67; p= 0.027).

	OR	CI-L	CI-U	p-value
Age	0.99	0.77	1.26	0.908 (NS)
Sex	1.13	0.91	1.41	0.262 (NS)
Preventive check-ups once a year	1.28	1.00	1.65	0.054 (NS)
Preventive check-ups low frequently	1.77	1.25	2.50	0.0013 (*)
Basic education, skilled	0.98	0.74	1.31	0.903 (NS)
High school	0.78	0.59	1.03	0.082 (NS)
Tooth brushing frequency once a day or less frequently	1.27	0.9	1.79	0.177 (NS)
Smoking associated illnesses	1.13	0.81	1.57	0.479 (NS)
Illnesses without association with smoking	1.11	0.82	1.51	0.497 (NS)
Eating after evening tooth brushing	1.68	1.12	2.51	0.011 (*)
Smoking	1.23	0.99	1.54	0.061 (NS)
- smoking to 10 cig./day	0.99	0.69	1.41	0.941 (NS)
- smoking 11 and more cig/day	1.23	0.84	1.81	0.293 (NS)

Table 13. Impact of selected variables on number of decayed teeth (reference value D= 0)
OR = odds ratio, CI-L = lower 95% confidence interval, CI-U = upper 95% confidence interval
NS (non-significant) = p ≥ 0.05; * = p < 0.05; ** = p < 0.01; *** p < 0.001

	OR	CI-L	CI-U	P value
Age	2,63	1,92	3,59	< 0,001 (***)
Sex	0,93	0,69	1,26	0,654 (NS)
Preventive check-ups once a year	1,45	1,04	2,02	0,03 (*)
Preventive check-ups less frequently	1,8	1,17	2,76	0,0073 (**)
Basic education, skilled	1,33	0,9	1,99	0,157 (NS)
High school	0,92	0,61	1,37	0,679 (NS)
Tooth brushing frequency once a day or less frequently	2,18	1,45	3,27	< 0,001 (***)
Smoking associated illnesses	1,39	0,94	2,07	0,102 (NS)
Illnesses without association with smoking	0,97	0,65	1,46	0,894 (NS)
Eating after evening tooth brushing	1,07	0,66	1,74	0,793 (NS)
Smoking	1,33	0,98	1,79	0,066 (NS)
- smoking to 10 cig./day	1,67	1,06	2,61	0,027 (*)
- smoking 11 and more cig/day	1,98	1,24	3,16	0,0043 (**)

Table 14. Impact of selected variables on necessity of complex therapy (TN III)
OR = odds ratio, CI-L = lower 95% confidence interval, CI-U = upper 95% confidence interval
NS (non-significant) = $p \geq 0.05$;   * = $p < 0.05$; ** = $p < 0.01$; *** $p < 0.001$

5. Discussion

Our study confirmed the differences in attitudes of smokers and non-smokers to oral health. The percentage of subjects with basic education was significantly higher among regular smokers and percentage of those with a university degree was highest among non-smokers. These findings are consistent with the results of previous studies conducted in other developed countries. Researchers of a study performed in Australia noted that those living in low socio-economic status areas were more likely to smoke (Najman et al., 2006). A study published in the Journal of Canadian Dental Association stated that a higher percentage of current smokers had education less than high school (Millar & Locker, 2007) and a study conducted in America stated that inequalities in smoking exist, as evidenced by persistent class-based disparities and the growing number of smokers in the lower socio-economic groups (Sorenson et al., 2004).

It has been undoubtedly documented, that after the first Surgeon General's report in 1964, the profile of cigarette smokers in U.S.A., and consequently in the other developed countries, has reversed. Cigarette smokers nowadays are more likely to be poor and less educated. The well educated people may have higher levels of health literacy, and were more responsive to messages of health-promoting and disease-prevention behaviours and beliefs. Additionally, the poor ones may have lower information on the health risks of smoking, the fewest resources, and the least access to cessation services. Socio-economic disadvantage is associated with persistent smoking, and consequently the burden of smoking-related disease falls disproportionately on those with lower social-economical status (Harwood et al., 2007). In contrary to this, we have found high prevalence of current smokers in the group of respondents with highest income in Czech Republic. This fact reflects great underestimation of generally well-known health risks of smoking by smokers, as well as high social tolerance to this negative habit in our country.

Smokers and non-smokers also differ in participation in dental prevention. Majority of Czech respondents visit the dentist for preventive check-ups twice a year. This can be explained by the fact that the regular preventive dental check-ups are covered by the Health Insurance in Czech Republic. Nevertheless, despite free dental preventive check-ups, smokers participate in these check-ups less frequently than the non-smokers do.

The differences according to the smoking habits were found also in chosen oral hygiene habits. The non-smokers had better brushing habits (brushed their teeth more frequently, used inter-dental tooth brush, dental floss and mouth wash more often and were more consistent in not eating anything after evening tooth brushing) compared to smokers. Non-smokers also abstained from eating anything after evening brushing more consistently than smokers.

Significant difference between smokers and non-smokers has been found in eating and drinking habits. Current smokers, mainly occasional smokers, consumed sweetened drinks more frequently in comparison with non-smokers or ex-smokers. In case of consumption of fruits and vegetables the trend was opposite. Non-smokers consumed fruits and vegetables more often than smokers, who, on the contrary, had higher alcohol intake.

Majority of factors mentioned above explains the differences in clinical findings in smokers and non-smokers. Smoking is considered to be an independent and most potent risk factor for chronic periodontal disease. The social and behaviour factors, which are typical among the population group of smokers, can aggravate the clinical findings.

Taking the gender of the respondents into consideration, we did not find the influence of gender on the highest (maximum) CPITN outcome. On the contrary, it has been reported that although there is no established, inherent difference between men and women in their susceptibility to periodontitis, men have been shown to exhibit worse periodontal health than women and this difference has been documented in different populations. Several periodontal diseases have been found to be more prevalent among males, even after oral hygiene, socio-economic status and age were considered, and hormonal conditions have been proposed which may explain this difference (Grossi et al., 1994).

The age of Czech respondents significantly influenced the maximum CPITN outcome. Early evidence demonstrated that both the prevalence and severity of periodontitis increases with aging, suggesting that age may be a marker for periodontal tissue support loss. A national survey conducted in 1986 in Brazil using CPITN methodology to assess the periodontal status estimated that 5.2 % and 7.4 % of subjects in the age groups 35 to 44 and 50 to 59 years had one or more teeth with probing depth of $\geq$ 5.5 mm (CPITN 4) (Sorenson et al., 2004) and another national survey in the United Kingdom using CPITN estimated that 42 % of 35 to 44 year olds and 70 % of 55 to 64 year olds had CAL > 3.5 mm (Morris et al., 2001). The fact that older age group (50-69 years) of the Czech study population having a higher percentage of maximum CPITN scores 3 and 4, indicating pathological pockets, may have been caused by the cumulative effect of prolonged exposure to external risk factors including cigarette smoke rather than an age-related, intrinsic abnormality. Although there is no established, inherent difference between men and women in their susceptibility to periodontitis, periodontal disease is often reported in epidemiological studies to be more prevalent and severe in males than in females at comparable ages (Gamonal et al., 1998; (Borrell & Papapanou, 2005), and similar results were found in the Czech population.

Education significantly influenced the maximum CPITN outcome in Czech study population. Previous studies have documented differences in periodontal health by socio-economic indicators, i.e., income and education, but these indicators have rarely been investigated as independent variables of main interest.

Socio-economic indicators are robust markers of periodontitis. Their role in periodontal disease can be attributed to differential access to resources and opportunities that may influence preventive behaviours. Evidence also suggests that education has a greater influence than income in favourably affecting the level of periodontitis in the population (Borrell & Papapanou, 2005). University and mainly vocational school graduates of Czech population having a higher percentage of maximum CPITN score 0, indicating healthy periodontium, can be attributed to the factors mentioned above.

Preventive dental visits and brushing frequency significantly influenced the maximum CPITN outcome of the Czech population. A general principle in preventive efforts towards chronic diseases is to focus on changeable causal or modifying factors. Regarding periodontal diseases, such factors are those related to life style, such as oral hygiene, regularity of dental visits and tobacco use. Comparative studies between the Eastern European countries and the Western societies showed that socio-economically less-developed Eastern European countries displayed a higher fraction with mild-to-moderate periodontitis than the Western well-developed societies. Particularly the Scandinavian countries, where a comprehensive public dental health care system with emphasis on prevention and regular dental visits has existed for more than 100 years, displayed high proportions of healthy subjects and even a low prevalence of severe periodontal disease (Gjermo, 2005). One study reported, that the subjects, who had a dental check-up at least once a year, had a significantly less gingivitis, calculus and periodontal pockets compared to those, who made less frequent visits (Lang et al., 1994). However, the same group of authors failed to find a relationship between dental insurance and improved periodontal health (Lang et al., 1995), although those with insurance were more likely to visit the dentist (Jack & Bloom, 1988). Differences among the populations of the world in terms of periodontal status, oral cleanliness and oral health behaviour probably reflect the social and economic development of the various regions. Cultural differences may also affect the attitudes towards dental health and dental care in populations (Gjermo, 2005). Lack of use of preventive care may reflect a general attitude toward preventive care, differences in willingness or ability to pay for dental services or differences in the availability of dental care.

The findings from this study concerning the fact that non-smokers exhibited a higher percentage of healthy periodontium compared to smokers, corroborates the results of several previous studies (Beck et al., 1997; Kelbauskas et al., 2003; Tanner et al., 2005; Torrungruang et al., 2005; Winn, 2001). This study also reconfirmed the relationship between smoking and a reduced gingival bleeding on probing, which has been well documented in previous studies (Dietrich et al., 2004; Müller et al., 2002; Tomar & Asma, 2000). This may be due to vasoconstrictive action of nicotine and as a result of a profound influence on vascular dynamics and cellular metabolism (Bergström & Bergström, 2001).

Smoking, as a strong and consistent risk indicator for periodontitis in the presence of calculus, an indicator of oral hygiene, has been documented in logistic regression model (Do, 2003), and smokers have been reported to exhibit a low awareness of their health (Gjermo, 2005). From this study it was evident that smokers had a higher prevalence of supragingival and/or subgingival calculus compared to non-consumers.

6. Conclusion

In conclusion, the present study shows that despite good access to dental care in Czech Republic, cigarette smoking exerts a strong and chronic effect on periodontium and reduces bleeding on probing. The current understanding of the importance of tobacco smoking as the most potent risk factor for chronic periodontal disease now has to be applied to the clinical management of the disease. Treatment of smoking patients not including corrective measures against the smoking habits should be regarded as unethical. The outcomes of this particular survey proves that it is mandatory to implement a more rigorous anti-smoking campaign in the dental practice.

7. Acknowledgement

Project was supported by the Ministry of Health Grant Agency No. NR 8781-3/06.

8. References

Ainamo, J. (1971). The Seeming Effect of Tobacco Consumption on the Occurrence of Periodontal Disease and Dental Caries. *Suom Hammaslaak Toim.* Vol. 67, No. 2, pp. 87-94, ISSN 0039-551X.

Ainamo, J. & Ainamo, A. (1994). Validity and Relevance of the Criteria of the CPITN. *International Dental Journal,* Vol. 44, pp. 527-532. ISSN 0020-6539

Alabandar, J.M.; Streckfus, C.F.; Adesanaya, M.R. & Winn DM. (2000). Cigar, Pipe and Cigarette Smoking as Risk Factors for Periodontal Disease and Tooth Loss. *J Periodontol.,* Vol. 71, pp.1874-1881, ISSN 0022-3492

Amarasena, N.; Ekanayaka, A.N.I.; Herath, L. & Miyazaki, H. (2003). Tobacco Use and Oral Hygiene as Risk Indicators for Periodontitis. *Community Dent Oral Epidemiol.* Vol. 31, pp. 158-160. ISSN 0301-5661

Axelsson, P., Paulander, J. & Lindhe, J. (1998). Relationship Between Smoking and Dental Status in 35-, 50-, 65-, and 75-Year-Old Individuals. *J Clin Periodontol.* Vol. 25, No. 4, (Apr 1998), pp. 297-305, ISSN 0303-6979

Beck, J.D.; Cusmano, L.; Green-Helms, W.; Koch, G.G. & Offenbacher, S. (1997). A 5 Year Study of Attachment Loss in Community-Dwelling Older Adults: Incidence Dentistry. *J Periodontal Res.* Vol. 32, pp. 506-515, ISSN 0022-3484

Bergström, J. & Boström, L. (2001). Tobacco Smoking and Periodontal Hemorrhagic Responsiveness. *J Clin Periodontol,* Vol. 28, pp. 680-685, ISSN 0303-6979

Borrell, L.N. & Papapanou, P.N. (2005). Analytical Epidemiology of Periodontitis. *J Clin Periodontol.* Vol. 32 (Suppl. 6), pp. 132-158, ISSN 0303-6979

Bruno-Ambrosius, K., Swanholm, G. & Twetman, S. (2005). Eating Habits, Smoking and Toothbrushing in Relation to Dental Caries: a 3-year Study in Swedish Female Teenagers. *Int J Paediatr Dent.* Vol. 15, No. 3, (May 2005), pp. 190-196, ISSN 0960-7439

Calsina, G.; Ramón, J-M. & Echeverrí, J-J. (2002). Effects of Smoking on Periodontal Tissues. *J Clin Periodontol.* Vol. 29, pp. 771-776, ISSN 0303-6979

Darby, I.B.; Hodge, P.J.; Riggio, M.P. & Kinane, D.F. (2005). Clinical and Microbiological Effect of Scaling and Root Planning in Smoker and Non-smoker Chronic Aggressive Periodontitis Patients. *J Clin Periodontol.* Vol. 32, No.2, pp.200, , ISSN 0303-6979

Dietrich, T., Bernimoulin, J.P. & Glynn, J.R. (2004). The Effect of Cigarette Smoking on Gingival Bleeding. *J Periodontol.* Vol. 75, pp. 16-22, ISSN 0022-3492

Do, G.L.; Spencer, A.J.; Roberts-Thomson, K.; Ha, H.D. (2003). Smoking as a Risk Indicator for Periodontal Disease in the Middle-aged Vietnamese population. *Community Dent Oral Epidemiol.* Vol. 31, pp. 437-446. ISSN:

Fagerström, K. (2002). The Epidemiology of Smoking: Health Consequences and Benefits of Cessation. *Drugs.* Vol. 62, No. 2, pp. 1-9. ISSN 0012-6667

Gamonal, J.A.; Polez, N.J. & Aranda W. (1998). Periodontal Conditions and Treatment Needs, by CPITN, in the 35 44 and 65-74 Year Old Population in Santiago, Chile. *Int Dent J.* Vol 48, pp. 96-103, ISSN 0020-6539

Genco, R.J. (1996). Current View of Risk Factors for Periodontal Diseases. *J Periodontol.* Vol. 67, pp. 1041-1049, ISSN 0022-3492

Gibbs, M.D. (1952). Tobacco and Dental Caries. *J Am Coll Dent.* Vol. 19, pp. 365-367, ISSN: 0002-7979.

Gjermo, P.E. (2005). Impact of Periodontal Preventive Programmes on the Data from Epidemiologic Studies. *J Clin Periodontol,* Vol. 32 (Suppl.6), pp. 294-300, ISSN 0303-6979

Grossi, S.G., Zambon & J.J., Ho, A.W. (1994). Assessment of Risk for Periodontal Disease. 1. Risk Indicators for Attachment Loss. *J Periodontol.* Vol. 65, pp. 260-267, ISSN 0022-3492

Hart, A.C. (1899). Prevention of Decay of the Teeth. *Dent Items Interest.* Vol. 21, No. 3, pp. 153-163. ISSN 0382-8514

Harwood, G.A., Salsberry, P., Ferketich, A.K. & Wewers, M.E. (2007). Cigarette Smoking, Socioeconomic Status, and Psychological Factors: Examining a Conceptual Framework. *Public Health Nurs.* Vol. 24, No. 4, pp. 361-371. ISSN 0737-1209

Heng, C.K; Badner, V.M. & Freeman, K.D. (2006). Relationship of Cigarette Smoking to Dental Caries in a Population of Female Inmates. *J Correct Health Care.* Vol. 12, No. 3, pp. 164-174. ISSN 1078-3458

Hirsch, J.M.; Livian, G.; Edward, S. & Noren, J.G. (1991). Tobacco Habits among Teenagers in the City of Goteborg, Sweden, and Possible Association with Dental Caries. *Swed Dent J.* Vol. 15, No. 3, pp. 117-123. ISSN 0347-9994

Hyman, J.J. & Reid, B.C. (2003). Epidemiological Risk Factors for Periodontal Loss Among Adults in the United States. *J Clin Periodontol.* Vol. 30, pp. 230-237, ISSN 0303-6979

Jack, S. & Bloom, B. (1988). Use of Dental Services and Dental Health. United States, 1986. Washington, DC: National Centre for Health Statistics, DHHS pub no (PHS) 88-1953. (Vital and Health Statistics; series 10; no 165).

Jacob, V.; Vellappally, S. & Smejkalova J. (2007). The Influence of Cigarette Smoking on Various Aspects of Periodontal Health. *ACTA MEDICA (Hradec Kralove).* Vol. 50, No. 1, pp. 3-5. ISSN 1211-4286

James, J.A.; Sayers, N.M.; Drucker, D.B. & Hul,l P.S. (1999). Effect of Tobacco Products on the Attachment and Growth of Periodontal Ligament Fibroblasts. *J Periodontol.* Vol. 70, pp. 518-525, ISSN:0022-3492

Jette, A.M., Feldman, H.A. & Tennstedt, S.L. (1993). Tobacco Use: A Modifiable Risk Factor for Dental Disease Among the Elderly. *Am J Public Health*. Vol. 83, No. 9, (Sep 1993), pp. 1271-1276. ISSN 0090-0036

Johnson, N.W. & Bain, C.A. (2000). Tobacco and Oral Disease. EU-Working Group on Tobacco and Oral Health. *Br Dent J*. Vol. 189, No. 4, (Aug 2000), pp. 200-206. ISSN 0007-0610

Johnson, G.K. & Hill, M. (2004). Cigarette Smoking and the Periodontal Patient. *J Periodontol*. Vol. 75, pp. 196-209, ISSN 0022-3492

Kassirer, B. (1994). Smoking as a Risk Factor for Gingival Problems, Periodontal Problems and Caries. *Univ TorDent J*. Vol. 7, No.1, pp. 6-10. ISSN 0843-5812

Kelbauskas, E., Kelbauskiene, S.& Paipaliene, P. (2003). Factors Influencing the Health of Periodontal Tissue and Intensity of Dental Caries. Stomatologija, *Baltic Dent Maxilo J*, Vol. 5, pp.144-148. ISSN 1392-8589

Kelbauskas, E.; Kelbauskiene, S. & Paipaliene, P. (2005). Smoking and Other Factors Influencing the Oral Health of Lithuanian Army Recruits. *Mil Med*. Vol. 170, No. 9, (Sep 2005), pp. 791-796. ISSN 0026-4075

Krejci, C.B. & Bissada, N.F. (1999). Periodontitis - The Risk of its Development. *Academy Gen Dent.*, pp. 430-436. ISSN 0363-6771

Lang, W.P., Farghaly, M.M., Ronis, D.L. (1994). The Relation of Preventive Dental Behaviours to Periodontal Health Status. *J Clin Periodontol*, Vol. 21, pp.194-198, ISSN 0303-6979

Lang, W.P., Ronis, D.L., Farghaly, M.M., (1995). Preventive Behaviours as Correlates of Periodontal Health Status. *J Public Health Dent*, Vol. 55, pp.10-17. ISSN 0022-4006

Lie, M.A.; Loos, B.G.; Henskens, Y.M.; Timmerman, M.F.; Veerman, E.C.; van der Velden, U. & van der Weijden, G.A. (2001). Salivary Cystatin Activity and Cystatin C in Natural and Experimental Gingivitis in Smokers and Nonsmokers. *J. Clin. Periodontol*. Vol. 28, No. 10, pp. 979-984, ISSN 0303-6979

Locker, D. (1992). Smoking and Oral Health in Older Adults. *Can J Public Health*. Vol. 83, No. 6, (Nov-Dec 1992), pp. 429-432. ISSN 0008-4263

Ludwick, W. & Massler, M. (1952). Relation of Dental Caries Experience and Gingivitis to Cigarette Smoking in Males 17 to 21 Years Old (at the Great Lakes Naval Training Center). *J Dent Res*. Vol. 31, No. 3, (Jun 1952), pp. 319-322. ISSN 0022-0345

Macgregor, I.D. (1985). Survey of Toothbrushing Habits in Smokers and Nonsmokers. *Clin Prev Dent*. Vol. 7, No. 6, (Nov-Dec 1985), pp. 27-30. ISSN 0163-9633

Mackay, J. & Amos, A. (2003). Women and Tobacco. *Respirology*. Vol. 8, pp. 123-130. ISSN 1323-7799

Millar, W.J. & Locker, D., (2007). Smoking and Oral Health Status. *J Can Dent Assoc*, Vol. 73, No. 2, pp.155a-155g. ISSN 0709-8936

Morris, A.J., Steele, J. & White DA. (2001). The Oral Cleanliness and Periodontal Health of UK Adults in 1998. *Br Dent J*, Vol. 191, pp.186-192. ISSN 0007-0610

Müller, H.-P.; Stadermann, S. & Heinecke, A. (2002). Gingival Recession in Smokers and Non-smokers with Minimal Periodontal Disease. *J Clin Periodontol*. Vol. 29, pp. 129-136, ISSN 0303-6979

Najman, J.M., Toloo, G. & Siskind, V. (2006). Socioeconomic Disadvantage and Changes in Health Risk Behaviours in Australia: 1989-90 to 2001. *Bull World Health Organ*, Vol. 84, No.12, pp.976-984. ISSN 0042-9686

Nunn, M.E. (2003). Understanding the Etiology of Periodontitis: An Overview of Periodontal Risk Factors. *Periodontology 2000*. Vol. 32, pp. 11-23. ISSN 0906-6713

Peter, S. (1999). Essentials of Preventive and Community Dentistry, 1st edition. New Delhi. Arya (medi) publishing house.

Razali, M.; Palmer, R.M.; Coward, P. & Wilson, R.F. (2005). A Retrospective Study of Periodontal Disease Severity in Smokers and Non-smokers. *British Dent Journal*. Vol. 198, pp. 495-498. ISSN 0007-0610

Reibel, J. (2003). Tobacco and Oral Diseases. Update on the Evidence, with Recommendations. *Med Princ Pract*. Vol. 12, Suppl 1, pp. 22-32. ISSN 1011-7571

Schmidt, H.J. (1951). Tobacco Smoke and the Teeth. *Stoma (Heidelb)*. Vol. 4, No. 2, (May 1951), pp. 111-125. (In German.) ISSN 0039-1697

Sgan-Cohen, H.D.; Katz, J.; Horev, T.; Dinte, A. & Eldad, A. (2000). Trends in Caries and Associated Variables Among Young Israeli Adults over 5 Decades. *Community Dent Oral Epidemiol*. Vol. 28, No. 3, (Jun 2000), pp. 234-240. ISSN 0301-5661

Sorenson, G., Barbeau, E., Hunt, M.K. & Emmons, K. (2004). Reducing Social Disparities in Tobacco Use: A Social Contextual Model for Reducing Tobacco Use among Blue-Collar Workers. *Am J Public Health*, Vol. 94, No. 2, pp. 230 - 239. ISSN 0090-0036

Spickerman, C.F.; Hujoel, P.P. & DeRouen, T.R. (2003). Bias Induced by Self-Reported Smoking on Periodontitis - Systemic Disease Associations. *J Dent Res*. Vo. 82, No.5, pp. 345-349. ISSN 0022-0345

Talhout, R.; Opperhuizen, A. & van Amsterdam, J.G. (2006). Sugars as Tobacco Ingredient: Effects on Mainstream Smoke Composition. *Food Chem Toxicol*. Vol. 44, No. 11, (Nov 2006), pp. 1789-1798. ISSN 0278-6915

Tanner, A.C.R.; Kent, R.Jr.; Van Dyke, T.; Sonis, S.T. & Murray, L.A. (2005). Clinical and Other Risk Indicators for Early Periodontitis in Adults. *J Periodontol*. Vol. 76, pp. 573-81, ISSN 0022-3492

Telivuo, M.; Kallio, P.; Berg, M.A.; Korhonen, H.J. & Murtomaa, H. (1995). Smoking and Oral Health: A Population Survey in Finland. *J Public Health Dent*. Vol. 55, No. 3, pp. 133-138. ISSN 0022-4006

Tomar, S.L. & Asma, S. (2000). Smoking-Attributable Periodontitis in the United States: Findings from NHANES III. *J Periodontol*. Vol. 71, pp.743-51, ISSN 0022-3492

Torrungruang, K., Nisapakultorn, K.& Sutdhibhisal, S. (2005). The Effect of Cigarette Smoking on the Severity of Periodontal Disease among Older Thai Adults. *J Periodontol*, Vol. 76, pp. 566-72, ISSN 0022-3492

Van Winkelhoff, A.J.; Bosch-Tijhof, C.J.; Winkel, E.G. & Van der Reijden, W.A. (2001). Smoking Afects the Subgingival Microflora in Periodontitis. *J Periodontol*. Vol. 72, pp. 666-71, ISSN 0022-3492

Vellappally, S.; Fiala, Z.; Smejkalova, J.; Jacob, V. & Shriharsha, P. (2007). Influence of Tobacco Use in Dental Caries Development. *Centr. Eur. J. Public Health*. Vol. 15, No. 3, pp. 116-121, ISSN 1210-7778

Winn, D.M. (2001). Tobacco Use and Oral Diseases. *J Dent Edu*. Vol. 65, No. 4, pp. 306-10. ISSN 0022-0337

Zitterbart, P.A.; Matranga, L.F.; Christen, A.G.; Park, K.K. & Potter, R.H. (1990). Association between Cigarette Smoking and the Prevalence of Dental Caries in Adult Males. *Gen Dent*. Vol. 38, No. 6, (Nov-Dec 1990), pp. 426-431. ISSN 0363-6771

Part 4

Clinical Oral Health Care

16

The Importance of Final Irrigation with Mineralolithic Effect Agents During Chemomechanical Treatment of Tooth Root Canal

Aleksandar Mitić[1], Nadica Mitić[1], Slavoljub Živković[2], Jelena Milašin[3],
Jovanka Gašić[1], Vladimir Mitić[4], Tatjana Tanić[4] and Jelena Popović[1]
[1]*Department of Restorative Dentistry and Endodontics, Clinic of Dentistry,
Medical Faculty, University of Nis, Nis,*
[2]*Department of Restorative Dentistry and Endodontics, Faculty of Dentistry,
University of Belgrade, Belgrade,*
[3]*Institute of Genetics, Faculty of Dentistry, Univesity of Belgrade,*
[4]*Department of Jaw Orthopaedics, Dental Hospital, Niš
Serbia*

1. Introduction

In primary tooth root canal infections, the largest number of microorganisms can be found in main root canal. However, a considerable portion of infection is located deeper, in the lateral canals, apical ramifications and dentinal tubules (Hülsmann et al., 1997; Matuse et al., 2003; Živković et al., 2005). It is precisely those anatomic variabilities and physiological specificities of endodontic and periodontal tissues that make impeding factors in endodontic infection resolving (Gašić et al., 2003; Mitić et al., 2009; Chacker 1974; De Deus, 1975). All chemomechanical techniques of canal preparation leave considerable amounts of debris and smear layer (Živković et al., 2005; Mitić, 2008).

Smear layer is a layer of debris remaining on dentin during instrumentation, and consists of dentin particles, remnants of vital or necrotic pulp tissues, bacteria and their components (Nešković & Živković, 2009; Abdullah et al., 2005; Calt & Serper, 2002; Fouad et al., 2002; Jacinto, 2003; Love, 2001; Portenier et al., 2001, 2003; Spratt et al., 2001; Shabahang et al., 2003.)

In clinical practice, instrumentation and irrigation of canal within endodontic treatment is time-consuming and the most demanding treatment phase (Mitić et al., 2011; Živković et al., 2005; Morazin et al., 1994; Baumgartner & Mader, 1987).

Smear layer is an ideal medium for growth and proliferation of microorganisms, and therefore should be removed before the final root canal obturation to reduce the microorganisms present in the root canal, to improve the adhesion of root canal sealers to the root canal walls and to reduce the apical and coronal microleakage (Hülsmann et al., 1997; Takeda et al., 1999; Mitić, 2010.).

Medication aspect of chemomechanical root canal treatment involves the irrigation of root canal and removal of smear layer by the application of various preparations. The efficacy of irrigants is determined by numerous factors: concentration, pH value, root canal length, "age" of dentin tissue and time of application. One should bear in mind the fact that dentin tissue reduces the antimicrobial effect of various irrigants. Dentin hydroxyapatite possesses a buffering capacity, as it can donate protons, cause a pH change, and reduce the effects of various chemical agents when making contact with the dentinal wall (Haapasalo et al., 2000). The most frequently used irrigants with organolithic effects are sodium hypochlorite, hydrogen peroxide, chloramines, chlorhexidine. The final irrigants with mineralolithic effect are 17% NaEDTA, 10% citric acid, and the solution of recent date - MTAD (Biopure, Tulsa Dentsply, Tulsa OK, USA) – a combination of tetracyclines containing weak organic acids and anion-active substances (Torabinejad et al., 2002, 2003; Kando et al., 1991; Di Lenardda, 2000; Mitić et al., 2009; Yamaguchi et al., 1996; Haapasalo et al., 2005; Mitić, 2010).

The purpose of the present research was to analyze the surface of intracanal dentin after instrumentation and irrigation by organolithic agents (2.5% sodium hypochlorite, 3% hydrogen peroxide, 2% chlorhexidine) and final irrigation by mineralolithic effect solutions (17% NaEDTA, 10% citric acid and MTAD solution).

2. Methods

2.1. Materials

In the research, 145 freshly extracted single-rooted and double-rooted maxillary and mandibular human teeth were used. The teeth were extracted for orthodontic reasons in children of both sexes, aged 9-12 years.

The preparation of biomaterial involved storing of teeth in the sterile isotonic saline solution at 4°C, without the use of fixatives. All samples were prepared by one operator. The preparation of root canal was carried out by hand K-files, sized # 15-40 (Display, Maillefer, Ballaigues, Switzerland) and rotary instrumentation. Root canals were instrumented using a standard step-back technique, while the apex third was enlarged up to # 30. For canal irrigation, we used special irrigation needles with lateral perforations. They ensured an immediate contact between solution and intracanal dentin even in the apical region, improving thus the debridement of the entire root canal wall.

Teeth were divided into two groups. A control group (n=40) was divided into four sub-groups (a, b, c, d) for the purpose of quantitative assessment of smear layer on the samples after manual and rotary root canal instrumentation without irrigation (a, b) and after rinsing with sterile saline solution solution (c, d) (positive control).

The second, experimental group (n=105) was divided into seven subgroups (A,B,C,D,E,F,G), in which process the samples from the subgroups A,B,C were rinsed only with solutions with organolithic effect, while the samples from the subgroups D,E,F and G, besides irrigation with organolithic solutions (2.5% sodium hypochlorite, 3% hydrogen peroxide, 2% chlorhexidine – 2ml), were finally rinsed by mineralolithic effect solutions (17% NaEDTA, 10% citric acid and MTAD - 2ml). The samples rinsed with 5.25% NaOCl and 17% NaEDTA served as (negative control).

After chemomechanical root canal preparation, teeth crowns were removed with a diamond disk at the cement - enamel junction. All the samples were irrigated with distilled water to remove the superficial debris accumulated during cutting. Canals were dried with compressed air. Using the separation pliers, tooth roots were longitudinally grooved, into the mesial and distal halves. Each half of a sample was further fixed to a bed, coated with gold and viewed under the a scanning electron microscope JEOL-JSM-5300. The apex, middle and coronal thirds of all samples were analyzed; photomicrographs were taken at different magnifications.

According to the crictria specified by Hülsmann (1997), the smear layer of the root canal dentin was scored as:

- Score 1 - No smear layer, dentinal tubules open;
- Score 2 - Small amount of smear layer, several dentinal tubules open;
- Score 3 - Homogenous smear layer covering the root canal wall, only few dentinal tubules open;
- Score 4 - Dentinal wall completely covered by smear layer, no dentinal tubules open;
- Score 5 - Heavy, non-homogenous smear layer completely covering the root canal wall.

Statistical analysis included the comparison of the mean scores for the seven groups of analyzed samples; Kruskal Wallis nonparametric test was also used. Post hoc analysis was performed by Mann Whitney U test to determine single, intergroup differences among the mean scores.

For statistical analysis, Software SPSS 15.0 was used. Statistical significance was taken at $p < 0.05$.

Diagnosis was established based on the anamnesis, objective examination and additional diagnostic methods (examination of vitality by electrotest and radiography). The patients were aged 29-56 years. All the examined teeth were diagnosed with primary apical periodontitis, with destructed tooth crowns but without fillings and prosthetic restorations. All interventions were performed maintaining a dry working field using a rubber dam.

Disinfection of crowns and cavities was done by 3% natrium hypochlorite.

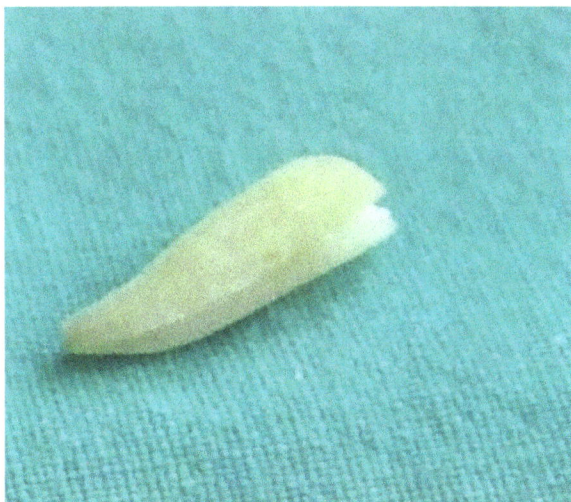

Fig. 1. Tooth roots notched with diamand discs

Subgroups/number of samples	Instrumentation	Irrigation during treatment			Final irrigation			Total time
		Irrigants	Amount	Time	Irrigants	Amount	Time	
A/10	Hand K file	*	*	*	*	*	*	*
B/10	Rotary Ni-Ti files	*	*	*	*	*	*	*
C/10	Hand K file	Saline solution	5 x 2 ml	3 min	Saline solution	5 ml	3 min	6 min
D/10	Rotary Ni-Ti files	Saline solution	5 x 2 ml	3 min	Saline solution	5 ml	3 min	6 min

*Without irrigation

Table 1. Experimental protocol for control group samples

The Importance of Final Irrigation with Mineralolithic Effect Agents During Chemomechanical
Treatment of Tooth Root Canal

277

Subgroups/ number of samples	Instrumentation	Irrigation during treatment			Final irrigation			Total time
		Irrigants	Amount	Time	Irrigants	Amount	Time	
A/ 15	Hand K file	$3\% H_2O_2$	$5 \times 2ml$	3 min	2,5% NaOCl	2 ml	3 min	6 min
B/ 15	Rotary Ni-Ti file	$3\% H_2O_2$	5×2 ml	3 min	2% CHX	2 ml	3 min	6 min
C/ 15	Hand K file	2,5% NaOCl	5×2 ml	3min	17% NaEDTA	2 ml	1 min	4 min
D/ 15	Rotary Ni-Ti file	2,5% NaOCl	5×2 ml	3 min	2% CHX	2 ml	1 min	4 min
E/ 15	Rotary Ni-Ti file	2,5% NaOCl	5×2 ml	3 min	10% citric acid	5 ml	1 min	4 min
F/ 15	Hand K file	$3\% H_2O_2$ + 2% CHX	5×2 ml alternatively	2×3 min	MTAD	5 ml	1 min	7 min
G/ 15	Hand K file	$3\% H_2O_2$	5×2 ml	3 min	MTAD	5 ml	1 min	4 min

Table 2. Experimental protocol for group II (experimental) samples

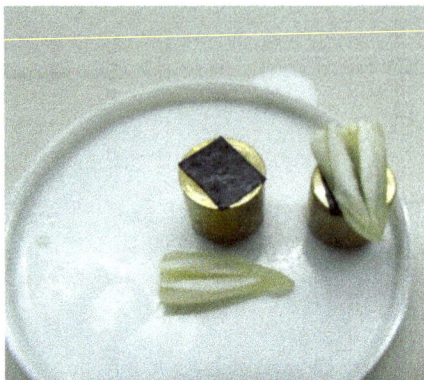

Fig. 2. Sample prepared for evaporation

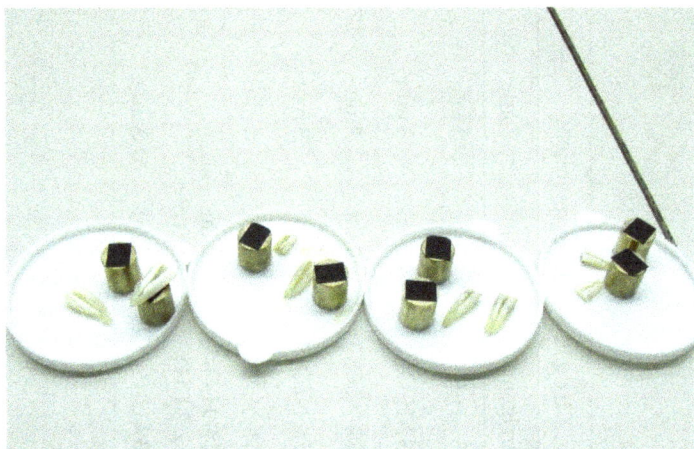

Fig. 3. Placing samples on appropriate supporter

3. Result

The results obtained in this study are presented in tables 1-7 and figures 1-15. In the first group of control samples subgroups (A, B, C, D), it was observed that root canal walls were covered with substantial amounts of dentin debris, where smear layer completely closed the openings of dentinal tubules. Such presentation of dentin surface is described in literature as "bark tree". Eight samples were scored 5, while two samples were scored 4.

In the experimental group, the poorest results were obtained after the irrigation of walls with organolithic effect solutions. The most favorable outcome of the procedure was observed in the group where canal irrigation during instrumentation was done with organolithic effect solutions, and final irrigation with mineralolithic effect irrigating agents, in which process the most optimal combination of irrigation solutions was 3% H_2O_2 + 2% CHX + MTAD (1.10±0.31), which is a good choice of irrigants in endodontic clinical practice.

Statistical analysis showed that the experimental group treated with MTAD as the final irrigation had significantly cleaner walls compared to control group samples (p<0.001).

The analysis of results showed that there was statistically significant difference in the mean scores among the examined groups of samples (χ^2=50.674; p<0.001). The lowest score, and therewith the most favorable outcome, was found in the group F (Tab. 2).

Mann Whitney U test determined statistically significant differences in scores among the groups, and the best results were obtained in the teeth in which MTAD was used as the final irrigation (p<0.001).

Group/subgroup	N	Chemomechanical treatment	5	4	3	2	1
I/A	10	Manual treatment without irrigation	8	2	0	0	0
I/B	10	Engine driven treatment without irrigation	9	1	0	0	0
I/C	10	Manual treatment + Saline solution	3	7	0	0	0
I/D	10	Engine driven treatment + Saline solution	4	4	2	0	0

Table 3. Values of quantitative estimation of smear layer and dentin debris for group I (control group) samples – subgroups A, B ,C and D

	N	$\overline{X}$	SD	95%C.I.	Min	Max	Sig.
I/A	10	4.80	0.42	4.50-5.10	4	5	A
I/B	10	4.90	0.32	4.67-5.13	4	5	B, C
I/C	10	4.30	0.48	3.95-4.65	4	5	B
I/D	10	4.20	0.79	3.64-4.76	3	5	A, C

A (I/A vs I/D); B (I/B vs I/C); C (I/B vs I/D);

Table 4. Comparison of values of quantitative estimation of smear layer and dentin debris in group I (control samples - subgroups A,B,C and D: ANOVA test

By comparing the quantitative estimation values obtained for smear layer and dentin debris in the group I (control) samples – subgroups A, B, C and D using the ANOVA test, a statistically significant difference was found in the mean values among the groups I/A and I/D, I/B and I/C, I/B and I/D.

3.1. Ultrastructural presentation of intracanal dentin
3.1.1 Ultrastructural presentation of intracanal dentin surface after manual treatment without irrigation

After tooth root canal treatment using the hand driven instruments, canal walls were covered with large particles of dentin debris and smear layer of irregular surface found at all levels of intracanal dentin. The size of dentin debris particles was 2-6 μm. Dentinal tubule openings were not visible; dentin debris with a „tree bark" configuration was observed at the level of the apical third.

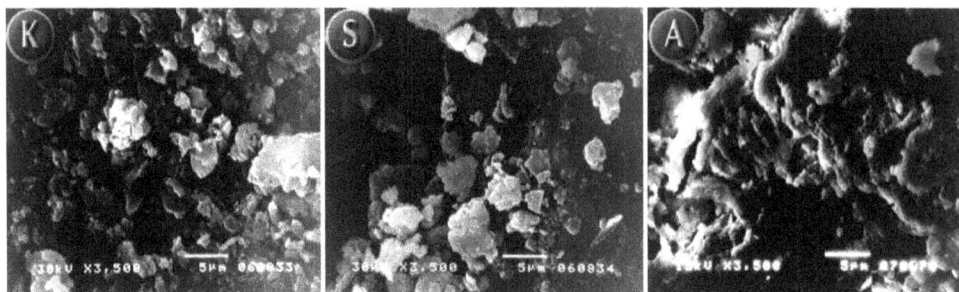

Fig. 4. SEM micrographs of coronal (K), middle (S) and apical (A) thirds of canal walls after manual treatment using K files without irrigation. Massive accumulation of dentin debris with large particles, with the underlying smear layer. Dentinal tubules invisible

3.1.2 Ultrastructural presentation of intracanal dentin surfaces after engine driven treatment without irrigation

Intracanal engine driven treatment of tooth root canal using NiTi instruments, without irrigation, leaves massive accumulation of dentin debris, with the underlying smear layer of thicker, more compact structure having large dentin particles distributed throughout the root canal. Dentinal tubules are completely closed. In the apical regions, there is a large amount of dentinal debris in the form of „plug".

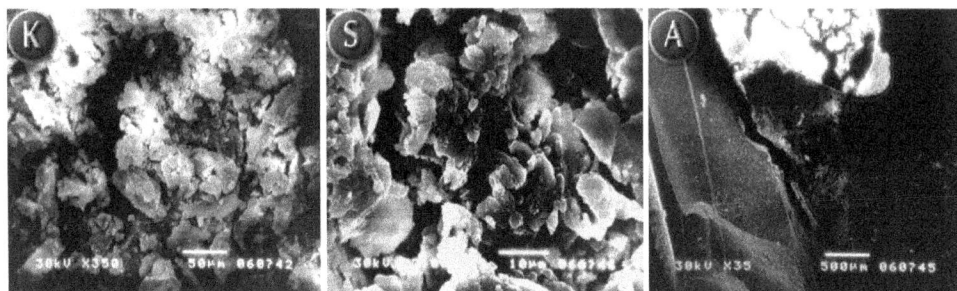

Fig. 5. SEM micrographs of coronal (K), middle (S) and apical thirds(A) of the canal walls after engine driven treatment using NiTi files without irrigation. Massive accumulation of dentinal debris

3.1.3 Ultrastructural presentation of intracanal dentinal surfaces following manual treatment using saline solution

After manual root canal treatment with K files and irrigation with saline solution during instrumentation, a smaller amount of superficial debris can be noted as well as the presence of inhomogeneous smear layer in all root regions. Only a few dentinal canal openings can be seen, completelly or partially covered with smear layer and debris (coronal and middle root regions), while the apical region contains larger amounts of surface debris and smear layer.

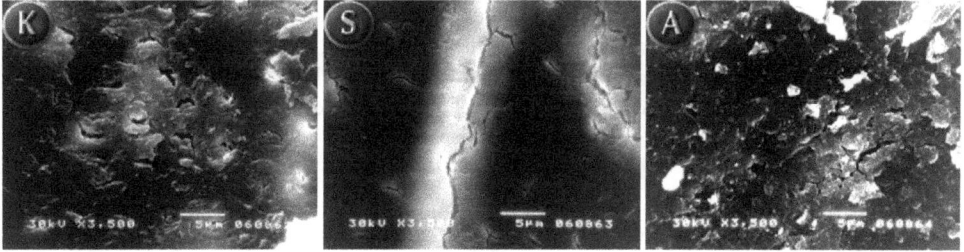

Fig. 6. SEM micrographs of coronal (K), middle (S) and apical (A) regions of canal walls after manual treatment (using K files) and irrigation with saline solution. A smaller quantity of superficial debris and inhomogeneous smear layer distributed in all root regions

3.1.4 Ultrastructural presentation of intracanal dentin surfaces after engine driven treatment and irrigation with saline solution

After intracanal engine driven treatment using NiTi instruments and irrigation during instrumentation with saline solution, smaller particles of dentinal debris and abundant smear layer can be seen.

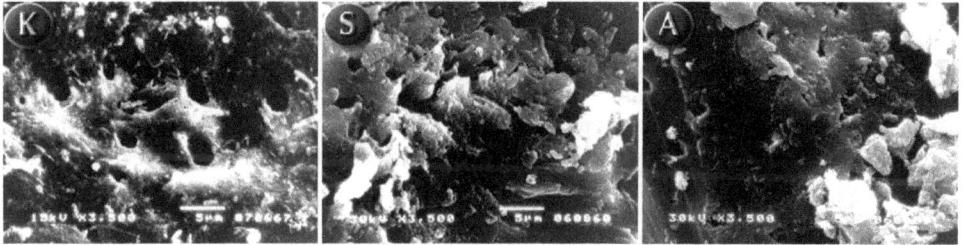

Fig. 7. SEM micrographs of coronal (K), middle (S) and apical (A) thirds of canal walls following engine driven treatment and irrigation with saline solution. Small particles (K) of dentinal debris, as well as larger ones (S, A), and abundant smear layer can be observed. Dentinal tubule openings of irregular diameters and infundibular shape

3.1.5 Ultrastructural presentation of intracanal dentin surfaces after the irrigation with 3% H$_2$O$_2$ and final irrigation with 2,5% NaOCl

After manual treatment and irrigation during instrumentation using 3% H$_2$O$_2$ and final irrigation with 2,5% NaOCl, it can be noted that larger amount of debris in the coronal

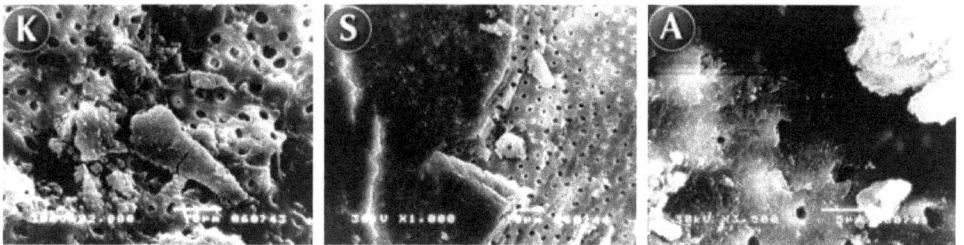

Fig. 8. SEM micrograps of coronal (K), middle (S) and apical (A) thirds of canal walls following the treatment and irrigation with 3% H$_2$O$_2$ and final irrigation with 2,5% NaOCl

region was removed; however, the smear layer is present. The open dentinal tubules show irregular shape and diameter. In the middle and apical thirds of the coronal region considerable amounts of surface debris attached to smear layer can be observed, which largely blocks the openings of dentinal tubules. There is a lack of mineralolithic effect, which results in impure intracanal dentin surface.

3.1.6 Chlorhexidine (CHX) as intracanal irrigants

Chlorhexidine is gluconate salt, and as an intracanal irrigants it is used in the form of bisbiguanide. This biocide has prolonged antibacterial efficacy at pH - 5.5-7.0. Ultrastructural presentation of intracanal dentinal surfaces after the irrigation with 3% H_2O_2 and final irrigation with 2% CHX.

After the manual root canal treatment and irrigation during instrumentation using 3% H_2O_2 and final irrigation with 2% CHX, the largest part of debris was removed. However, small particles of the smear layer, sized 1-2 μm, can be noted in all the samples, which results in not so smooth surface of the intertubular dentin. Dentinal tubule openings are not clearly limited, and inside the tubules some small particles of precipitate can be seen, produced during the reaction between hydrogen peroxide and chlorhexidine.

Having observed the dentinal wall from the coronal to the apical third, it was found that the amount of the smear layer was increased from the middle towards the apical third. In the middle third, the openings of dentinal tubules are of uneven diameter and irregular shape. The largest quantity of the smear layer in the form of „plug " is in the apical thid, wherein the created precipitate is incorporated into the dentinal tubules. In the apical third, the openings of dentinal tubules cannot be seen.

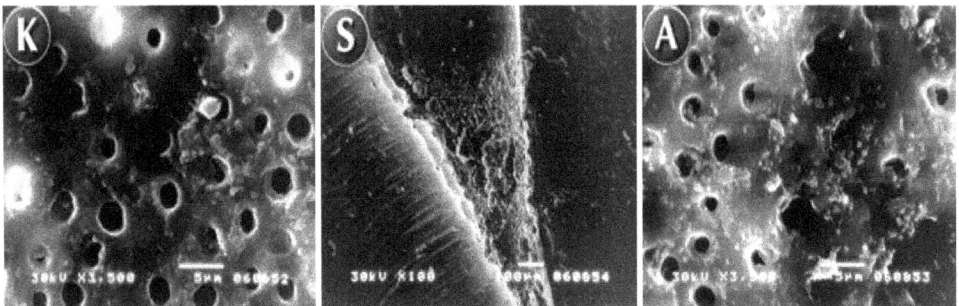

Fig. 9. SEM micrographs of the coronal (K), middle (S) and apical (A) thirds of the canal wall after the treatment and irrigation with 3% H_2O_2 and final irrigation with 2% CHX solution. Only small particles of dentinal debris can be partly seen as well as the smear layer on intertubular dentin; precipitates present inside the dentinal tubules

3.1.7 Ultrastructural presentation of intracanal dentin surfaces after treatment, irrigation with 2,5% NaOCl and final irrigation using 17%Na EDTA

Intracanal dentin surfaces in all regions, after the treatment and irrigation with 2,5% NaOCl and final irrigation with 17% NaEDTA solution, show preserved and clean structural dentin surface, open dentinal tubules of regular and even lumen.

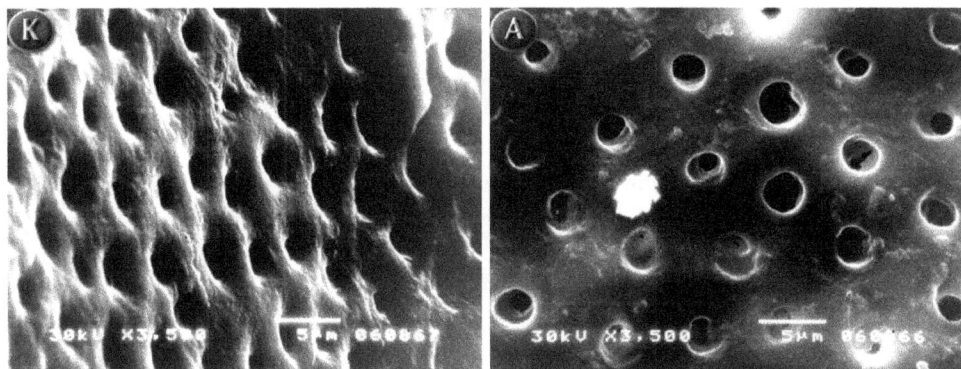

Fig. 10. SEM micrographs of canal walls after treatment and irrigation with 2,5% NaOCl and final irrigation using17% NaEDTA solution. Dentinal debris and smear layer comletely removed. Dentinal tubules clearly open, of regular shape; preserved, smooth dentinal structure

3.1.8 Ultrastructural presentation of intracanal dentin surfaces after treatment and irrigation with 2,5% NaOCl + 10% citric acid

Citric acid (10%) is efficient in removing the smear layer from the root canal walls and complete cleansing of the canal system, and, therefore, can be used as a final irrigant during endodontic treatment. In order to avoid agressive etching and potential erosion of dentin, the time of citric acid action must be limited from 20 seconds to 1 minute. The basic problem when applying the citric acid in the intracanal irrigation is the acidity of solution and a possibility of accidental contact with the mouth cavity soft issues. Combined application with NaOCl can bring about sudden neutralization, pH changes and releasing the chloride

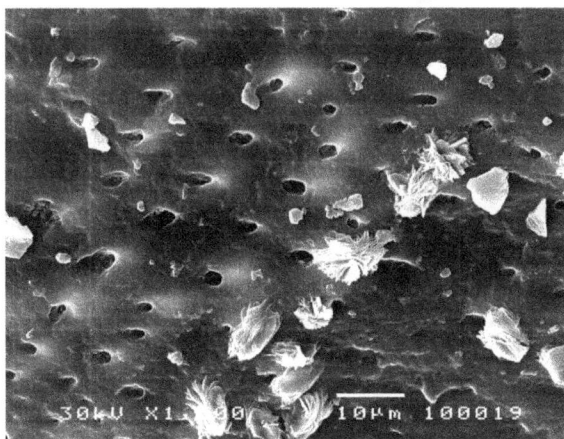

Fig. 11. SEM micrographs of intracanal dentine after irrigation with 2,5% NaOCl and 10% citric acid in duration of 60 sec. Small dentin particles present with the underlying smear layer. Dentinal tubules open, of eneven diameter and shape. Because of chelating Ca+ from dentin, formations of calcium citrate are produced

gases. Higher concentration of citric acid can chelate Ca^{2+} from dentin and cause the formation of calcium citrate crystals in the root canal. Industrial products are: 19% citric acid solution – canal Clean (Ognapharma, Italy); 10% citric acid solution – Citric acid solution (Ultradent) for canal application, Cetrimide.

3.1.9 Ultrastctural presentation of intracanal dentin surface after the irrigation with 3% H_2O_2 i 2% CHX and final irrigation with MTAD solution

After the canal system instrumentation and irrigation with 3% H_2O_2 i 2% CHX and final irrigation with MTAD solution in duration of 1 minute, the results obtained are ideal in the coronal, middle and apical thirds of the tooth root canal. Dentinal debris and smear layer compley removed. Dentinal tubules open, of regular shape and even diameter (coronary third 3,5 µm, middle third 2,5-3 µm, apical third 2-2,5 µm). Dentinal structure preserved.

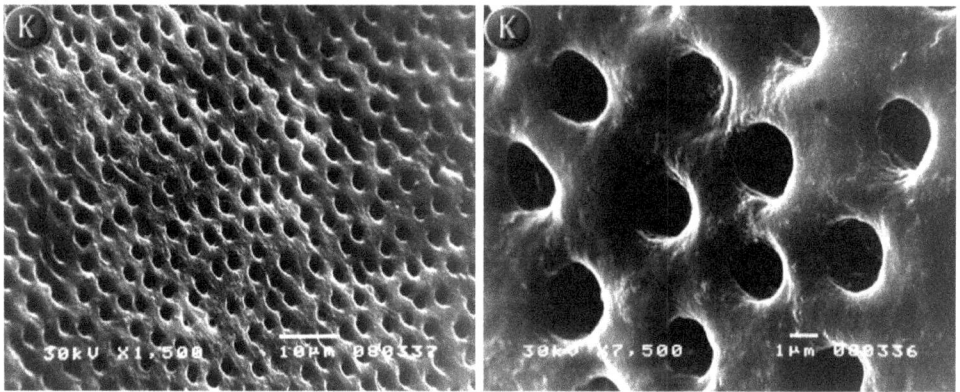

Fig. 12. SEM presentation of coronal third of intracanal dentin after manual treatment and irrigation with 2% CHX + 3% H_2O_2 and final irrigation with MTAD solution

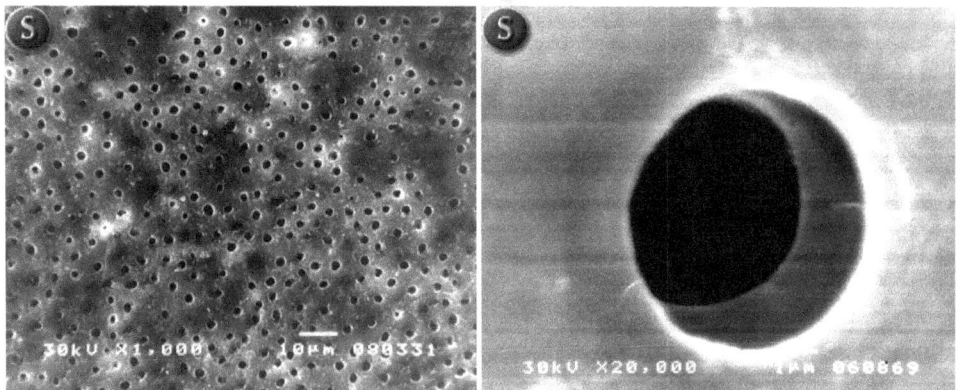

Fig. 13. SEM presentation of middle third of intracanal dentin after manual treatment and irrigation with 2% CHX + 3% H_2O_2 and final irrigation with MTAD solution

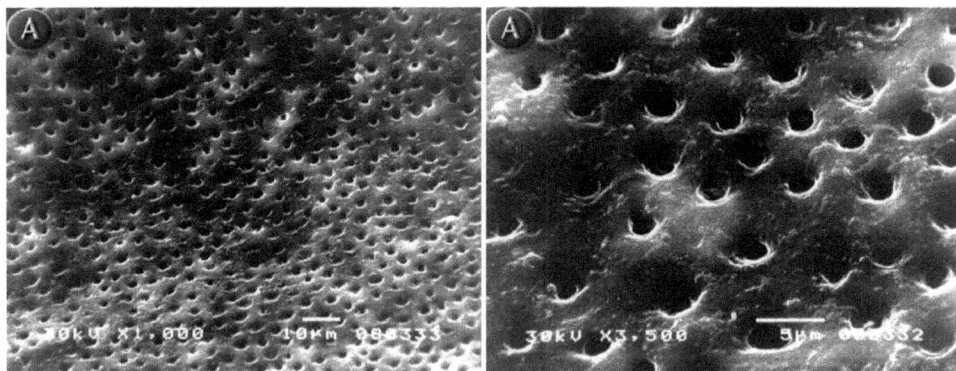

Fig. 14. SEM presentation of apical third of intracanal dentin after manual treatment and
irrigation with 2% CHX + 3% H_2O_2 and final irrigation with MTAD solution

Group/subgroup	N	Irrigants	5	4	3	2	1
II/A	15	3%H_2O_2+2,5% NaOCl	0	2	3	8	2
II/B	15	3%$H_2O_2$2% +CHX	0	1	3	9	2
II/C	15	2,5%NaOCl+17%NaEDTA	0	0	0	2	13
II/D	15	2,5%NaOCl	4	4	7	0	0
II/E	15	2,5%NaOCl +10% citric acid	0	0	0	4	11
II/F	15	3%H_2O +2%CHX +MTAD	0	0	0	1	14
I/G	15	3%H_2O_2 + MTAD	0	0	0	0	15

Table 5. Values of quantitative estimation of smear layer and dentinal debris for the
samples of group II (experimental) – subgroups A, B, C, D, E, F and G

Group/subgroups	N	$\overline{X}$	SD	95%C.I.	Min	Max	Sig.
II/A (3%H_2O_2+2,5%NaOCl)	15	2.66	0.89	2.16-3.16	1.00	4.00	A,B,C,D,E,F
II/B (3%H_2O_2 +2%CHX)	15	2.73	0.88	2.24-3.22	1.00	4.00	A,G,H,I,J,K
II/C (2,5%NaOCl+17%NaEDTA)	15	1.20	0.41	0.97-1.42	1.00	2.00	A,G,L
II/D (2,5%NaOCl)	15	3.80	0.86	3.32-4.27	3.00	5.00	C,H,L,M,N,O
II/E (2,5%NaOCl +10% citric acid	15	1.26	0.45	1.01-1.52	1.00	2.00	D,I,M
II/F (3%H_2O_2+2%CHX +MTAD)	15	1.06	0.25	0.92-1.20	1.00	2.00	E,J,N
II/G (3%H_2O_2+MTAD)	15	1.00	0.00	1.00-1.00	1.00	1.00	F,K,O

A (II/A vs II/B); B (II/A vs II/C); C (II/A vs II/D); D (II/A vs II/E); E (II/A vs II/F); F (II/A vs
II/G);G (II/B vs II/C); H (II/B vs II/D); I (II/B vs II/E); J (II/B vs II/F); K (II/B vs II/G);L (II/C vs
II/D); M (II/D vs II/E); N (II/D vs II/F); O (II/D vs II/G)

Table 6. Comparison of quantitative estimation values of smear layer and dentinal debris on
the samples of group II (experimental) – subgroups A, B, C, D, E, F, and G: ANOVA

By comparison of the quantitative estimation values of smear layer and dentinal debris on
the samples of group II (experimental) – subgroups A, B, C, D, E, F and G, using the
ANOVA test, it was found that the values obtained in the group II/A are statistically

significantly different from the results obtained in all other groups. Mean value obtained in the group II/A was statistically significantly lower compared to the values in the groups II/B and II/D. The values obtained in the group II/B are statistically significantly higher compared to the values obtained in the groups II/C, II/E, II/F and II/G, but lower than the values obtained in the group II/D. The values of group II/d are statistically significantly higher than the values obtained in all other groups. The values of groups II/F and II/G are lower compared to the values obtained in the groups II/A, II/B and II/D.

3.2 Analysis of antimicrobial effect with MTAD in infected canal system using PCR technique

With the aim to determine the antibacterial efficacy of MTAD solution using the PCR method, several most common endopathogenic microorganisms were identified in the

Bacterial species	Number of infected root canals				χ^2	p
	Before therapy		After therapy			
	N	%	N	%		
Agregatibacter	8	32	4	16	1.72	0.185
Prevotella intermedia	9	36	0	0		0.002
Porphyromonas gingivalis	4	16	0	0		0.11
Tanerella forsythenis	6	24	0	0		0.022
Enterococcus faecalis	15	60	5	20	8.17	0.004
Treponema denticola	7	28	3	12	1.96	0.161

Table 7. Prevalence of microorganisms in infected root canals prior and after MTAD therapy

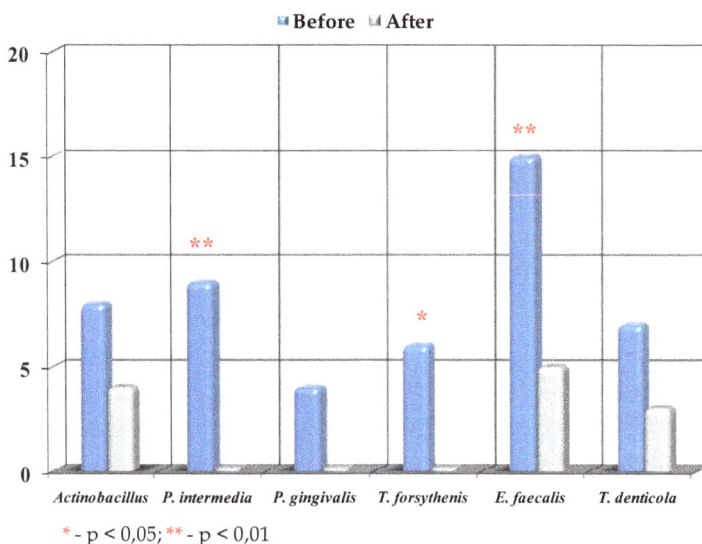

* - p < 0,05; ** - p < 0,01

Fig. 15. Prevalence of microorganisms in infected root canals before and after therapy with MTAD

infected canal system (*Porphyromonas gingivalis, Acgregatibacter actinomycetemcomitans, Tanerella forsythensis, Prevotella intermedia, Treponema denticola* and *Enterococcus faecalis*) before and after the irrigation with MTAD solution. Analysis of results and estimation of antibacterial efficacy of MTAD solution gives the clinical reference to this final irrigant in the treatment of infected root canals.

By comparing the frequency of occurrence of certain bacteria in root canals, before and after the irrigation with MTAD solution, statistically significant decrease of *Prevotella intermedia* (36% vs 0%),*Tanerella forsythenis* (24% vs 0%) and *Enterococcus faecalis* (60% vs 20%) was found. The presence of other bacteria was also decreased, but not statistically significant.

4. Conclusion

Based on the results obtained by SEM and statistical data processing, it can be concluded that the final irrigation of root canal system with mineralolithic effect irrigations must be a mandatory part of endodontic protocol. The best results and outstanding efficacy were demonstrated with MTAD solution. In combination with CHX and H_2O_2, it completely removes the smear layer from root canal walls, where the dentin surface structure remains preserved and openings of dentinal tubules are of even diameters and regular shapes. All mineralolithic solutions for final irrigation are used in duration of one minute, as longer exposure of dentin to these agents can bring about unwanted erosive changes and compromise the entire endodontic procedure. By regular use of final irrigating agents, complete efficacy in removal of smear layer from root canal system could be achieved.

5. Clinical recommendations

- When performing the manual and endgine driven instrumentation of the root canal, dentinal debris and smear layer are produced at all the levels of the intraradix region; they are not different in respect to the amount but presentation and structure.
- Saline solution applied as an irrigant exerts only the mechanical effect of removal and parial evacuation of debris.
- Irrigation by using organolithic agents alone cannot completely remove the smear layer.
- The combination of organolithic with mineralolithic agents has shown as the most efficient in the removal of smear layer at all the levels of the intraradix region.
- The combined application of hydrogene peroxide (and clorehexidine) during instrumentation and final irrigation with MTAD solution in duration of 1 minute results in complete removal of the smear layer.
- MTAD solution as the final irrigant meets all the standards for good irrigant proscribed by the endodontic protocol, which means that it preserves the structure of dentine, removes the smear layer and possesses the satisfactory antimicrobial properties.
- After the chemomechanic treatment and irrigation of the root canal using the MTAD solution, statistically significant decrease of *Enterococcus faecalis, Prevotella intermedia* and *Tanerella forsythenis* was found, while in cases of *Treponema denticola, Actinobacillus actinomycetemcomitans and Porphyromonas gingivalis* the antibacterial efficacy of MTAD solution was considerable but not statistically significant.
- MTAD solution, used as the final intracanal antiseptic in duration of 1 minute, efficiently removes the smear layer, in the case of which the intracanal structure

remains intact and morphologically unchanged, eliminating thus the majority of microorganisms.

6. References

Abdullah, M.; Ng, Y-L.; Gulabivala, K, Moles, D. & Spratt DA. (2005). Susceptilies of Two Enterococcus Faecalis Phenotypes to Root Canal Medications. *Journal of Endodontics,* Vol. 31, pp. 30-36. ISSN 0099-2399

Baumgartner, JC. & Mader, CL. (1987). A scanning Electron Microscopic Evaluation of Four Root Canal Irrigation Regimens. *Journal of Endodontics,* Vol. 13, pp. 147-157. ISSN 0099-2399

Calt, S. & Serper, A. (2002). Time-dependet Effects of EDTA on Dentine Structures. *Journal of Endodontics,* Vol. 28, pp. 17-29. ISSN 0099-2399

Chacker, FM. (1974). The Endodontic-periodontic Continuum. *Dental Clinics of North America,* Vol. 18, pp. 393-414. ISSN 0011-8532

De Deus, QD. (1975). Frequency Location and Direction of the Latheral Secondary and Accessory Canals. *Journal of Endodontics,* Vol. 1, pp. 361-366. ISSN 0099-2399

Di Lenardda, R.; Cadenaro, M. & Sbaizero, O. (2000). Effectiveness of 1 mol L^1 Citric Acid and 15%EDTA Irrigation on Smear Layer Removal. *International Endodontic Journal,* Vol. 33, pp. 46-52. ISSN 1365-2591

Fouad, AF.; Barry, J.; Caimano, M.; Clawson, M.; Zhu, Q.; Carver, R.; Hazlett, K. & Radolf JD. (2002). PCR-based Identification of Bacteria Associated with Endodontic Infections. *Journal of Clinical Microbiology,* Vol. 40, pp. 3223-3231. ISSN 0095-1137

Gašić, J.; Simonović, D.; Radičević, G.; Mitić, A.; Stojilković, G. & Daković, J. (2003). Scanning Electron Microscopy Of Root Canal Walls After Removing The Smear Layer. *Serbian Dental Journal,* Vol. 50, pp. 65-68. ISSN 0039-1743

Haapasalo, HK.; Siren, EK.; Waltimo, TM.; Ørstavik, D. & Haapasalo, MP. (2000). Inactivation of Local Root Canal Medicaments by Dentine: an In Vitro Study. *International Endodontic Journal,* Vol. 33, No. 2, pp. 126-131. ISSN 0143-2885

Haapasalo, M.; Endal, U.; Zandi, H. & Coil, JM. (2005). Eradication of Endodontic Infection by Instrumentation and Irrigation Solutions. *Endodontic Topics,* Vol. 10, pp. 77-102. ISSN 1601-1538

Hülsmann, M.; Riimmelin, C. & Schafers, F. (1997). Root Canal Cleanliness After Preparation with Different Endodontic Handpieces and Hand Instruments. A comparative SEM Investigation. *Journal of Endodontics,* Vol. 23, pp. 301-306. ISSN 0099-2399

Jacinto, RC.; Gomes, BP.; Ferraz, CC.; Zaia AA. & Filho FJ. (2003). Microbiological Analysis of Infected Root Canals From Symtomatic Teeth with Periapical Periodontitis and the Antimicrobial Susceptibility of Some Isolated Anaerobic Bacteria. *Oral Microbiology and Immunology,* Vol. 18, pp. 285-292. ISSN 0902-0055

Kando, J. (1991). A Method for Bonding to Tooht Structure Using Phosphoric Acid as a Dentin-Enamel Conditioner. *Quintessence International,* Vol. 22, pp. 285-290. ISSN 0033-6572

Love, RM. (2001) Enterococcus Faecalis-a Mechanism for its Role in Endodontic Failure. *International Endodontic Journal* Vol. 34, pp. 399-405. ISSN 0143-2885

Matsuo, T.; Shirakami, T.; Ozaki, K.; Nakanishi, T.; Yumoto, H. & Ebisu, S. (2003). An Immunohistological Study of the Localization of Bacteria Invading Root Pulpal Walls of Teeth with Periapical Lesions *Journal of Endodontics,* Vol. 29, No. 3, pp. 194-200. ISNN 0099-2399

Mitić A, Mitić N, Živković S, Tošić G, Savić V. Dačić S. & Stojanović M. (2009). Efficiency of Final Irrigation of Root Canal in Removal of Smear Layer. *Serbian Archives for the Whole Medicine*, Vol. 9-10, pp. 482-489. ISSN 0370-8179

Mitić A. (2009). Ultrastructural research of the dentine surface of the tooth root canal after the appliance of chemomechanical, ultrasound and laser technique (PhD Thesis). Niš, Serbia: University of Niš.

Mitić, A. *Chemomechanical treatment of infected tooth root canal*. (2011). Monograph, ISBN 978-86-7757-189-4, Studentski kulturni centar, Niš, Serbia

Mitić, A.; Mitić, N.; Muratovska, I.; Stojanovska,V.; Popovska, L. & Mitić, V. (2008). Ultrastructural Investigation of Root Canal Dentine Surface After Application of Active Ultrasonic Method. *Serbian Archives for the Whole Medicine*, Vol. 5-6, pp. 226-231. ISSN: 0370-8179

Morazin, AD.; Vulcain, JM. & Mallet, MB. (1994). An Ultrstructural Stady of the Smear Layer; Comparative Aspects Using Secondary Electron Image and Backscattered Electron Image. *Journal of Endodontics*, Vol. 20, pp. 531-534. ISSN 0099-2399

Nešković, J. & Živković, S. (2009). Possibilities of Endodontic Therapy of Endodonic- Periodontal Lesions. *Serbian Archives for the Whole Medicine*, Vol. 137, No. 7-8, pp. 351-356. ISSN 0370-8179

Portenier, I.; Haapasalo, H.; Rye, A.; Waltimo, T.; Ørstavier, D. & Haapasalo, M. (2001). Inactivation of Root Canal Medicaments by Dentine, Hydroxilapatite and Bovine Serum Albumin. *International Endodontic Journal*, Vol. 34, No. 2, pp. 184-188. ISSN 0143-2885

Portenier, I.; Waltimo, TMT. & Haapasalo, M. (2003). Enterococcus Faecalis–the Root Canal Survivor and ´star´ in Post-treatment Disease. *Endodontic Topics*, Vol. 6, pp. 135-159. ISSN 1601-1538

Shabahang, S.; Pouresmail , M. & Torabinejad, M. (2003). In Vitro Antimicrobial Efficacy of MTAD and Sodium. *Journal of Endodontics,* Vol. 29, No. 7, pp. 450-452. ISSN 0099-2399

Siqueira, JF Jr.; Rôças, IN.; Abad, EC.; Castro, AJ.; Gahyva, SM. & Favieri A. (2001). Ability of Three Rod – End Filling Materials to Prevent Bacteria Leakage. *Journal of Endodontics*, Vol. 27, No.11, pp. 673-675. ISSN 0099-2399

Spratt, DA.; Pratten, J.; Wilson, M. & Gulabivala K. (2001). An In Vitro Evaluation of the Anti Microbial Efficacy of Irrigants on Biofilms of Root Canal Isolates. *International Endodontic Journal*, Vol. 34, pp. 300-307. ISSN 0143-2885

Takeda, FH.; Harashima, T.; Kimura, Y. & Matsumoto, K. (1999). A comparative Study of the Removal of the Smear Layer by Three Endodontic Irrigants and Two Types of Laser. *International Endodontic Journal*, Vol. 32, pp. 32-39. ISSN: 1365-2591.

Torabinejad, M.; Cho, Y.; Khademi , AA.; Bakland, LK. & Shabahang, S. (2003). The Effect of Different Concentrations of Sodium Hypochlorite on the Ability of MTAD to Remove the Smear Layer. *Journal of Endodontics*, Vol. 29, pp. 233-239. ISSN 0099-2399

Torabinejad, M.; Handysides, R.; Ali Khademi, A. & Bakland, LK. (2002). Clinical Implications of Smear Layer in Endodontic: a Review. *Oral Surgery, Oral Medicine, Oral Pathology, Oral Radiology and Endodontology*, Vol. 94. pp. 658-666. ISSN 1079-2104

Torabinejad, M.; Khademi, AA.; Babagoli, J.; Cho, Y.; Johnson, WB.; Bozhilov, K.; Kim, J. & Shabahang, S. (2003). A New Solution for the Removal of the Smear Layer. *Journal of Endodontics,* Vol. 29, pp. 170-175. ISSN 0099-2399

Torabinejad, M.; Shabahang, S.; Aprecio, RM. & Kettering, JD. (2003). The Antimicrobial Effect of MTAD: an In Vitro Investigation. *Journal of Endodontics*, Vol. 29, pp. 400-403. ISSN 0099 2399

Yamaguchi, M.; Yoshida, K.; Suzuki, R. & Nakamura, H. (1996). Root Canal Irrigation with Citric Acid Solution. *Journal of Endodontics*, Vol. 22, pp. 27-29. ISSN 0099-2399

Živković, S.; Brkanić, T.; Dačić, D.; Opačić, V. & Pavlović, V. (2005). Smear Layer in Endodontics. *Serbian Dental Journal* Vol. 52, pp. 7-19. ISSN 0039-1743

17

Tooth Autotransplantation

Eduardo Santiago, Germano Rocha and João F. C. Carvalho
Oporto School of Dentistry, University of Oporto
Portugal

1. Introduction

Teeth autotransplantation is an alternative treatment for single tooth oral rehabilitation, and it is possible that it becomes more frequent if the technique respects protocol. It is important to choose patients with prognostic factors that may provide a favorable condition for success. (Tsukiboshi 2001) The main reason for failure of this technique is a bad selection of patients, and this can be overpast by previous planning and the knowledge of all prognostic factors that are a part of the process.

Follow-up studies for 3 to 14 years indicate that either the transplantation is placed in a natural or artificial alveolus, teeth vitality is preserved in 90-96% of all cases. (Donado 2007) (Ahlberg, Bystedt et al. 1983) The ideal condition for success, according to the literature seems to be a donor tooth with 3/4s of root development, with open apex. (Akiyama, Fukuda et al. 1998; Josefsson, Brattstrom et al. 1999; Czochrowska, Stenvik et al. 2002; Kallu, Vinckier et al. 2005; Donado 2007)

When planning a surgery such as this, it is important to study the patient's age, the existence of a natural alveolus and the root development. (Tsukiboshi 2001) It seems well defined by the literature that the preference for selection of clinical cases is young and cooperative patients, without any systemic diseases. (Tsukiboshi 2001) It is also shown that in teeth with incomplete root formation, vitality is preserved in 90-96% of all cases in 3-14 year follow-up studies, and the preference is also for natural alveolus. (Ahlberg, Bystedt et al. 1983; Donado 2007) The best case scenario seems to be when root formation is in its 3/4s, with open apex. (Akiyama, Fukuda et al. 1998; Josefsson, Brattstrom et al. 1999; Tsukiboshi 2001; Czochrowska, Stenvik et al. 2002; Kallu, Vinckier et al. 2005; Donado 2007)

The success rate must be detached from the survival rate in tooth autotransplantation. The survival rate refers to the presence of the transplanted tooth, even if its function, esthetics or development, are compromised. (Aslan, Ucuncu et al. 2010) On the other hand, to say that success has been achieved, there must be good esthetics and positioning, ability to chew without restrictions, pulpar vitality, and good dentofacial development. (Aslan, Ucuncu et al. 2010) This success rate is influenced by surgical technique, experience of the surgeon, the patient's age or root development. (Aslan, Ucuncu et al. 2010)

According to Andreasen et al, in 1990, survival rate of transplanted teeth after 13 year follow-up is 95-98%. (Aslan, Ucuncu et al. 2010) In 1999, Josefsson found a 82% survival rate after shorter follow-up time - 4 years follow up (Josefsson, Brattstrom et al. 1999). The main reason for high rates is case selection. It is important to note that literature shows higher percentage of survival rate for immature teeth, in adolescents with natural alveolus. (Akiyama, Fukuda et al. 1998; Josefsson, Brattstrom et al. 1999; Czochrowska, Stenvik et al. 2002; Kallu, Vinckier et al. 2005, Donado 2007)

Literature also tells us that if the tooth is transplanted to an artificial alveolus, it lowers survival rates more than in natural alveolus. (Akiyama, Fukuda et al. 1998; Josefsson, Brattstrom et al. 1999; Czochrowska, Stenvik et al. 2002; Kallu, Vinckier et al. 2005; Donado 2007) Even so, Ahlberg et al tell us that maxillary canines transplanted into artificial alveolus may have similar survival rates than those transplanted into natural alveolus. (Ahlberg, Bystedt et al. 1983; Donado 2007) That is, artificial alveolus normally have worse prognosis than natural ones. At best, survival rates may be equal in both types of alveolus.

Cases submitted to orthodontic treatment are an indicator that transplanted teeth may be a viable solution and the most natural one for replacing missing teeth. These teeth can even be moved and serve as anchorage in orthodontic treatment and still allow bone remodeling around them. (Andreasen, Paulsen et al. 1990; Paulsen 2001)

To achieve the complete root formation, it is important that during the surgery, periodontal ligament is preserved as much as possible, and it needs to be a technique as little invasive as possible, because that may compromise root development, leading to anchylosys or root reabsorptions. (Thomas, Turner et al. 1998; Aslan, Ucuncu et al. 2010) Most authors conclude that immature teeth are preferable for better outcomes. (Andreasen, Paulsen et al. 1990; Paulsen, Andreasen et al. 1995; Paulsen 2001; Paulsen, Shi et al. 2001) On the other hand, the fact that a considerable percentage of teeth completed root formation indicates an important factor of normal and physiological process. (Paulsen, Shi et al. 2001) Root development can go on with no impediments, but even so, it may end with an unfavorable crown-root relation. (Aslan, Ucuncu et al. 2010) The root may close its apex, but may not continue to grow apically. According to Andreasen, if the root development is very low when the tooth is transplanted, that is, less than 3/4s of its complete formation, the root growth is also inferior, and may end-up with closed apexes, but with small length. (Andreasen, Paulsen et al. 1990; Andreasen, Paulsen et al. 1990; Andreasen, Paulsen et al. 1990; Northway 2002; Tsukiboshi 2002; Aslan, Ucuncu et al. 2010)

Andreasen also reveals a higher incidence of pulpar necrosis in teeth with completed root development at the time of the transplant, but claims that, with adequate root canal treatment, survival rates may be assured, and, in some cases, endodontic treatment may even be unnecessary, because of partial pulpar obliteration that may be present in teeth with pulpar regeneration and healing. (Andreasen, Paulsen et al. 1990; Andreasen, Paulsen et al. 1990; Andreasen, Paulsen et al. 1990; Czochrowska, Stenvik et al. 2000; Jonsson and Sigurdsson 2004)

In sum, vital teeth are most frequent in immature teeth transplanted. Tooth with complete root formation, normally present endodontic treatment and may achieve some success if there is an adequate root canal treatment.

Predicting the prognosis for tooth autotransplantation is important to evaluate the ability of this technique for replacing a missing tooth. A large number of cases are needed to predict the prognosis before surgery and to eliminate most doubts. Literature shows us that having this knowledge allows the clinician to select transplanted teeth cases very carefully and with a high level of stringency.

2. History in a glance

Teeth autotransplantation have been considered, since the middle of the 20th century, as viable rehabilitation alternatives, and have been usually a part of treatment planning. In several occasions, good results were obtained and registered, with clinical viability, either esthetics or functional. (Ahlberg, Bystedt et al. 1983; Akiyama, Fukuda et al. 1998; Josefsson, Brattstrom et al. 1999; Czochrowska, Stenvik et al. 2002; Kallu, Vinckier et al. 2005) However, a considerable percentage seemed to develop complications, turning this option into a controversial one. (Ahlberg, Bystedt et al. 1983; Czochrowska, Stenvik et al. 2002; Kim, Jung et al. 2005)

Teeth autotransplantation technique is well supported by documentation. According to historic evidence, populations from over 1000 years back have used it, reaching a more frequent use during the middle ages. They would use animal, ivory, bone or even human teeth extracted from corpses, but the problem was that, because of discoloration, bad odor and lack of resistance, it didn't achieve a good public opinion. (Magheri, Grandini et al. 2001; Tsukiboshi 2001)

The first known documented reference of this surgical procedure is in Ambroise Paré's work (1561), a Renascence French Surgeon that describes a noble woman in who, after extracting a tooth, was placed another tooth that belonged to one of hers maid, stating that after some time, the lady could chew perfectly. Two centuries later, Pierre Fauchard (1725), the founder of Modern Medicine, wrote about re-implants and dental transplantation, claiming that they could be performed in the same individual, or between 2 individuals. John Hunter (1728-1793), in England, described a vascular and periodontal regeneration after a transplantation of animal or human teeth in crests of cocks, therefore preserving the tooth vitality, and if a painful tooth was to be extracted, it could be boiled and re-implanted. These were the first laboratory investigations towards teeth transplantations. (Marzola 1968; Tsukiboshi 2001)

The same investigator, however, also introduces the problem of diseases' transmission, such as syphilis. In 1827, Emile Blaise Gardette recorded the impossibility of teeth autotransplantation success if case selection was not taken as an important issue. This author studied the results of 170 transplants in function for only 1 or 2 years, analyzing that good results were only obtained with careful selection of cases.

In 1935, the microscopic investigation started, with Lundquist. Apfel, in 1950, advised the use of the tooth transplantation technique, but only according to rules he described, such as planning according to the patients' age, donor tooth germ size, and good intra-oral x-rays. He also presents the surgical technique, in which he maintains the pericoronal sac and the gum that covers it. This technique was later abandoned by Marzola in 1988, claiming it was unnecessary to preserve the gum that covered the pericoronal sac. (Marzola 1968) But it was only in 1956, with Fong, Apfel and Miller that scientific relevance was achieved, with 50% success rates, justifying the not successful cases with lack of root development and presence of external and internal root reabsorptions. (Magheri, Grandini et al. 2001) During that same year, a world symposium defined specific rules for the tooth transplantation success:

- Lack of discomfort of the patient,
- soft and hardtissue regeneration and
- Functional retention for at least 2 years.

Ten years later, Metro presented a variation from the previous surgical technique, with simultaneous bilateral teeth transplantation, and stated that he was not in favor of teeth splinting, because of the food accumulation, because of difficulties in hygiene, and because of epithelial adherence inhibition as a result. He reported using simple sutures of the dental papillae, placing the tooth germ in occlusion and instructed that no chewing in the first 3 days should exist, just liquid diet. This would allow total success. (Marzola 1968) In the 70s of the 20th century, this technique was re-evaluated by Andreasen and his works on biological principles, the causes of failure and the periodontal healing after tooth transplantation. (Kim, Jung et al. 2005) This was a major reference for tooth transplantations. Immunological research has also been reported and documented. However, this field still needs more investigation. In the meantime, several works are presented regularly, showing the success rates of this technique, its precise indications and follow-up periods.

3. Concepts

Teeth autotransplantion can be defined as the placement of a tooth or tooth germ, with or without vitality, in a natural alveolus corresponding to another tooth, or in an artificially created alveolus for this end. (Escoda 1999; Donado 2007)

A natural alveolus is already physiologically formed, and previously occupied by another tooth. On the other hand, an artificial one is created by the surgeon, that is, in a place where a tooth was not present at the time of, or previously to the transplantation. (Escoda 1999; Donado 2007)

The main purpose of this specific technique is to substitute a tooth, that has been lost or that has indication for extraction, because of a bad prognosis, by another tooth that presents more advantages for being in the receptor area, and/or that has no function in its primary location. (Czochrowska, Stenvik et al. 2000; Donado 2007)

It can be considered, in a wider concept of tooth autotransplantation for some authors such as Tsukiboshi, 3 distinct situations: First, when a tooth is extracted from a location and reimplanted in a different one, which is named tooth transplantation; Second, when a tooth is repositioned in its own alveolus, as in verticalization of 3rd molars or surgical extrusion of a tooth; Third, and finally, when an extracted or avulsed tooth is treated and reimplanted in its own location sometimes as an alternative to periapical surgery. (Tsukiboshi 2001) This is a more global concept including intra-alveolar transplantation and intentional reimplantation, because all are characterized by a similar healing process. (Aslan, Ucuncu et al. 2010)

Autotransplantation of teeth are an alternative as any other and should be considered when planning a treatment. This technique can give some advantages, such as a possibility for a fixed bridge (where before it would only be possible to place a dental implant or removable prothodontics), the reposition of teeth without orthodontics, the use in helping to solve agenesis problems and the surgical extrusion of fractured teeth (to allow dentistry/fixed crowns). (Aslan, Ucuncu et al. 2010)

This technique usually requires one surgery. Besides all this advantages, one of the biggest is the fact that the patient regains a proprioceptive feeling in the transplanted tooth, with normal periodontal healing, allowing a natural feel during chewing. (Aslan, Ucuncu et al. 2010) But the main advantage is the use in children and adolescents, because of its continuous induction on the alveolar bone, and therefore allowing for the normal physiological alveolar growth. (Aslan, Ucuncu et al. 2010)

It also presents some disadvantages, such as being less predictable when using teeth with complete root development, the possibility of pulpar necrosis, and the need for endodontic treatment, very frequently. It also demands a strong collaboration and motivation from the patient. If this does not happen, the success rate falls abruptly.

4. Prognostic factors

The first and most important prognostic factor is case selections. Therefore, indications and counter-indications are of major relevance to achieve success.

The main indication is the existence of a risk/benefit more favorable than for any other kind of treatment, when a tooth must be maintained for esthetics and functional demands. (Josefsson, Brattstrom et al. 1999; Kallu, Vinckier et al. 2005) The best patients for this treatment are motivated youngsters, with impossibility to be subjected to dental implants. (Aslan, Ucuncu et al. 2010)

The 3rd molar when used to substitute a 1st or 2nd molar, the use of an extracted premolar for orthodontic reasons to substitute a central incisor or the placement of a retained canine in its correct position are the most frequent situations for teeth transplantations. (Paulsen, Andreasen et al. 1995; Escoda 1999; Donado 2007) It is also common to use this technique in trauma patients, with avulsed teeth that can be re-placed in their own location. (Aslan, Ucuncu et al. 2010)

For all this, it is essential to obtain a complete and thorough clinical history, a detailed x-ray exam, to measure the donor tooth and the receptor location, and to determine the root form.

The counterindications are the ones that all surgical intervention are subjected to, but the lack of bone in the reception area, and complicated extractions for donor teeth can also lead to non-successful cases. (Ahlberg, Bystedt et al. 1983; Escoda 1999) Compromised teeth with periodontal disease, in which epithelial adherence is lost in more than one 3rd of the root should be considered as inadequate as donor teeth for autotransplantation because of the lack of periodontal ligament. This characteristic favors anchylosis and root reabsorptions. (Tsukiboshi 2001)

Literature shows that a tooth autotransplantation has better prognosis when performed in younger patients, with immature donor teeth. Follow-up studies of 3 to 14 years report that pulpar vitality is preserved in 90 to 96% of immature donor teeth cases. Although it has also been shown that teeth transplantation works at any age, and even with artificially created alveolus, the ideal situation, and with the best prognosis, seems to be when the transplanted tooth has 3/4s of root development, and an open apex. (Akiyama, Fukuda et al. 1998; Josefsson, Brattstrom et al. 1999; Czochrowska, Stenvik et al. 2002; Kallu, Vinckier et al. 2005; Donado 2007)

The technique success has been presented throughout the years, approaching different factors. Fleming, back in 1956 suggested that, for a transplanted tooth to be considered successful, it should:

- Have no inflammatory reaction in the alveolus,
- the dental germ should be maintained in its new position,
- the periodontium should be preserved,
- There should be no root reabsorption,
- the color of the transplanted tooth should suffer no changes, and
- it should maintain its vitality. (Fleming 1956)

The success rate seems to vary with the surgical technique, the experience and capability of the surgeon, and several pre and post operative factors, such as age of the patient, root development, the type of transplanted tooth, the extra-oral time, the placement of the donor tooth and the receptor location. (Kallu, Vinckier et al. 2005; Aslan, Ucuncu et al. 2010) Besides all this, we should be careful with the amount of space needed, the occlusion and the size and shape of the donor tooth. (Aslan, Ucuncu et al. 2010)

The surgical technique must be as non-traumatic as possible, with minimum handling of the donor tooth in order to preserve the periodontal ligament and maintain the Hertwig Epithelial Sheath, so that root development is not compromised, avoiding anchylosis, root reabsorptions and loss of epithelial adherence. (Thomas, Turner et al. 1998; Aslan, Ucuncu et al. 2010)

The transplanted tooth can be placed in the receptor location and maintained only by simple sutures or by a crossed suture over the crown, or even by a non rigid splint. It seems clear that a prolonged rigid splitting of the transplanted tooth has adverse effects in pulpar and periodontal healing, and that there should be a relative immobilization period of 2 weeks to 2 months, depending on the accommodation of the donor tooth in the receptor alveolus. (Aslan, Ucuncu et al. 2010)

The ideal receptor alveolus must have sufficient height and width to shelter the donor tooth, and it can be improved increasing its measurements surgically, for example, with an non-traumatic sinus lift, similar to the technique used in dental implants placement. (Tsukiboshi 2001) In the specific case of 3rd molars transplanted to the contiguous 2nd molar alveolus, the prognosis is worse when the wisdom tooth is positioned more apically according to the 2nd molar, becoming harder to achieve epithelial adherence in the distal surface of the transplanted tooth. (Tsukiboshi 2001) The donor tooth must be placed, according to the literature, slightly under the occlusal plan, but not forced into the alveolus, with no pressure on the apexes, to allow root development. (Aslan, Ucuncu et al. 2010)

The root development of the transplanted tooth can, therefore, continue with no impediment, but may also be disrupted leading to a unfavorable crown/root relation. (Aslan, Ucuncu et al. 2010) Andreasen showed that although they have higher success rates, more immature roots present less root growth after transplant, than immature but in a more advanced growth stage roots. (Andreasen, Paulsen et al. 1990; Andreasen, Paulsen et al. 1990; Andreasen, Paulsen et al. 1990) This is the reason why the literature shows that the ideal stage for tooth transplant is when the root has 3/4s of its development, and an open apex of more than 1 mm. (Northway 2002; Tsukiboshi 2002)

The periodontal healing is normally achieved after 2 months, in most cases, (Andreasen, Paulsen et al. 1990; Andreasen, Paulsen et al. 1990; Andreasen, Paulsen et al. 1990; Andreasen, Paulsen et al. 1990) and it is characterized by no root reabsorption and the x-ray presence of lamina dura. (Aslan, Ucuncu et al. 2010) In x-rays, the periodontium shows himself as a continuous space throughout the root surface. (Cohen, Shen et al. 1995; Akiyama, Fukuda et al. 1998) The root reabsorption by substitution, that is, anchylosis, happens in teeth with injured cement, which suggests the importance of this structure for the periodontal regeneration. (Akiyama, Fukuda et al. 1998) Anchylosis is normally diagnosed in the 1st year, in x-rays, or clinically by a metallic percussion sound, and after 1 year, it is usually seen external root reabsorption, that may also appear, according to Andreasen, because of lack of oral hygiene. (Andreasen, Paulsen et al. 1990; Andreasen, Paulsen et al. 1990; Andreasen, Paulsen et al. 1990; Thomas, Turner et al. 1998)

Revascularization normally occurs 4 days after the surgery, and advances in a 0.1mm/day rate. Immature teeth most often do not need endodontic treatment, and normally finish their root development and maintain vitality. One of the main factors for revascularization is the extra-oral time of the donor tooth and its handling during surgery. Teeth re-implants are more likely to be successful if performed immediately after tooth lost or up to 30 minutes of extra-oral time. The extra-oral time of the donor tooth is also consensual to be of no more than 7-8 minutes, but there hasn't been no relation between this factor and root reabsorptions or anchylosis. (Kim, Jung et al. 2005)

5. Treatment sequence

The sequence for an autotransplantation, in an ideal and complete version, implicates thorough clinical and radiographic exams, treatment plan, surgical procedure, endodontic treatment, if needed, rehabilitation treatment if needed and follow-up. (Tsukiboshi 2002)
As in any surgical intervention, protocol must begin with clinical data collection, with the patient's age, medical and dental history, and with a clinical examination and radiographic study of the donor tooth, its root development, and finally with the clinical and radiographic examination of the receptor location. This clinical exam allows the identification of the periodontal biotype, important to predict gingival retractions, for example, and more importantly, the measurement of the available space in the receptor area. On the other hand, the radiographic study, with a panoramic x-ray, periapical and occlusal x-rays, make it possible to determine the shape of the donor tooth and the receptor location, root development, the alveolar bone, the position and placement of the tooth, the degree of inclination and the relationship with nearby noble anatomic structures. (Tsukiboshi 2002)
If we find 2 teeth that are suitable to be used as donors, the choice should be the made looking at the tooth's crown, because 3rd mandibular molars are more similar to 1st and 2nd mandibular molars, and the same happens for 3rd maxillary molars, that are similar to the neighbor teeth. (Tsukiboshi 2001)
The treatment plan is all about case study and selection, so that the best time for tooth transplantation is chosen. For example, if a tooth in the receptor area needs to be extracted, the transplantation must be done within 2-6 weeks after, to avoid extended bone reabsorption. (Tsukiboshi 2002) If possible, the tooth transplantations is best when performed immediately after extraction in the receptor area, and if there is predictable need for endodontic treatment, based on root development grade, it can be done before transplantation is complete, extra-orally, or it can be started within 2 weeks after surgical intervention. (Tsukiboshi 2002) Transplanted teeth restorations should take in account the preference to avoid tooth reduction, that is, there is no absolute indication for fixed prosthodontics after tooth transplantation. (Tsukiboshi 2002)
The treatment plan also needs good radiographic study, and the image of the donor tooth must be measured mesio-distally at the crown and at the roots, and the root length must also be evaluated. (Tsukiboshi 2002)

5.1 Surgical technique – Fase 1
The surgical technique is perfectly accepted and present in the literature, with references to some important particularities, with some different points of view.
The surgical material needed is:
- Intra-oral mirror
- probe
- Dissection tweezers

- Carpule
- Disposable needles
- Local anesthetics
- N.er 12 and n.er 15 blade
- Retractors
- Levers
- Forceps
- Curette
- Bone file
- Hand piece
- Surgical drills
- Supramide suture 3/0 and 4/0
- Needle holders
- Scissors

To lower the risk of infection of the operative field, the patient should first perform mouth rinse with clorohexidine before surgery. Secondly, the peri-oral structures should be cleansed with clorohexidine and some authors suggest starting taking systemic antibiotics orally a few hours before surgery. (Tsukiboshi 2002)

5.2 Surgical technique – Fase 2

The anesthetics technique is conventional, with loco-regional blockage complemented with suprabone infiltrative anesthetic bucally and lingually, using if possible, anesthetic with adrenaline to potentiate the effect in the donor tooth area. In the receptor region, it usually is enough to anesthetize with suprabone infiltrative anesthetic bucally and lingually.

The incision on the donor tooth can include vertical release if needed because of the difficulty degree for extracting it. If not needed, an intrasulcular incision should be enough.

Mucoperiosteum retraction starts in the interdental papillae, following to the gingiva, releasing the soft tissues and preserving the periosteum membrane integrity, for better posterior regeneration.

The donor tooth luxation should be controlled, allowing the tooth to stay in the alveolus, but also making it possible for an easy and fast extraction. Sometimes, osteotomy with bone drills is necessary to expose the donor tooth and to allow a support surface for the elevator. Just then, the elevator can leave the tooth in the alveolus but with mobility and small retention forces. Some authors suggest an intra-crevicular incision before luxation, to preserve as much as possible, the periodontium of the root. (Tsukiboshi 2002)

Some also defend the donor tooth extraction before the receptor location is prepared, to confirm anatomy, size and periodontal ligament condition. They then suggest replacement of the donor tooth in the original alveolus, while the receptor site is being prepared. (Tsukiboshi 2002) If a delay is predicted on the preparation of the receptor site, the tooth should be placed according to a few authors, in a saline Hank solution, to maintain periodontal ligament cells viability, and never be placed in water, because of it hypotonic characteristic that would implicate having no viability that is needed for the periodontal ligament regeneration. (Tsukiboshi 2002)

The receptor site preparation, with the extraction of the tooth, if present, should also include removal of the inter-root septum, and all the inflammatory tissue that may be present. If possible, it is better to extract without using curettes at the end, because it allows periodontal ligament cells to be maintained. If there is no tooth present, a surgical bone drill should be used to create or adapt an artificial alveolus for the donor tooth, with slightly more than enough space vertically, mesio-distally, and bucal-lingually. A saline solution embed compress should be placed in the alveolus. (Tsukiboshi 2002)

5.3 Surgical technique – Fase 3

The previously luxated donor tooth is now extracted, removing the pericoronal sac. The transplant is then performed, verifying the adaptation to the receptor site, without forcing its entry so that there is no apical pressure in any way. Obstacles in the alveolus are removed if found. The perfect adaptation needs a similar biologic space to the one in a normally erupted tooth.

The donor tooth needs at this time, to be maintained on the chosen position. Literature seems to show that the semi-rigid technique for keeping the tooth in position is the best. A rigid fixation of the tooth can originate dental tissue reabsorption and anquilosys, and some mobility stimulates periodontal ligament cells to regenerate. So, a crossed suture over the crown of the tooth slightly in infra-occlusion, allows good adaptation of the wound and protects the clot, and, on the other hand, avoids entrance of bacteria. (Tsukiboshi 2002) Some authors recommend simple papillae suture before the placement of the donor tooth, so that a better adaptation of the tooth in the alveolus and marginal gingiva is achievable, especially in those cases where a 3rd molar is placed in the contiguous 2nd molar place and there is no distal bone structure for perfect adaptation. (Tsukiboshi 2002) Literature also reveals an important detail: 2 loose ends in the mesial and distal sutures should be left free, so that those ends are tied over the crown of the transplanted tooth. (Tsukiboshi 2002) In some cases, a thin orthodontic wire can be used to splint the tooth, with no rigidity, but allowing to release pressure from the root apex. Occlusion must be "spot on".

At this time, an x-ray should be taken to evaluate the position of the donor tooth and to have a perspective to compare with future controls.

Some authors use surgical cement for 2-3 days after surgery.

At the end of the surgery, a revision and suture of the donor tooth original area has to be performed, to be possible to eliminate bone fragments and regularize bone edges. Suture has to allow repositioning of soft tissues.

5.4 Surgical technique – Fase 4

After the surgery, the patient must be advised to do soft and cold feeding for 1 week. He must apply ice locally to reduce swelling and pain, and avoid intense physical exercise for 2-3 days.

A systemic antibiotic via orally for 1 week, an AINE's and an analgesic must be considered. Clorohexidine must also be advised in gel and mouthrinse.

The transplanted tooth should be controlled clinically and radiographically after 2 days, 1 week, 1 month, 3 months, 6 months and annually, and suture removal should be on the 10th day after surgery. These controls allow a close monitoring of the tooth's position, the oral hygiene of the patient and the occlusion.

If needed, endodontic treatment is to be started after 2 weeks of the surgery. If the tooth is immature, with open root apexes, it is normally not necessary because of the high possibility of revascularization of the pulp. In those cases, it should be controlled by cold and hot tests, to identify pulpar necrosis. (Tsukiboshi 2001)

If the case is a re-implant, the process is similar:
- Localization of the tooth, if it is retained
- Osteotomy if needed
- Luxation of the tooth and placement on the correct position
- Endodontic treatment if there is pulpar necrosis 7-14 days after surgery
- Non rigid fixation with suture and/or orthodontic wire
- X-ray control

6. Tooth autotransplantation vs. dental implants

Dental implants have been gaining use in Oral rehabilitation, with very high survival rates, and teeth autotransplantations have been set aside because of its higher technical demands, and its slightly lower success rates that leave some doubts towards its prognostic. (Tsukiboshi 2001) Implants and bone regeneration techniques have shown a high predictability, and that is why autotransplantations have lost their value has a rehabilitation alternative. (Magheri, Grandini et al. 2001)

Evolution still continues in implant and bone regeneration industry, but, at this time and besides all their high success rates, both have advantages and disadvantages that cannot be forgotten or set aside. (Tsukiboshi 2001)

The decision on the rehabilitation option should come from the informed patient, together with the clinician, considering the factors such as the patient's age, the possible donor tooth and the receptor location condition, and , of course, considering the possibility of long term function and esthetics. (Tsukiboshi 2001)

The young age of a patient is the main reason to consider not using dental implants. (Aslan, Ucuncu et al. 2010) Due to facial residual growth in young patients, infra-oclusion of the dental implant may occur, because it is normal anchylosed to the alveolar bone, named osteointegration.

However, dental implants can also be an alternative to autotransplantation disadvantages, such as the higher and more complex surgical needs on the latter, the higher prognostic difficulties, possible root reabsorptions complications or lost of epithelial adherence that may lead to autotransplanted tooth loss, and the possibility to have to perform endodontic treatment few days after the intervention. (Tsukiboshi 2001)

So, implants are more likely to be a first choice in oral rehabilitation than autotransplantations, in those cases where patients have extended edentulous areas, if they do not present a donor tooth or if its extraction seems to be complicated, if there is limit of space, if there is tooth avulsion history and the tooth cannot be re-implanted by any reason, or if the patient is not motivated to have a tooth autotransplant, among other options. (Tsukiboshi 2001)

On the other hand, teeth autotransplantation should become the first option if all the requirements previously discussed are fulfill, having in mind that the more prognostic factors are respected, the higher the success rate can be achieved. (Tsukiboshi 2001) Implants also have limitations when compared to autotransplantation. The placement of an implant does not induce alveolar bone formation, the gingival papillae has to be created or manipulated if possible, passive eruption is not achievable, dental implant cannot be moved orthodontically, it is confined to adults or young adults with finished bone growth, and it is more expensive to the patient. (Tsukiboshi 2001)

So, both dental implants and tooth transplantation have their specific indications, and must be considered has treatment options, not overcoming one another but complementing each other on the clinician rehabilitation treatment plan.

7. Conclusion

Tooth autotransplantation has a very long history, with numerous non-successful cases, but also many good results are described. As all surgical techniques, it is hard to predict, and needs thorough case studying. But, in a general point of view, literature shows that it should be in the oral surgeon's long rehabilitation list of solutions to present to patients in need. Sometimes, the technique is forgotten, but should be reawaked and even investigated again, using more modern investigation techniques to improve the work that we do on our patients.

8. References

Ahlberg, K., H. Bystedt, et al. (1983). Long-term evaluation of autotransplanted maxillary canines with completed root formation. *Acta Odontol Scand* 41(1): 23-31.

Akiyama, Y., H. Fukuda, et al. (1998). A clinical and radiographic study of 25 autotransplanted third molars. *J Oral Rehabil* 25(8): 640-644.

Andreasen, J. O., H. U. Paulsen, et al. (1990). A long-term study of 370 autotransplanted premolars. Part I. Surgical procedures and standardized techniques for monitoring healing. *Eur J Orthod* 12(1): 3-13.

Andreasen, J. O., H. U. Paulsen, et al. (1990). A long-term study of 370 autotransplanted premolars. Part IV. Root development subsequent to transplantation. *Eur J Orthod* 12(1): 38-50.

Andreasen, J. O., H. U. Paulsen, et al. (1990). A long-term study of 370 autotransplanted premolars. Part II. Tooth survival and pulp healing subsequent to transplantation. *Eur J Orthod* 12(1): 14-24.

Andreasen, J. O., H. U. Paulsen, et al. (1990). A long-term study of 370 autotransplanted premolars. Part III. Periodontal healing subsequent to transplantation. *Eur J Orthod* 12(1): 25-37.

Aslan, B. I., N. Ucuncu, et al. (2010). Long-term follow-up of a patient with multiple congenitally missing teeth treated with autotransplantation and orthodontics. *Angle Orthod* 80(2): 396-404.

Cohen, A. S., T. C. Shen, et al. (1995). Transplanting teeth successfully: autografts and allografts that work. *J Am Dent Assoc* 126(4): 481-485; quiz 500.

Czochrowska, E. M., A. Stenvik, et al. (2000). Autotransplantation of premolars to replace maxillary incisors: a comparison with natural incisors. *Am J Orthod Dentofacial Orthop* 118(6): 592-600.

Czochrowska, E. M., A. Stenvik, et al. (2002). Outcome of tooth transplantation: survival and success rates 17-41 years posttreatment. *Am J Orthod Dentofacial Orthop* 121(2): 110-119; quiz 193.

Donado, M., Ed. (2007). *Cirugia Bucal*, Masson.

Escoda, G., Ed. (1999). *Cirugía Bucal*. Madrid, Ediciones Ergon, S.A.

Fleming, H. S. (1956). Experimental transplantation of teeth in lower animals. *Oral Surg Oral Med Oral Pathol* 9(1): 3-17.

Jonsson, T. and T. J. Sigurdsson (2004). Autotransplantation of premolars to premolar sites. A long-term follow-up study of 40 consecutive patients. *Am J Orthod Dentofacial Orthop* 125(6): 668-675.

Josefsson, E., V. Brattstrom, et al. (1999). Treatment of lower second premolar agenesis by autotransplantation: four-year evaluation of eighty patients. *Acta Odontol Scand* 57(2): 111-115.

Kallu, R., F. Vinckier, et al. (2005). Tooth transplantations: a descriptive retrospective study. *Int J Oral Maxillofac Surg* 34(7): 745-755.

Kim, E., J. Y. Jung, et al. (2005). Evaluation of the prognosis and causes of failure in 182 cases of autogenous tooth transplantation. *Oral Surg Oral Med Oral Pathol Oral Radiol Endod* 100(1): 112-119.

Magheri, P., R. Grandini, et al. (2001). Autogenous dental transplants: description of a clinical case. *Int J Periodontics Restorative Dent* 21(4): 367-371.

Marzola, C. (1968). [Dental reimplantation. Surgical, clinical and radiographic considerations]. *Rev Bras Odontol* 25(153): 254-269.

Northway, W. (2002). Autogenic dental transplants. *Am J Orthod Dentofacial Orthop* 121(6): 592-593.

Paulsen, H. U. (2001). Autotransplantation of teeth in orthodontic treatment. *Am J Orthod Dentofacial Orthop* 119(4): 336-337.

Paulsen, H. U., J. O. Andreasen, et al. (1995). Pulp and periodontal healing, root development and root resorption subsequent to transplantation and orthodontic rotation: a long-term study of autotransplanted premolars. *Am J Orthod Dentofacial Orthop* 108(6): 630-640.

Paulsen, H. U., X. Q. Shi, et al. (2001). Eruption pattern of autotransplanted premolars visualized by radiographic color-coding. *Am J Orthod Dentofacial Orthop* 119(4): 338-345.

Thomas, S., S. R. Turner, et al. (1998). Autotransplantation of teeth: is there a role? *Br J Orthod* 25(4): 275-282.

Tsukiboshi, M., Ed. (2001). *Autotransplantation of teeth.*

Tsukiboshi, M. (2002). Autotransplantation of teeth: requirements for predictable success. *Dent Traumatol* 18(4): 157-180.

Permissions

The contributors of this book come from diverse backgrounds, making this book a truly international effort. This book will bring forth new frontiers with its revolutionizing research information and detailed analysis of the nascent developments around the world.

We would like to thank Professor Dr. Mandeep Singh Virdi, for lending his expertise to make the book truly unique. He has played a crucial role in the development of this book. Without his invaluable contribution this book wouldn't have been possible. He has made vital efforts to compile up to date information on the varied aspects of this subject to make this book a valuable addition to the collection of many professionals and students.

This book was conceptualized with the vision of imparting up-to-date information and advanced data in this field. To ensure the same, a matchless editorial board was set up. Every individual on the board went through rigorous rounds of assessment to prove their worth. After which they invested a large part of their time researching and compiling the most relevant data for our readers. Conferences and sessions were held from time to time between the editorial board and the contributing authors to present the data in the most comprehensible form. The editorial team has worked tirelessly to provide valuable and valid information to help people across the globe.

Every chapter published in this book has been scrutinized by our experts. Their significance has been extensively debated. The topics covered herein carry significant findings which will fuel the growth of the discipline. They may even be implemented as practical applications or may be referred to as a beginning point for another development. Chapters in this book were first published by InTech; hereby published with permission under the Creative Commons Attribution License or equivalent.

The editorial board has been involved in producing this book since its inception. They have spent rigorous hours researching and exploring the diverse topics which have resulted in the successful publishing of this book. They have passed on their knowledge of decades through this book. To expedite this challenging task, the publisher supported the team at every step. A small team of assistant editors was also appointed to further simplify the editing procedure and attain best results for the readers.

Our editorial team has been hand-picked from every corner of the world. Their multi-ethnicity adds dynamic inputs to the discussions which result in innovative outcomes. These outcomes are then further discussed with the researchers and contributors who give their valuable feedback and opinion regarding the same. The feedback is then collaborated with the researches and they are edited in a comprehensive manner to aid the understanding of the subject.

Apart from the editorial board, the designing team has also invested a significant amount of their time in understanding the subject and creating the most relevant covers. They scrutinized every image to scout for the most suitable representation of the subject and create an appropriate cover for the book.

The publishing team has been involved in this book since its early stages. They were actively engaged in every process, be it collecting the data, connecting with the contributors or procuring relevant information. The team has been an ardent support to the editorial, designing and production team. Their endless efforts to recruit the best for this project, has resulted in the accomplishment of this book. They are a veteran in the field of academics and their pool of knowledge is as vast as their experience in printing. Their expertise and guidance has proved useful at every step. Their uncompromising quality standards have made this book an exceptional effort. Their encouragement from time to time has been an inspiration for everyone.

The publisher and the editorial board hope that this book will prove to be a valuable piece of knowledge for researchers, students, practitioners and scholars across the globe.

List of Contributors

Mandeep S. Virdi
PDM Dental College and Research Institute, Bahadurgarh, Haryana, India

Agim Begzati, Ajtene Begzati,Teuta Kutllovci and Blerta Xhemajli
Department of Pedodontics and Preventive Dentistry, School of Dentistry, Medical Faculty, University of Prishtna, Prishtina, Republic of Kosovo

Kastriot Meqa
Department of Periodontology and Oral Medicine, School of Dentistry, Medical Faculty, University of Prishtina, Prishtina, Republic of Kosovo

Mehmedali Azemi
Department of Pediatric, Medical Faculty, University of Prishtina, Prishtina, Republic of Kosovo

Merita Berisha
National Institute of Public Health of Kosovo, Department of Social Medicine, Medical Faculty, University of Prishtina, Prishtina, Republic of Kosovo

Shani Ann Mani
University Sains Malaysia, Malaysia

Wei Yen Ping
Formerly University Sains Malaysia, Malaysia

Jacob John
University of Malaya, Malaysia

Noorliza Mastura Ismail
Melaka Manipal Medical College, Malaysia

Folakemi Oredugba and Patricia Ayanbadejo
Faculty of Dental Sciences, College of Medicine, University of Lagos, Nigeria

Jalaleddin Hamissi
Department of Periodontics & Preventive Dentistry, Faculty of Dentistry, Qazvin University of Medical Sciences, Qazvin, Iran

Patrícia Del Vigna de Ameida, Aline Cristina Batista Rodrigues Johann, Luciana Reis de Azevedo Alanis, Antônio Adilson Soares de Lima and Ana Maria Trindade Grégio
Pontifícia Universidade Católica do Paraná & Universidade Federal do Paraná, Brazil

Rafael da Silveira Moreira
Centro de Pesquisas Aggeu Magalhães, Fundação Oswaldo Cruz, Recife, Pernambuco, Brazil

M. Larmas, H. Vähänikkilä, K. Leskinen and J. Päkkilä
University of Oulu, Finland

Harini Priya Vishnu
Department of Pedodontics and Preventive Dentistry, Vydehi Institute of Dental Sciences and Research Centre, Bangalore, India

Eftekharalsadat Hajikazemi and Fatemeh Haghdoost Osquei
Tehran University of Medical Sciences (TUMS), Center for Nursing Care Research, Iran

Kadriye Peker
Department of Basic Sciences, Faculty of Dentistry, Istanbul University, Turkey

Kristian Hellgren
Specialistkliniken, Helsingborg, Sweden

José Roberto de Magalhães Bastos
University of São Paulo/ Faculty of Dentistry at Bauru, Brazil

Febronia Kokulengya Kahabuka
Muhimbili University of Health and Allied Sciences, School of Dentistry, Tanzania

Flora Masumbuo Fabian
International Medical and Technological University, Tanzania

Jindra Smejkalova, Vimal Jacob, Lenka Hodacova, Zdenek Fiala, Radovan Slezak and Sajith Vellappally
Charles University in Prague, Medical Faculty in Hradec Kralove, Czech Republic

Aleksandar Mitić, Nadica Mitić, Jovanka Gašić, and Jelena Popović
Department of Restorative Dentistry and Endodontic, Clinic of Dentistry, Medical Faculty, University of Nis, Nis, Serbia

Slavoljub Živković
Department of Restorative Dentistry and Endodontic, Faculty of Dentistry, University of Belgrade, Belgrade, Serbia

Jelena Milašin
Institute of Genetics, Faculty of Dentistry, University of Belgrade, Serbia

Vladimir Mitić and Tatjana Tanić
Department of Jaw Orthopedics, Dental Hospital, Niš, Serbia

Eduardo Santiago, Germano Rocha and João F. C. Carvalho
Oporto School of Dentistry, University of Oporto, Portugal

THE INTELLIGENCE WITHIN

How Smart Organizations Align, Plan, and Decide Faster in a Complex Tech World

RICHARD TARITY

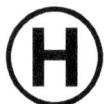

TESTIMONIALS

"The Intelligence Within doesn't just challenge how organizations think—it rewires how they move. In an era of AI acceleration, this book delivers the missing blueprint: how to harness discovery as a system, not a stall. It's bold, brilliant, and long overdue."

— **Geoffrey A. Best**,
AI Strategist & Bestselling Author of the *42 Rules trilogy for Using, Planning, and Managing AI in Your Contact Center*

"Rich captures what so many in CX and AI leadership have been feeling but couldn't articulate—discovery is broken, and speed is the new superpower. This book doesn't just call for transformation; it gives us the framework to lead it. Essential reading for every modern CX leader serious about impact, not theory."

— **Dave Zimmerman**, 2018/2024 Top 50/100 CX
Professional & CX AI Leader

"Rich is the consummate entrepreneur. He thinks about business, strategy in particular, with a focus that we should all emulate. As a result, he has led his teams to discover the latest trends and formulate novel ideas in the technology industry. Rich is also a student of business. His impressive

experience is continually complemented by his drive to learn, creative acumen, and mastery of disrupting the status quo."
— **Frank Powers**, Co-Founder & Managing Partner, Elevate, Co.

"This book really resonated with me. We've all experienced the bloated assessments, analysis paralysis, endless debates resulting in inability to make progress. I guarantee you, as you read this book you will be shaking your head "yes". In clear, simple terms this book presents deep insights into the problems we've all been frustrated with and an extraordinary and graceful solution. Rich has built the playbook every executive and manager needs – one that replaces noise with clarity, speed, and precision."
— **Todd Matters**, Co-Founder & CTO, Rackware, Inc.

"Speed is the new competitive advantage, and no one understands that better than Rich. His consulting expertise has helped businesses rethink discovery, accelerate decision-making, and adopt technology at record speed. If you want to future-proof your company and lead with confidence, this book is essential reading."
— **Shailesh Goswami**, Chief Executive Officer, Foyr

DEDICATION

For the visionaries, builders, and risk-takers who challenge the norm and create what others never dared to imagine.

To my parents, my loving wife Layne, and the two who first taught me the depth of a father's love, Madison and Gavin, my beautiful daughter and son, and Joseph and Tyler, who've brought their own special joy into my life.

CONTENTS

EPIGRAPH

"The difference between extinction and evolution is simple: one clings to the past, the other builds the future."

— Richard Tarity

FOREWORD

Why am I introducing this book to you?

Because I've had the privilege to coach and work with some of the brightest, most driven minds in business over the past five decades. I've worked with leaders who have transformed industries, built billion-dollar enterprises, and redefined the way we think about innovation. They've changed our approach to technology adoption, industry leadership, and CX (customer experience).

Among those high achievers I've had the privilege to mentor, there are a few who stand out—not just for their intelligence (every one of them was intelligent) but for their unwavering commitment to destroying barriers, challenging the "same old-same old," and creating sustainable impact in their arenas.

Rich Tarity is one of those few. I met Rich when he was in his early 20s, applying for his first sales job. The owner of the business didn't want to hire him (I think he was intimidated by Tarity's quick mind and his confidence).

I told the owner: "If you want to build a sales team and you won't hire Tarity, you're not committed to your own success. If you don't make a better decision, I'll resign."

He relented.

We hired Rich. He sold. And led. He helped transform his first company. He went from rookie to rising star, graduated to star, and was on his way to superstardom when he realized he could not achieve his personal goals in that company. He left and started his own company, doing it his way. He succeeded. It set the stage for what would come later.

For almost 3 decades, I've watched this extraordinary leader rearrange boundaries, challenge outmoded thinking, and build solutions that have transformed the way organizations conduct business. He has never been satisfied doing things the way they have always been done. He has dedicated his career to discovering smarter, faster, more effective ways for businesses to succeed. Not just marginally, exponentially!

This book is the result of years of his relentless pursuit. He is obsessed with solving one of the most costly and frustrating problems in modern business: How so many quality organizations remain stuck while others break free, then dominate! His experiential knowledge, combined with cutting-edge research and a deep understanding of customer experience, has led him to develop the industry's first CX discovery platform.

Why?

So, you can transform your business and your life! Most importantly, it's practical…and it's powerful!

Companies were drowning in molasses-slow decision-making, crippling bureaucracy, and ancient methodologies. Now, they become innovators in their industries. They go from uncertainty to clarity, stagnation to acceleration, struggling to thriving. They don't just talk about transformation, they demand it. And they make it happen! They do it with a precise strategy and creative insight, which only comes from years of dig-deep experience. What happens? The business optimization that we all dream of, the customer experience which creates raving fans, the enterprise technology decision-making which accelerates progress and profits!

This book isn't about the history of other's success. It's dedicated to your success, your transformation, your life!

If you're a business leader, a CX stakeholder, or an operations or information technology executive who knows that your organization is capable of more but can't quite figure out how to break free, here's your road map! It's a clear, structured path to accelerated, smarter decision-making, true companywide alignment, and continuous and never-ending innovation. I am certain, if you absorb what's in these chapters—if you apply the design thinking outlined here, your business will be transformed! You'll move with more clarity and speed. You'll make bolder, more confident decisions. You'll see results, not someday, immediately! Business transformation! What a concept!

This is not theory. These techniques have been tested, refined, re-tested, and proven! They help businesses unlock their true potential technologically, accelerate business decision-making to warp speed, and create a customer experience that leaves competitors scrambling in your dust.

Finally, these strategies are now in your hands!

I've had the privilege to observe this author's journey from relentless young innovator to an accomplished industry leader. He sets the standard for how businesses should operate in this century. His insights, their frameworks, and his clear vision for the future of customer experience aren't just changing the way you'll operate; they'll disrupt your entire industry! You'll change how you think. More importantly, you will change how you act. And you will lead by example!

I have only two questions:

1. Will you take these proven strategies and run with them?
2. Will you be one of the leaders who breaks free?

If your answers are Yes to both, everything in your business, in your career, and in your life, is about to be transformed.

Make it happen! Best wishes for your transformation!

Bruce Morrow, Founder and Head Coach,
Lead.Sell.Grow, Inc., www.leadsellgrow.com.

INTRODUCTION

The Intelligence Within

For years, businesses have been operating with blinders on and stuck in outdated operating models. They are slowed by bloated decision cycles and held back by a status quo disguised as "best practice." Nowhere is this inertia more dangerous than in how organizations approach customer experience and technology innovation.

The world isn't changing, it's accelerating. New Customer Experience (CX) platforms, AI tools, and automation technologies are emerging daily, yet most companies remain locked in legacy behaviors and motions. Instead of enabling transformation, these advancements overwhelm already overstretched teams. IT leaders struggle to gather cross-functional input fast enough to drive meaningful change for the business. Departments stay siloed, conversations stall, and decisions drag while customer expectations evolve in real-time.

The operating environment has changed. Once, businesses had time to explore options, pilot solutions, and deliberate before committing to technology investments. The pace was linear and predictable. But not anymore. Today's customers demand more, faster. They expect connected, intelligent, personalized experiences. And the brands that deliver—Amazon, Tesla, Apple—aren't waiting around. They're redefining industries by moving with speed, precision, and relentless customer obsession.

Yet many organizations still operate with outdated discovery processes that rely on slow, consultant-heavy, manual approaches. Workshops, interviews, spreadsheets—months of back-and-forth before anyone even knows what the real problem is. In the time it takes to gather internal input, the market shifts, budgets disappear, and urgency dissolves.

The result? Paralysis. Momentum dies. Innovation never launches.

This book is your way out. It's about **breaking free** from legacy thinking, paralyzing indecision, and processes that no longer match the speed of business. It introduces a new model: one that enables rapid, aligned, insight-driven decisions. A model that empowers teams to move forward with confidence, not because everything is perfect, but because clarity beats caution in a world that moves this fast.

The truth is technology isn't the bottleneck. The real problem is how companies evaluate, align around, and act on the technology they need. If you're using 20th-century decision-making models to adopt 21st-century tech, you're already behind. Today, speed, alignment, and insight aren't competitive advantages; they're survival requirements.

This book offers a new blueprint—a way to transform how decisions are made and how innovation is delivered. It's for leaders who want to move faster, with less friction and more impact. It's for organizations ready to stop defaulting to "how we've always done it" and start building systems that evolve as fast as the customers they serve.

What's at stake?

Everything. The companies that can't adapt will be left behind by competitors who execute faster, by customers who demand more, and by employees who refuse to stay trapped inside slow-moving machines.

But the opportunity?

It's enormous. For those bold enough to change, the future is wide open. With the right frameworks, alignment tools, and intelligence-driven platforms, companies can eliminate delay, increase clarity, and unlock a new rhythm of innovation and execution.

This isn't a warning. It's a wake-up call.

This isn't a critique. It's a call to reinvention.

The time for patchwork solutions is over.

The time to rethink everything starts now.

Let's begin.

CHAPTER 1

The Trap of the Status Quo: When Intelligence Is Ignored

Businesses aren't stuck because they lack technology. They're stuck because they ignore their internal intelligence—the insights locked inside their people, systems, and operations. While technology evolves at an unprecedented pace, most organizations fail to activate what they already know.

Instead of accelerating transformation, businesses are caught in a cycle of hesitation, analysis paralysis, and ineffective execution. That's the real trap of the status quo.

This chapter sets the stage for why so many organizations are paralyzed in the face of change and why traditional approaches to innovation are no longer working. We'll explore the root causes of this stagnation, the high cost of remaining stuck, and why the time to break free from outdated models has never been more urgent.

The Illusion of Progress

Many businesses believe they are moving forward simply because they are adopting new tools and platforms. They point to their investments in artificial intelligence, digital transformation initiatives, and cloud-based customer engagement platforms as proof that they are innovating. The reality, however, is that many of these organizations are simply spinning their wheels, confusing motion with progress. Progress isn't about what you buy; it's about what you unlock.

The other missed opportunity that happens most often is when *businesses migrate from an older technology platform to a newer one and just simply repeat the same programming, turning on the same features as the older legacy platform. They miss a window to innovate and make changes inside the organization, and it happens all the time. Sound familiar?*

In today's fast-moving business landscape, investing in technology is not the same as leveraging it effectively. A company can have the most advanced contact center software, AI-powered analytics, and automated customer journey tools yet still fail to deliver the experiences that customers expect. Transformation isn't about piling on more tools. It's about activating the dormant intelligence already present across your organization.

Instead of enabling change, many businesses unintentionally layer new technology on top of outdated processes. They pour millions of dollars into digital upgrades without truly evolving the way they operate. They replace old software with new software, but they don't reimagine the workflows that drive customer interactions.

They implement AI-powered chatbots but fail to integrate them in a way that enhances—not frustrates—the customer experience. They launch data-driven initiatives but don't establish a framework to translate that data into actionable strategies.

Why Technology Alone Won't Fix the Problem

Technology is a tool, nothing more. Just as a scalpel in the hands of an untrained individual does not make them a surgeon, an AI-powered customer engagement platform in an organization with a broken CX strategy will not create a better customer experience. In fact, in many cases, it can make things worse. Instead of streamlining operations, new tools layered onto old problems create more complexity, inefficiency, and frustration.

Consider a company that implements an advanced omnichannel customer support platform. On the surface, this looks like progress; customers now have multiple ways to reach the company, from chatbots to self-service portals to social media messaging and so on. But beneath the surface, nothing has changed. The customer service agents are still following the same rigid scripts, the backend data remains siloed, and the escalation process remains just as frustrating as before. The result? The company invested in technology but failed to transform the experience.

Now, customers are even more frustrated. They expected seamless service, but instead, they encountered AI that couldn't understand them—agents who still lack access to their full history and a system that feels more robotic than ever before. What happened? The company confused implementation with innovation.

New Tools, Old Mindsets: The Hidden Barrier to Change

Technology alone does not create transformation. Organizations must change how they **think, decide, and implement** technology. But too often, they fall into the trap of using new tools with legacy thinking, failing to adapt their processes, workflows, and approach to customer insights, as well as their internal decision-making structures. The intelligence within is not a mystery. It's a mirror. If you know where to look, it will tell you everything you need to move forward.

I remember working with a major North American retailer with over 700 stores in the mid-2000s. At the time, they were operating on a 15-year-old phone and contact center system. To modernize their technology, the CIO brought in an external consultant to lead the discovery process. Over six months, the consultant gathered extensive data from their existing infrastructure, culminating in a comprehensive RFP document, roughly 70 pages long.

Our company was one of three technology providers invited to bid. We represented a top-tier solution capable of handling both their phone and contact center needs, along with advanced capabilities that far exceeded their current system. On our first call, I asked the CIO what mattered most to him in this process. His priorities were clear: new features, ease of administration for his IT staff, and enhanced contact center functionality, a common response from executives at the time. But I knew we needed to dig deeper, beyond just the technology, to uncover the real opportunities for transformation.

Instead of simply responding to the RFP, my team and I took a different approach. We decided to experience the brand as customers. On separate trips, one in Texas and one near our headquarters, we visited two of their retail locations. We walked the aisles, observed interactions, and even engaged with store managers. What we discovered was eye-opening: challenges with scheduling alterations, delivery logistics, bandwidth constraints, and call-in inefficiencies, all pain points that directly impacted store operations but weren't accounted for in the RFP.

Armed with this firsthand insight, we refined our presentation. While other vendors focused on the HQ phone system and contact center software, we aimed to reframe the conversation. After all, in retail, the point of sale is the heartbeat of the business—why not innovate around how stores are supported?

The day of the presentation arrived. We had two hours to demonstrate our solution and walk through our RFP response. As we entered the room, the CIO smirked and complimented our suits, an unexpected but telling moment. About halfway through, we shifted the discussion to the stores, revealing the insights we had gathered from our field visits.

The room fell silent. The CIO, initially speechless, looked at his team and said, "None of you went this far in uncovering these opportunities." He was astonished that we had taken the initiative to experience the brand firsthand, something even his internal teams had not done or stopped doing. We didn't just bring technology. We revealed the intelligence the brand already had but had stopped listening to.

A month later, we won the contract. That decision led to a long-standing partnership with the brand, built on trust, insight, and a shared commitment to innovation. The lesson? True transformation doesn't start with a vendor demo. It starts by tuning into the intelligence within.

This misunderstanding is why so many transformation efforts fail. Many business leaders believe technology itself will drive innovation rather than recognizing that technology is an enabler, not the solution.

Consider the following:

- A company adopts AI-driven analytics but still relies on gut feelings instead of data to make decisions.
- A brand builds a new self-service portal but never studies customer behaviors to understand what issues customers actually want to resolve themselves.
- An enterprise integrates an automated customer journey mapping tool but fails to update its service design to reflect new customer expectations.

These examples illustrate a painful truth: Without a fundamental shift in mindset and approach, new technology will only amplify and replicate old designs and problems. Instead of accelerating transformation, it reinforces the status quo.

The Comfort of Familiarity: Why Organizations Resist Real Change

One of the biggest reasons businesses struggle to break free from this illusion of progress is comfort. Even when leaders recognize that their current approach isn't working, familiarity feels safer than uncertainty. While the traditional ways of evaluating technology, making decisions, and getting consensus across key stakeholders involved in the decision-making process may be inefficient, they are known, and that makes them comfortable.

This resistance to change is often subconscious. Organizations don't deliberately sabotage themselves; rather, they fall into deeply ingrained patterns:

- **They focus on short-term fixes instead of long-term reinvention.** Many businesses opt for small, incremental improvements instead of true transformation because it feels less risky. They choose to "optimize" or "upgrade" their current platforms and processes rather than rethinking them entirely.
- **They mistake busyness for progress.** Teams are constantly engaged in software implementations, vendor meetings, and system upgrades, but none of these efforts fundamentally change how the organization operates and innovates.
- **They fear the unknown.** Leaders worry that if they abandon the traditional ways of doing things, they'll make a costly mistake. They hesitate to experiment with new decision-making frameworks or more agile approaches to technology adoption.

So, instead of making meaningful progress, businesses remain trapped in a cycle of surface-level change, one in which new technology enters the organization, but the underlying inefficiencies, misalignments, and decision-making barriers remain intact.

How to Break Free from the Illusion of Progress

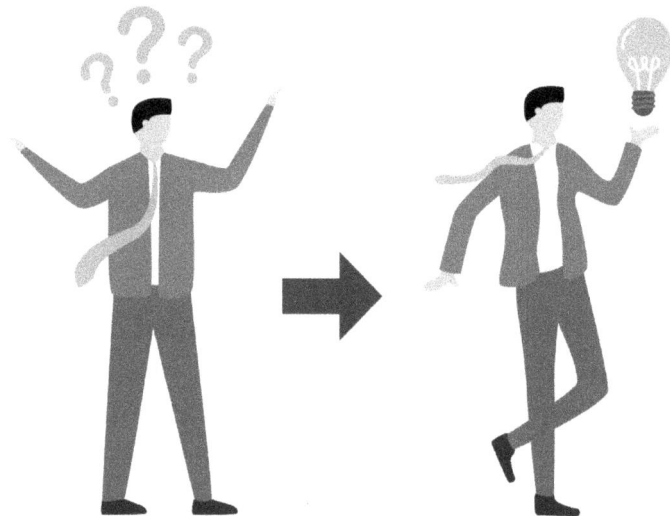

The first step to escaping this cycle is recognizing that true progress requires more than just new technology; it demands a new way of thinking, deciding, and implementing change. Organizations that successfully transform their customer experience do three things differently:

1. **They challenge their assumptions.** Instead of assuming that upgrading technology equals innovation, they ask, "Are we changing the way we operate or just changing our tools?"

2. **They rethink decision-making.** Instead of relying on slow, manual discovery processes, they use structured, data-driven frameworks that bring clarity and alignment across teams.
3. **They build a culture of continuous improvement.** Instead of treating technology transformation as a one-time initiative, they embed it into their DNA, ensuring that innovation is ongoing and iterative. They can measure ongoing improvement through trending and comparisons.

The organizations that understand this are the ones that truly break free from the status quo. They stop mistaking motion for progress. They stop layering new technology onto old problems. Instead, they embrace a **new model of decision-making—one that prioritizes speed, clarity, and alignment.** And that is the difference between companies that thrive and those that remain stuck.

A Case Study in Stagnation

Consider a global retail brand that embarked on a multi-million-dollar digital transformation initiative. They invested in a new customer experience platform, hired consultants, and restructured their CX department. Yet, after two years, customer satisfaction scores had barely improved, employees were frustrated with the complexity of the new systems, and leadership was questioning whether the transformation had been worth it.

What went wrong?

1. **Fragmented Decision-Making** – The company had no structured process to align internal stakeholders on the real

problems that needed solving and no way to surface their priorities and needs.

2. **Consultant-Driven Dependency** – Instead of taking ownership of discovery, they relied on external consultants to tell them what they needed, creating delays and misalignment, which also comes with a bias at times toward certain outcomes.

3. **Lack of Agility**—By the time they implemented their technology roadmap, customers' needs had already changed.

This outcome is a classic case of an organization that mistook activity for progress. They had the right intentions but the wrong execution model.

The Overwhelming Flood of Technology: Why More Choices Are Slowing Businesses Down

For businesses today, technology should be a catalyst for progress. It should make decisions easier, operations smoother, and customer experiences more seamless. Yet, in many organizations, the opposite is happening. Instead of accelerating transformation, the explosion of new technology is paralyzing business leaders, leaving them uncertain about where to invest, what to prioritize, and how to align their decisions with real customer needs.

This overwhelming flood of technology is one of the biggest roadblocks preventing companies from making meaningful progress. Organizations are bombarded with options: AI virtual assistants and chatbots, journey orchestration tools, predictive analytics, workforce optimization solutions, customer data platforms, and automation software, each promising to be the key to unlocking better customer experiences.

The irony? The more choices companies have, the harder it becomes to make a decision.

The Paradox of Too Many Choices

In psychology, there's a well-known concept called the **paradox of choice**, which suggests that while people crave options, an overabundance of choices can lead to anxiety, decision paralysis, and dissatisfaction. This is not just a consumer issue, it's a massive challenge for business leaders tasked with selecting the right technology for their organizations.

Think about the last time you went out for dinner and got a massive menu packed with options on every page. With so many choices in front of you, you probably felt overwhelmed, unsure of where to start. Instead of deciding quickly, you likely asked your server for more time so you could sift through all the possibilities before making a choice. Ever been there?

A decade ago, IT, Operations, and CX leaders had a relatively limited number of major vendors to choose from when selecting their contact center and related technology, customer relationship management (CRM) software, or workforce management solutions. The decision-making process was still complex, but at least it was manageable. Vendors had clear differentiation, and companies could dedicate the necessary time and resources to evaluating their options.

"This book really resonated with me. We've all experienced the bloated assessments, analysis paralysis, endless debates resulting in inability to make progress. I guarantee you, as you read this book you will be shaking your head "yes". In clear, simple terms this book presents deep insights into the problems we've all been frustrated with and an extraordinary and graceful solution. Rich has built the playbook every executive and manager needs – one that replaces noise with clarity, speed, and precision." Todd Matters, Co-Founder & CTO, Rackware, Inc.

Today, the landscape has changed dramatically.

Technology solutions flood organizations, each claiming to be the ultimate game-changer. As a result, many business leaders find themselves overwhelmed, unable to confidently determine which solutions will truly drive measurable improvements and which are simply shiny distractions.

Here's how the landscape has evolved and how it has made decision-making more difficult than ever before:

1. **AI and Automation Have Exploded**

   Artificial intelligence has become one of the most hyped technologies in the business world. While it holds enormous potential, it has also complicated the decision-making process for IT and business leaders alike.

- In AI-powered customer service alone, organizations must evaluate solutions ranging from chatbots and virtual agents to speech recognition engines, AI-powered agent assistance, and real-time sentiment analysis tools.

- In predictive analytics, businesses now have access to AI models that promise to forecast customer churn, predict call volumes, and recommend the next best actions for agents. However, integrating them into existing workflows can be a major challenge.

- In automation, companies must decide between robotic process automation (RPA), AI-driven self-service platforms, and hyper-automation suites, each with its strengths, weaknesses, and compatibility concerns.

The choices are endless, and the fear of picking the wrong solution oftentimes leads to indecision and inaction.

2. The Contact Center Platform Market Has Become Hyper-Specialized

Ten years ago, selecting a contact center platform was a relatively straightforward decision. Organizations had a handful of major providers to choose from, each offering similar core functionalities—call routing, Interactive Voice Response (IVR), and basic reporting. While customization was available, the platforms were largely built around traditional voice-based customer service operations.

Today, the landscape has completely changed. The contact center market has fractured into highly specialized solutions, making the selection process far more complex:

- Industry-Specific Contact Center Platforms now cater to verticals such as healthcare, financial services, and retail, each offering tailored compliance, customer engagement models, and workflow automation designed for their unique regulatory and operational needs.
- Omnichannel Contact Center Solutions go far beyond voice, integrating seamlessly with chat, SMS, email, social media, and video—offering cross-channel continuity and AI-driven customer engagement.
- Workforce Engagement and Optimization Platforms now embed AI-driven scheduling, real-time performance analytics, and predictive workforce management, making agent productivity and experience a key differentiator.
- Cloud-Native vs. Hybrid vs. On-Premises Solutions adds another layer of complexity, requiring organizations to evaluate scalability, security, compliance, and total cost of ownership before making a choice.

With so many vendors and specialized platforms available, organizations often find themselves **stuck in long evaluation cycles,** unsure of which solution best aligns with their evolving customer experience strategy. The complexity of integrations, pricing models, and AI capabilities only adds to the hesitation—leading to delayed decisions, lost opportunities, and outdated infrastructure that struggles to keep up with customer expectations.

3. The Customer Journey Tech Stack is Overwhelming

Customer journey orchestration was once a luxury that only a few large enterprises could afford. Today, it has become a critical capability for businesses of all sizes, but the sheer number of available platforms has made the selection process daunting.

- Journey mapping tools help visualize customer interactions, but they vary widely in depth, usability, and integration capabilities.
- Real-time journey orchestration engines promise to deliver personalized, context-aware experiences, but many struggle with data unification.
- Customer data and analytics platforms offer deep insights into customer behavior, but companies must choose between tools that focus on historical reporting, real-time engagement, or predictive modeling.

Each of these solutions claims to offer seamless personalization but without a structured approach to implementation. Many organizations end up with fragmented systems that fail to deliver on their promises.

4. **Workforce Optimization is More Complex Than Ever**

Workforce management (WFM) and optimization (WFO) used to be relatively straightforward—scheduling agents, tracking performance, and monitoring quality assurance.

Now, companies must evaluate solutions that:

- Leverage AI for dynamic scheduling and demand forecasting, reducing overstaffing and understaffing.
- Incorporate gamification to drive employee engagement, offering personalized coaching and incentives.

- Analyze sentiment and behavioral data to improve performance management, using AI-driven insights to identify top performers and those in need of training.
- Integrate with broader CX platforms, ensuring that WFO doesn't operate in isolation but actively enhances the customer experience.

The problem is that many of these platforms overlap in functionality, making it difficult for decision-makers to determine which best aligns with their needs.

5. **Digital Experience and Personalization Have Created a Data Chaos Problem**

With the rise of digital-first interactions, businesses have invested heavily in tools that allow them to track, analyze, and personalize customer experiences. But instead of creating a single source of truth, many companies find themselves drowning in disconnected data silos.

- Web analytics tools provide insights into digital behaviors, but they often operate separately from CRM and support platforms.
- AI-powered recommendation engines promise hyper-personalization, but many require advanced data modeling expertise to be effective.
- Personalization engines claim to improve engagement, but companies often struggle to integrate them with legacy systems.

The explosion of data and analytics tools has made it harder for companies to extract **clear, actionable insights instead of making customer experience easier to optimize.**

The Impact: Decision Paralysis and Poor Technology Adoption

With so many options, many businesses experience **decision paralysis,** a state where too many choices prevent them from making any decision at all.

The result?

- **Delays in technology adoption** because leadership teams struggle to reach a consensus.
- **Investments in the wrong platforms** lead to underutilization and wasted budgets.
- **Missed opportunities to improve CX**, as competitors who move faster gain a competitive advantage.

The paradox of too many choices means that companies don't need more options: they need a better way to evaluate the right solutions efficiently.

"Every great project starts with ambition, but most stall before they ever deliver real impact. The Intelligence Within shows exactly how to get unstuck, cut through complexity, and unlock the full potential of every initiative. It's not just about moving faster, it's about finally moving forward."

— Mike Sprague, Sr. Director of Enterprise Technology,
Swisher

How Organizations Can Break Free from the Choice Overload

Businesses must shift their approach in order to succeed in this overwhelming technology landscape. Instead of **relying on manual decision-making processes, endless meetings, and subjective opinions**, organizations need a **structured, data-driven framework** for evaluating, selecting, and implementing technology.

- **They must automate and streamline discovery** to surface business needs quickly and efficiently.
- **They must use real-time analytics** to prioritize technology investments based on impact, feasibility, and alignment with CX and business goals.
- **They must align stakeholders from day one**, preventing competing priorities from derailing progress.

Companies that embrace a structured, fast-moving approach to technology decision-making will dominate their industries. They will even have the time to pivot and make changes to their decisions before others get off go. Those who remain stuck in endless evaluation cycles will find themselves losing ground to competitors who **move with confidence and speed**.

The paradox of choice is real—but it does not have to be a roadblock. Businesses that break free from **traditional, slow-moving selection processes** will unlock a level of agility, clarity, and competitive advantage that others can only dream of.

The Chaos of Unstructured Decision-Making

The sheer volume of technology choices isn't the only problem; **it's the lack of a clear decision-making framework** that leads to confusion and stagnation.

Here's what typically happens inside organizations:

1. **A flood of vendor pitches:** Technology providers aggressively market their solutions, promising higher efficiency, better customer satisfaction, and cost savings. Business leaders get bombarded with sales meetings, presentations, and case studies, each one claiming to be the "must-have" solution.

2. **Internal misalignment:** IT leaders struggle to gather requirements from all their business units and teams. The contact center wants better automation, marketing wants improved customer insights, finance wants cost control, and operations wants seamless integration with existing systems. However, without a structured approach to gathering input, priorities remain unclear.

3. **Analysis paralysis:** With multiple vendors, conflicting internal needs, and uncertainty about ROI, organizations hesitate to move forward. Instead of making bold, confident decisions, they delay them, afraid of making the wrong choice or investing in technology that won't deliver on its promises.

The result? **Stagnation.** Businesses remain stuck, wasting valuable time and resources while competitors who have figured out a better decision-making approach move ahead.

The Hidden Cost of Indecision

Delaying a decision might feel like the safest move, but **indecision is one of the most expensive business problems today**. Every day spent evaluating tools without a clear path forward is a day lost in competitive advantage, customer experience improvement, and revenue growth.

- **Customer expectations are rising.** Customers don't wait for organizations, stuck in choice paralysis, to figure things out. They demand seamless, intuitive experiences, and they'll switch to competitors who provide them.
- **Technology is evolving faster than ever.** A solution that seems cutting-edge today can quickly become outdated. By the time a company finally decides, the landscape may have already changed.
- **Costs spiral out of control.** Organizations spend months— or even years—evaluating different tools, only to realize that the prolonged decision-making process its wasted millions in lost productivity, delayed innovation, and inefficiencies.

One of the most telling signs that an organization is stuck in this decision deadlock is when projects don't die—they just fade away. Teams continue discussing solutions in endless meetings, but no concrete action is taken. While the company remains trapped in this cycle, competitors who **embrace speed, clarity, and decisive action** leapfrog ahead.

How to Break Free from Technology Overload

As we covered, the problem isn't the technology itself; it's **how organizations evaluate, compare, and implement these tools.** Companies that successfully navigate the overwhelming flood of choices do things differently:

1. **They use a structured discovery process to surface real business needs.** Instead of mindlessly reacting to vendor pitches, they take the time to understand their true requirements, the needed outcomes, what problems need solving, and how success will be measured. They define success before they even engage with technology providers.
2. **They align internal teams before evaluating solutions:** Successful organizations ensure that IT, CX, sales, marketing, finance, and other key stakeholders are on the same page before they start evaluating vendors. This alignment prevents conflicts, miscommunications, and last-minute roadblocks. It also helps the organization to build momentum and consensus for the projects.
3. **They use data-driven decision-making:** Rather than relying on gut feelings or marketing hype, these companies use real insights, relevant categorical frameworks, CX baselining, and industry best practices to guide their choices.
4. **They embrace agile adoption:** Instead of spending years analyzing options, they test, iterate, and refine, allowing for flexibility and continuous improvement.

The organizations that take this approach don't just survive in a crowded technology landscape; they thrive. They make **faster, smarter decisions** and implement technology in a way that truly transforms their customer experience and business instead of just adding complexity.

The Future Belongs to Those Who Move with Clarity

The companies that win in the coming years will not be the ones that adopt the most technology; they will be the ones that adopt the **right technology in the right way and at the right time**.

The question is: Will your organization continue drowning in choices, or will it break free from the cycle of indecision?

> **The path forward is clear: businesses must move beyond outdated, manual discovery processes and embrace a new model for evaluating and adopting technology with speed, alignment, and confidence.**

Those who do will lead the next era of CX and technology transformation. Those who don't will find themselves stuck in **the illusion of progress**, watching as their competitors move forward without them.

The Flawed Approach to Discovery

At the heart of the problem is how organizations conduct discovery—the process of identifying what they need, why they need it, and how to execute it effectively. Traditionally, discovery has been done through manual, consultant, and internal-led processes that involve long interviews, workshops, and endless documentation.

This method is deeply flawed:

1. **It Takes Too Long**—Some organizations spend a year or more gathering requirements before they begin implementation. By then, market conditions and customer expectations have already shifted.

2. **It's Inefficient** – Business units and teams often provide conflicting priorities, leading to indecision and watered-down short-term solutions.

3. **It Relies Too Much on External Opinions** – Many organizations depend on third-party advisors who lack deep internal knowledge, causing disconnects between recommendations and real business needs. This reliance leads to inconsistent decisions, to no one's fault other than to the legacy process that just exists.

Without a better way to surface insights and align teams, businesses will continue making flawed decisions, or worse, no decisions at all.

The Cost of No Decision

Many organizations assume that delaying decisions is a safe approach, but the cost of no decision is often greater than the cost of a wrong decision. In a competitive landscape, hesitation translates to lost revenue, declining customer satisfaction, and an eroding brand reputation.

The Real Consequences of Staying Stuck:

- **Loss of Competitive Edge** – While one company debates its next steps, a competitor is already executing.

- **Declining Customer Loyalty** – Customers expect seamless, intelligent interactions. Brands that fail to deliver will lose them to those that do.
- **Employee Frustration** – Teams that deal with outdated technologies, processes, and ineffective tools become disengaged, leading to turnover and lower productivity.
- **Wasted Budget**—Millions of dollars are spent on research, pilots, and consultant fees without producing tangible results or real internal requirements.

Stalled at the Starting Line: Congested Technology Roadmaps

My friend Dave Zimmerman shared his insights on this matter. "For over twenty years, I led teams, projects, and initiatives that focused on improving the experience; it's what fills my cup. In that time, there has been no shortage of approaches on how to "get work done", the process. In most scenarios the methodology or framework either mirrored the C Suite leader or shiny trends with the same objective – move faster, accomplish more, and deliver better results. These project system changes can be frustrating, requiring more time and allowing the competition to claim or leapfrog our service standard. Two personal learnings:

Sometimes, service or experience priorities do not have a clear ROI benefit calculation and do not fit neatly into a financial P&L. There are times you need to take action when you are chasing parity or not meeting customer expectations. This reality resulted in many "go-backs." Can you size, measure, or look into this more? I've learned that once you encounter the "go back," the odds are stacked, and most likely, the initiative will not launch or will be severely delayed.

Congested technology roadmaps are a blueprint for experiencing disappointments or significant delays in progress. Over the years, I've heard countless times we agree with your strategy, but there are higher priorities that we need to focus on. Congested roadmaps lead to a chronic stall and time drag and the humbling reality that your initiative is not moving forward. I also acknowledge the need did not go away, and your customers continue with a mediocre experience, opening a window for your competition to win over your customers". Dave Zimmerman, 2018/2024 Top 50/100 CX Professional & CX AI Leader.

Breaking Free Starts Within

Technology isn't the answer. Alignment is. Speed isn't a goal. It's a result. Confidence doesn't come from knowing everything; it comes from knowing what matters.

The organizations that win aren't the ones with the flashiest tools. They're the ones who stop guessing, start listening, and let their internal intelligence lead.

The path forward is clear:

- Align before you invest.
- Discover before you decide.
- Plan with intelligence, not instinct.

This hidden intelligence within is how smart organizations break free.

Businesses do not have to remain stuck. There is a new way forward, a model that allows organizations and consultants to move faster, make confident decisions, and ensure alignment across all stakeholders. It's about shifting from **slow, manual-driven discovery** to a **data-driven, structured, and continuous improvement approach**.

The next chapter will explore how organizations can escape this trap and rethink the way they evaluate, adopt, and integrate new technologies. It's time to break free from outdated processes and embrace a future where decisions are made with speed, clarity, and confidence.

Let's begin.

CHAPTER 2

When Discovery Becomes a Dead End: Reclaiming the Intelligence Within

Discovery is supposed to illuminate. But for most organizations, it obscures. The irony? The insights leaders are externally chasing are already buried within their business, ignored, misaligned, and unexplored. We'll call this the discovery dilemma. It's not that we don't ask enough questions, but that we don't ask them in the right way, to the right people, at the right time.

Most organizations think they are making informed decisions when choosing technology solutions. They believe their processes are thorough, their discovery methodical, and their approach structured. After all, they hold workshops, conduct stakeholder interviews, and consult with industry experts, and in most cases, they do this over six months or more. On paper, it looks like due diligence.

But in reality? Most businesses are running in circles.

Rather than finding clarity, they are drowning in complexity. Instead of making progress, they get stuck in indecision. When they try to **accelerate** transformation, they slow themselves down.

Why? Because **traditional technology discovery processes are fundamentally broken**.

Manual, consultant, or internal-led discovery methods, those that rely on interviews, Q&A sessions, workshops, online meetings, and months of back-and-forth conversations, coupled with multiple technology demonstrations, are inefficient, expensive, and outdated. They may have worked in an era when change happened gradually, but in today's fast-moving digital economy, they are actively **killing progress.**

This chapter will expose why the traditional discovery process is failing organizations, how it creates more confusion than clarity, and what businesses must do to break free from this broken approach.

The Flawed Foundation of Traditional Discovery

Discovery is supposed to be the first and most crucial step in making a business decision, especially one as significant as investing in a new technology platform. It should provide leaders with deep insights into their organization's needs, helping them make informed, confident decisions.

But that's not what happens in most businesses today.

Instead, discovery is often:

- **Slow** – Taking months, sometimes years, to complete.
- **Inconsistent** – Different teams and stakeholders have conflicting opinions, creating internal misalignment.
- **Heavily reliant on consultants** – Companies pay external experts hundreds of thousands of dollars to interview stakeholders and compile reports, but they rarely deliver actionable insights and business justifications.
- **Too subjective** – Based on opinions, personal biases, and anecdotal evidence rather than data-driven insights and structured frameworks.

In short, businesses aren't discovering anything new. They are just collecting more archives.

And the result? **Paralysis.**

Companies get stuck in the discovery phase and are unable to move forward. The more time they spend gathering requirements, the more overwhelming the process becomes. Instead of building momentum, they get trapped in an endless cycle of meetings, interviews, and "stakeholder alignment" sessions that lead nowhere.

> **By the time they finally reach a decision, if they ever do, the landscape has already changed. Customer expectations have evolved. New competitors have entered the market. The technology they were evaluating is already outdated.**

Welcome to the discovery dilemma, a process designed to help businesses make better decisions but keeps them trapped in indecision and inefficiency.

The 5 Biggest Flaws in Traditional Discovery

1. It's Too Slow for the Speed of Business Today

Traditional discovery methods assume that people and businesses have time. They rely on long, drawn-out workshops, interviews, surveys, and consultant-driven analysis, which can last months or even years, as we've covered.

But today, business moves too fast for this approach to work.

- **Customer expectations evolve rapidly.** By the time a company finishes discovery, their customers' needs may have already changed.
- **Competitors aren't waiting.** Businesses that move faster will out-innovate those stuck in analysis paralysis.
- **Technology changes constantly.** A "best-in-class" solution today might be outdated tomorrow.

Companies that rely on slow, outdated discovery processes are constantly making decisions based on yesterday's reality, not today's opportunities.

2. It's Riddled with Subjectivity and Bias

Traditional discovery is often opinion-based, not data-driven.

- Stakeholders have different perspectives, and the goals of their departments shape their input, not necessarily what's best for the company as a whole.
- Business leaders rely on personal experience rather than objective insights.
- Consultants bring their own biases, often steering companies toward solutions that align with their past projects, partnerships, or preferred vendors.

Instead of uncovering the truth and the business's real "core" requirements, traditional discovery often reinforces existing biases and internal politics. Traditional discovery doesn't hold up a mirror; it holds up a microphone. It records opinions, not truths.

Manual Technology Discovery takes time and hinders momentum

CURRENT ASSESSMENT = 6+ MONTHS

Participant Selection	Rescheduling Meetings	Study Progress Checkpoint 3	
Manually Email Participants	Progress Report to Sponsors	Complete Follow Up Interviews	
Participant Kick Off	Survey Completion Checkpoint 2	Manual Interpretation of Gathered Data	Present Findings & Recommendations to Key Stakeholders
Training of Process	Survey Completion Checkpoint 1	Complete Business Case/ ROI Metric Collaboration	Present & Validate Preliminary Findings w/ Project Stakeholders

3. It Creates Internal Misalignment

Discovery should align teams, but in reality, it often creates more division.

- Different business units have conflicting priorities, making it difficult to reach a consensus.
- IT wants security and scalability, while Marketing and Sales want agility and personalization.

- The CFO wants cost and hard dollar savings, while Operations wants efficiency and automation.

Because traditional discovery lacks a structured, unified approach, it often turns into an internal power struggle, with decisions based on who argues the loudest, not what's best for the company.

4. It's Overly Dependent on External Resources

For decades, businesses have outsourced discovery and research to consultants, believing that external experts can provide better insights than their internal teams.

The reality?

Most consultants don't have a magic formula but simply follow the same outdated manual process that the industry possesses:

- **Conduct stakeholder interviews,** which are just conversations, not structured data collection, driven by key stakeholders within the entire organization, coupled with advanced analytics and insights that help justify initiatives.
- **Compile a report** that summarizes what they heard in various forms like Word, Excel, and PowerPoint.
- **Make recommendations** that are often based on generic industry best practices, not unique business needs.

This process is exhausting, lengthy, expensive, and rarely results in real innovation. Companies spend millions on consulting firms, only to receive PDF reports that sit in a drawer instead of accelerating decision-making and generating actionable outcomes. It is also based on a single point in time, so you cannot trend and compare for continuous improvement.

5. It Doesn't Lead to Confident Decisions

The biggest failure of traditional discovery is that **it doesn't produce clarity**.

- Too much data, not enough insight. Companies end up with hundreds of pages of notes, survey results, and interview transcripts, but they still don't know what to do next.
- Endless debates, no action. Teams spend more time arguing about options than implementing solutions.
- There is more confusion, not less. Even after months of research, businesses still feel uncertain about which technology choices will drive the best results or what to focus on first.

If a discovery process doesn't create clarity, alignment, and action, it's a failure.

The New Model: Fast, Data-Driven Insights, and Aligned Discovery

The solution isn't to abandon discovery; it's to **reinvent it** for businesses and consultants. I've seen brands spend over a million dollars over 18 months on external discovery, only to circle back to the same three options they were considering at the start, just now with a stack of PDFs and no stronger decision-making muscle.

Instead of **slow, subjective, and consultant-driven processes**, businesses need a **faster, more structured, and data-driven approach**, one that they own and that is representative of their data, scoring, and priorities.

Key Principles of Modern Discovery

1. **Automate Data Collection:** Instead of relying on manual interviews, use structured journeys to gather insights from stakeholders at scale.

2. **Focus on Alignment:** Use categorically relevant frameworks that surface areas of agreement and disagreement early so teams can resolve conflicts quickly and drive consensus across the business.

3. **Use Real-Time Analytics and Business Intelligence:** Replace static reports with live dashboards that provide continuous visibility into needs, priorities, scoring, and decision criteria.

4. **Reduce Time to Decision:** Move from months of exhaustive and long discovery to a process that delivers actionable insights in days and weeks, which drives momentum internally and captures the organization's real requirements.

Side by Side Comparison of Current Discovery Methods versus Next Gen Technology Discovery

NEXT GEN CX BASELINING = DAYS TO WEEKS

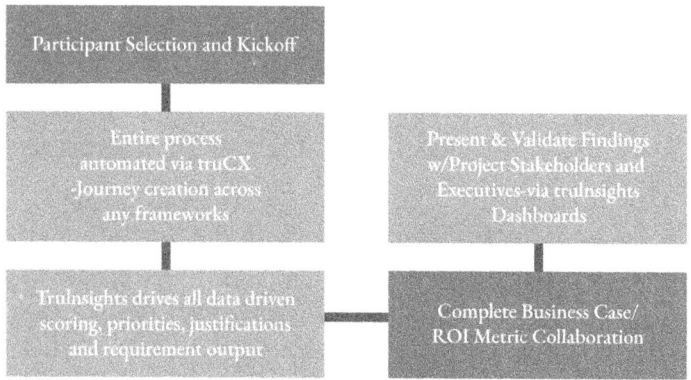

Participant Selection and Kickoff

Entire process automated via truCX -Journey creation across any frameworks

Present & Validate Findings w/Project Stakeholders and Executives via truInsights Dashboards

Trulnsights drives all data driven scoring, priorities, justifications and requirement output

Complete Business Case/ ROI Metric Collaboration

CURRENT ASSESSMENT = 6+ MONTHS

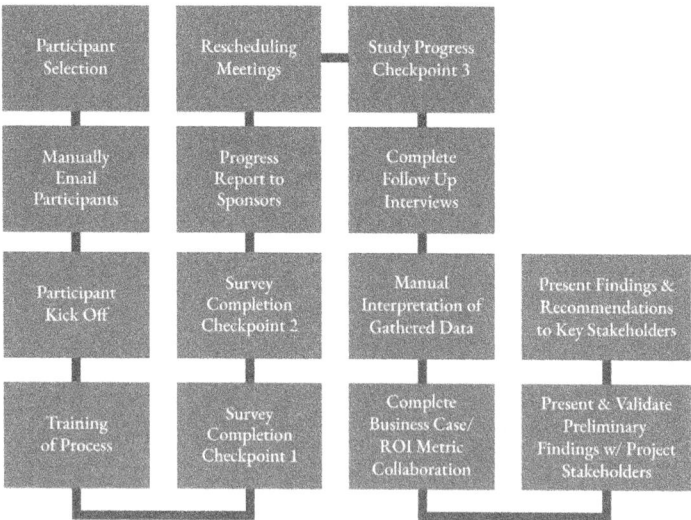

Participant Selection

Rescheduling Meetings

Study Progress Checkpoint 3

Manually Email Participants

Progress Report to Sponsors

Complete Follow Up Interviews

Participant Kick Off

Survey Completion Checkpoint 2

Manual Interpretation of Gathered Data

Present Findings & Recommendations to Key Stakeholders

Training of Process

Survey Completion Checkpoint 1

Complete Business Case/ ROI Metric Collaboration

Present & Validate Preliminary Findings w/ Project Stakeholders

Here's How the Intelligent Organization Discovers

Smart organizations don't wait for consultants to tell them who they are. They discover themselves.

They don't rely on meetings that drag or surveys that drift.

They surface their own truth, fast, structured, and scalable.

That's what activating the intelligence within looks like.

Not to guess. Not to debate.

But to know.

In the next chapter, we'll explore what modern discovery really looks like and how organizations are using it to align, plan, and decide faster than ever before.

Chapter 3

The High Cost of No Decision: When Silence Drowns Intelligence

Indecision is not neutral.

It's expensive.

It's silent.

And worst of all, it buries the intelligence your organization already has.

In a world moving at algorithmic speed, the cost of doing nothing isn't stability; it's surrender.

Indecision is one of the most expensive and destructive business problems today.

When organizations fail to make timely decisions, they don't just delay progress; they actively harm their customer experience, employee engagement, and competitive position.

Opportunities are lost—momentum stalls. Innovation dies.

Yet, many leaders don't even realize how much their hesitation is costing them. They believe that taking more time to decide is a prudent move, a way to ensure they're making the best choice. But in reality, delaying a decision is often worse than making the wrong one.

This chapter will examine the true cost of indecision, revealing the hidden ways it weakens businesses, frustrates employees, and drives customers into the hands of competitors. We'll explore real-world stories of organizations that failed to act in time and paid the price.

By the end, one thing will be clear: The riskiest move is standing still.

The Illusion of Playing It Safe

Many companies believe that waiting is a safe strategy.

> **They assume that postponing a decision gives them more time to gather data, weigh options, and avoid mistakes. This mindset is reinforced by traditional corporate culture, where decision-making is often slow and bureaucratic.**

Leaders hesitate because they fear:

- Choosing the wrong technology and wasting money
- Disrupting internal workflows and frustrating employees
- Embarrassment if the initiative fails
- Pushback from other executives or board members

But waiting leads to bigger problems than simply making a choice and course-correcting if necessary.

Here's why:

- **The world keeps moving, even if you don't.** While one company debates, competitors make bold moves, adopt new technology, and capture market share.
- **Customers expect continuous improvement.** A company that doesn't innovate is falling behind, even if it feels stable.
- **Waiting doesn't reduce risk—it increases it.** The longer a company hesitates, the more complex and costly the eventual decision becomes.

To put it simply: Indecision isn't harmless—it's a slow, silent killer of progress.

The Quiet Cost of a Stalled Brain: The Four Hidden Costs of Indecision

When an organization stalls, its brain does too.

The knowledge is still there in decks, dashboards, and domain experts. But it's not moving, connecting, or evolving. That's the true cost of indecision: It paralyzes intelligence.

1. Missed Opportunities That Competitors Capture

Every time a company delays a decision, it hands an opportunity to its competitors.

This pattern happens across industries:

- **Retail:** A company hesitates to implement a better e-commerce platform while a competitor does—and wins more customers.
- **Banking:** A financial institution drags its feet on adopting AI-driven fraud detection while a rival moves ahead and prevents millions in losses.
- **Healthcare:** A hospital delays implementing a more efficient patient scheduling system, forcing patients to endure long wait times while competitors offer seamless digital booking.

Example: Blockbuster vs. Netflix

Perhaps the most famous example of a missed opportunity is **Blockbuster's failure to act against Netflix**. Blockbuster didn't lose to Netflix because it lacked data. It lost because it ignored it. The intelligence was within—market signals, customer frustration, operational inefficiencies—but Blockbuster's leadership didn't act on it.

In 2000, a Netflix co-founder approached Blockbuster with an offer to **partner or sell Netflix for around $50 million**. At the time, Netflix was a small startup mailing DVDs, while Blockbuster dominated the video rental industry with thousands of stores.

Blockbuster's executives **hesitated**. They weren't sure if online streaming and DVD rentals by mail would ever be viable.

By the time they **realized their mistake**, Netflix had already disrupted the market.

The result?

- Netflix has a net worth of over **$484 billion**
- Blockbuster filed for **bankruptcy in 2010**

All because Blockbuster **failed to make a timely decision.**

2. Employee Frustration and Talent Drain

Employees want to **work for companies that take action.**

When leadership fails to make decisions, it creates **uncertainty, frustration, and disengagement.**

- Teams waste **hours in endless meetings** without making progress.
- Employees feel like **their work doesn't matter** because projects keep stalling.
- Top talent thrives in environments of **momentum and innovation** and leaves for companies that make decisions and move forward.

Example: The Case of a Tech Giant Losing Its Best Talent

A Fortune 500 tech company had an opportunity to **adopt a new AI-powered customer service platform** that would streamline interactions and reduce costs.

- The customer support team wanted it.
- IT had tested it and confirmed it could integrate with existing systems.
- The finance department approved the budget.

But the executive team **hesitated.**

They requested **more market research, more vendor presentations, and more internal meetings** to evaluate "every possible scenario."

Eighteen months later, they still hadn't made a decision.

- By then, **competitors had already adopted similar AI solutions** and were seeing huge improvements.
- Several **top employees left**, frustrated with the lack of leadership.
- The delay cost them **millions in operational inefficiencies.**

Had they acted sooner, they would have been a market leader. Instead, they **fell behind and never caught up.**

3. Customer Loss Due to Poor Experience

Customers don't wait for companies to get their act together. In a customer experience economy, indecision signals apathy. Customers interpret inaction as indifference, and they don't wait for permission to leave.

In today's world, customers expect immediate improvements, seamless experiences, and continuous innovation.

If a business fails to keep up, customers leave—quickly.

Example: The Hotel Chain That Refused to Modernize

A major hotel chain had an outdated online booking system. Customers:

- Struggled to make reservations on mobile devices
- Faced long wait times when calling customer support
- Found the process frustrating and confusing

The company **knew they needed to upgrade their digital experience.**

- Internal studies showed that an improved system would increase bookings by 20%.
- Competitors had already upgraded their platforms.
- Customers were complaining in their online reviews.

But leadership hesitated. They feared:

- The complexity of migrating systems
- The upfront investment cost
- The potential pushback from franchise owners

So as a result, **they delayed the decision for three years.**

By the time they finally upgraded, it was too late. Competitors had already built loyal customer bases with superior digital experiences.

Result?

- The **hotel chain lost market share** to more agile competitors.
- **Customer retention plummeted.**
- The delay in action **cost them millions in lost revenue.**

4. Financial Losses That Compound Over Time

Indecision drains money in ways companies rarely measure.

- **Operational inefficiencies stack up.** Employees spend time debating instead of executing.
- **Costs rise.** The longer a company waits, the more expensive solutions become.
- **Revenue declines.** Delays prevent organizations from launching new products or improving customer experience, resulting in lost sales.

Example: The Online Retailer That Waited Too Long to Adopt E-Commerce

A large national retailer saw competitors shifting to online shopping in the early 2010s.

They **considered launching their own e-commerce platform but kept delaying**:

- "We need more research."
- "Let's wait until next year's budget cycle."
- "We're not sure if customers will shop online."

When they finally launched their platform, Amazon, Walmart, and Target had already captured most of the online market.

The retailer never recovered.

The cost of their indecision?

- Hundreds of stores closed.
- Thousands of employees were laid off.
- **A once-thriving company reduced to irrelevance.**

Activate the Intelligence Within: Stop Waiting. Start Listening.

The most dangerous thing a company can do is wait to feel ready.

Readiness isn't a signal; it's a side effect of alignment, action, and momentum.

Inside your organization is the insight to decide, the experience to execute, and the clarity to move.

The intelligence within is already speaking. The question is, will you listen? Break Free. Decide Forward.

> **The companies that will win the future are not the ones that wait, they are the ones that align, plan, and decide faster.**

CHAPTER 4

The Breakthrough: Activating the Intelligence Within

A New Way Forward

You've seen how broken the old system is. You've lived it.

Now, it's time to break through it.

The smartest organizations aren't waiting for perfect clarity. They're unlocking it from within by adopting a faster, collaborative, data-powered approach to decision-making that aligns their teams and accelerates progress.

This isn't a tweak. It's a transformation. And it begins by activating what your organization already knows.

Now, it's time to shift gears.

This chapter introduces a new way forward, a modern decision-making model that is:

Faster – Gathering business requirements and aligning stakeholders in days, not months.

Collaborative – Breaking down internal silos and ensuring that all business units and teams have a voice without unnecessary delays.

Data-Driven – Replacing opinions and assumptions with objective, structured analysis that leads to confident decisions.

Say goodbye to lengthy, manually driven engagements, endless internal debates, and outdated discovery methods. This modern approach puts organizations in the driver's seat, streamlining decision-making and eliminating bottlenecks, silos, and uncertainty. It enables businesses to assess their technology and CX needs with clarity, speed, and alignment across teams. Imagine entering the market with all your internal technology requirements, spanning unified communications, contact centers, AI, and CX, fully defined before you even begin the vendor selection process.

By adopting this new approach, companies can move at the speed of business, ensuring that they don't just survive, but thrive in today's hyper-competitive, rapidly evolving landscape. We will talk more about this in Chapter 5.

The Three Core Principles of the New Decision-Making Model

To transform how organizations **align, plan, and decide new technology**, this model is built on **three essential principles**:

1. **Speed** – This isn't rushed decision-making. It's right-time decision-making, because your business already knows more than it thinks. You just need to give it structure, space, and speed.
2. **Collaboration as Clarity** – The new model doesn't just gather opinions. It orchestrates organizational intelligence. It gives every stakeholder a voice and builds consensus through data, not debate.
3. **Data-Driven Insights** – Moves away from gut-feeling decisions and replaces them with structured, evidence-based decision-making. Data is the great equalizer. It removes ego. It removes bias. And when applied in real-time, it becomes the compass that smart organizations use to move forward, together.

Let's explore each of these principles in detail.

1. Speed: Making High-Stakes Decisions in Days, Not Months

The most successful organizations today are the ones that make high-impact decisions quickly.

- Amazon launches innovations at breakneck speed, even if they aren't perfect. They iterate and refine continuously rather than waiting for a perfect plan.
- Tesla rolls out software updates to vehicles globally in real-time, adjusting performance on the fly, while competitors struggle with outdated, multi-year product cycles.
- Leading SaaS companies test, adjust, and deploy new features every week, not every year.

Contrast this with traditional enterprises, where decision-making can take months or even years:

- **Committees hold endless meetings**, reviewing the same information over and over without making a clear decision.
- **Stakeholders fail to align**, delaying progress because no one is willing to commit.
- **Fear of failure paralyzes leadership**, leading to indecision rather than bold, calculated action.

The Problem: The Business World Moves Too Fast for Slow Decisions

Today's business landscape is faster and more competitive than ever before. Companies don't have the luxury of waiting:

- **Customer expectations evolve rapidly.** If you're not innovating, you're already falling behind.
- **Competitors move aggressively.** The companies that act quickly capture market share before slower competitors even finalize their strategy.
- **Technology changes constantly.** A "best-in-class" solution today might be outdated in six months to a year.

Speed matters because delay is a competitive disadvantage.

The Solution: An Intelligence Activation Platform With Structured Time Boxed Technology Frameworks

The **new decision-making model eliminates unnecessary delays** by using:

- **Automated, structured discovery processes** instead of drawn-out interviews.
- **Clear prioritization frameworks** that surface real needs and priorities immediately.
- **A time-boxed approach** that ensures decisions happen in days or weeks—not months.

By reducing the time spent gathering business requirements and speeding up internal alignment, businesses can make decisions at the right time—before opportunities pass them by.

The Alignment Factor

Over the past year, we partnered with a large healthcare Business Process Outsourcing Provider (BPO) supporting 2,500 remote contact center agents. When we first engaged with their senior IT executives, they were convinced that aligning with the business, defining requirements, and transitioning from their legacy contact center platforms would take more than a year. The complexity of the task, combined with the challenge of gaining consensus across stakeholders, seemed like an insurmountable roadblock.

We introduced a structured, time-sensitive approach that not only accelerated the process but also ensured alignment across all decision-makers. By guiding their teams through a comprehensive evaluation framework, we enabled them to score every aspect of their existing technology landscape while simultaneously educating them on modern CX solutions. This process ensured that all 25 stakeholders had equal exposure to the same insights, methodologies, and decision-making criteria.

The impact was immediate. In just one week, our CX design thinking methodology facilitated structured scoring and data gathering, generating 1,625 critical data points. Using advanced intelligence and analytics, we distilled those insights into 123 core requirements—providing a clear blueprint for vendor selection.

Within a month, the team had narrowed their choices down to two best-fit suppliers. Just five weeks after kicking off the process, they were in contract negotiations with procurement. The best part? The speed of execution did not come at the expense of quality. Instead, it enabled them to move with confidence, precision, and alignment, turning what they expected to take over a year into a strategic, insight-driven decision in record time.

2. Collaboration: Creating Instant Alignment Across Teams

One of the biggest roadblocks to decision-making is internal misalignment.

- IT wants security and scalability.
- Marketing wants personalization and agility.
- Finance wants cost control.
- Operations wants seamless integration.

When business units fail to align, organizations fall into endless debates and delays.

The Problem: Lack of a Structured Optimization Framework
Without a structured decision-making process, most organizations experience:

- **Fragmented decision-making**, where each department prioritizes its own goals, which makes company-wide decisions impossible.
- **Meetings that go nowhere**, where stakeholders discuss but never resolve conflicting priorities.
- **Last-minute roadblocks** occur when decisions that seemed final are revisited because a key business unit was left out of the conversation.

Sound familiar?

The Solution: A Fast-Tracked Alignment Process
The new model solves internal misalignment by:

- **Gathering input** from all business units and teams in a structured way (no more timely ad hoc discussions that go nowhere).
- **Using real-time analytics** to surface the biggest priorities instantly.
- **Creating a shared decision-making framework** that makes trade-offs clear and transparent.

Instead of forcing every department to fight for its own agenda, this model ensures that every team is aligned without slowing progress.

3. Data-Driven Insights: Replacing Assumptions with Objective Decision-Making

Traditional discovery is **opinion-driven**, based on what executives **think** they need rather than what the **data proves** they need.

The Problem: Decision-Making Based on Opinions, Not Real Requirements

- Executives have their own biases about what technology the company needs.
- Different departments push their own agendas, creating misaligned priorities.
- Decisions are made based on historical trends, not real-time insights about what customers actually want today.

The Solution: Structured, Data-Driven Decision-Making
The new model **flips this approach** by using:

- **Real-time scoring mechanisms** that rank business needs objectively.
- **AI-powered analysis** that highlights key gaps and opportunities for improvement.
- **Benchmarking against industry standards** to see where the company stands.

Instead of endless meetings and gut-feeling decisions, organizations get clear, data-backed insights that point to the best path forward.

"Your team's priceless insights and forward-thinking approach around CX inspires confidence in us as a partner and with our customers. Your client-centric approach and optimization platform empowers organizations to take ownership, ensuring their decisions are expertly guided. Looking back, I cannot see how this level of success would have been realized with a traditional discovery process."

— Michael Kotze, CEO – SenderoCloud

Break the Loop, Build the Future

The traditional model isn't just slow. It's broken.

The organizations winning today are the ones that unlock their internal intelligence, create alignment in days, not months, and make decisions rooted in insight, not instinct.

Speed is clarity. Alignment is power. Insight is freedom.

That's what activating internal intelligence looks like.

In the next chapters, we'll unpack exactly how to do it, step by step.

> **The result? Organizations that move quickly capture opportunities first, adapt to change effortlessly, and continuously innovate, while others are still stuck in approval loops and lack sophisticated business justifications.**

CHAPTER 5

Step 1 – Redefining Discovery: From Gut Feel to Intelligent Action

Why Traditional Discovery is Fundamentally Flawed

Discovery isn't a checklist. It's the ignition switch for transformation.

When done right, it aligns stakeholders, reveals real needs, and creates the momentum every decision needs. But when done the old way, manual, slow, and subjective, it doesn't just delay progress. It damages trust, wastes time, and erodes confidence from the inside out.

This chapter introduces a modern discovery model, one designed to unlock the intelligence within your organization and move you from assumptions to alignment and from discussion to action.

Discovery is the most crucial step in making any high-impact business decision, whether selecting new technology, improving customer experience (CX), or realigning business strategy. It's the foundation upon which everything else is built. If the discovery process is slow, inaccurate, or misaligned, then every subsequent decision will be flawed, leading to wasted time, missed opportunities, and failed implementations.

And yet, traditional discovery methods are fundamentally broken.

Organizations that rely on manual, consultant-led discovery processes that:

- Take months or years to complete.
- Depend on subjective opinions instead of structured data and design thinking.
- Create conflicting priorities across business units.
- Often results in "no decision" or delayed action.

Most companies assume that taking longer to make decisions leads to better outcomes. In reality, the longer they take, the more they stagnate, the more opportunities they miss, and the more their competitors pull ahead.

The solution is not to abandon discovery, but to reinvent it.

This chapter introduces a structured, modern approach to discovery that allows organizations to:

Surface data-driven insights quickly (in days, not months).
Align stakeholders efficiently (without external bottlenecks).
Make confident, data-led decisions that lead to real transformation.

With the right frameworks, organizations can cut through complexity, eliminate uncertainty, and accelerate progress.

Imagine walking into a high-stakes meeting with a potential customer, armed with the usual arsenal of PowerPoint slides, case studies, and an over-caffeinated enthusiasm that screams, "We are the solution to your problems!" You sit down, exchange pleasantries, and dive headfirst into a discovery session that feels eerily familiar because it is. It's the same set of questions, the same vague answers, and the same awkward pauses where both sides pretend they know what the other is talking about.

And just like that, you're already losing.

If you're a vendor, partner, or supplier in the CX or technology industry, you've likely been guilty of the crime I call **"Death by Discovery."** What we call 'discovery' today is often just unstructured guessing masked in PowerPoint. It's not strategic. It's theatrical. You've unknowingly subjected your customers and prospects to an interrogation that could rival an FBI investigation, all in an attempt to piece together requirements that should have been clear before you ever walked into the room.

But here's the kicker: it's not just your fault. It's the industry's fault. We've built an entire ecosystem that treats discovery as a checkbox exercise rather than the foundation for real business transformation and opportunity to impact real change. We enter sales cycles woefully unprepared and, at times, somewhat prepared, assuming that the customer is just as eager to fill in our knowledge gaps as we are to close the deal. We assume they know what they want. We assume they have the data. We assume they have the internal buy-in, the budget, and the green light to move forward.

Spoiler alert: they don't.

I've spent almost thirty years consulting businesses of all sizes, from scrappy startups to Fortune 500 giants, and I've seen this broken system play out again and again. The problem isn't that salespeople, vendors, and suppliers don't care about their customers and prospects. It's that we don't actually understand them—not in the way that matters.

We think we're being consultative when we ask, "What are your biggest challenges?" or "What's keeping you up at night?" or my historical favorite, "If you had a magic wand, what would you wish for? "But let's be real, if they knew the answer to that, they wouldn't need us.

The truth is that most companies don't fully understand their gaps, inefficiencies, or even what they need to succeed. Yet, we continue to approach sales as if discovery is a one-time event rather than an ongoing, dynamic process.

And that's where everything falls apart.

"I have had the privilege of knowing (and learning) from Rich for many years and can clearly say that he is one of the most talented entrepreneurs that I've ever met. He has the unique ability to understand the economic drivers of a business and laser focus on helping organizations adopt technologies that drive their growth and technology adoption. All of that aside, he is a transparent, genuine leader."

— Scott Cohen, Partner, Quattro

When Discovery Becomes a Dead End

Discovery is supposed to be the first and most critical step in making informed business decisions, whether selecting new technology, improving customer experience, or refining operational strategies. However, traditional discovery methods are fundamentally broken. They were designed for a different era, one where businesses had the luxury of time, industries moved at a slower pace, and customer expectations weren't shifting overnight. Today, those conditions no longer exist.

A colleague of mine, a seasoned consultant working with large enterprise clients, once shared a story that perfectly illustrates this challenge. Several years ago, he and his team were tasked with conducting discovery for a Fortune 200 company, one that was already a client. Their goal? To define requirements for migrating from a **premise-based contact center** to a **cloud-based solution**.

What should have been a streamlined process quickly turned into an operational nightmare. Coordinating **interviews with over 80 stakeholders** and scheduling **countless one-on-one meetings, web calls, and follow-ups** stretched the discovery process **beyond 13 months**. After an additional month of compiling and analyzing the findings, they finally presented their report.

But instead of approval, the Global CIO delivered a sobering reality check: "Well, it's been more than 13 months, so we might as well start this process all over again; there are too many new features and capabilities in the market now."

The market had moved forward—their discovery had not.

Let's be clear: this isn't a failure of the consultant or the company; it's a failure of the traditional discovery process itself. The pace of innovation has outstripped the ability of legacy discovery methods to keep up. In today's world, where technology capabilities evolve month-to-month, taking a year to gather requirements is no longer just inefficient, it's obsolete.

For business leaders and consultants to remain effective, **discovery must evolve;** it needs to be **faster, more intelligent, and continuously adaptive**. The old way of doing things is no longer viable. The modern business leader doesn't have **13 months to wait**—they need insights **now** to make decisions that keep them ahead, not playing catch-up.

Instead of helping businesses move forward, these outdated processes often do the opposite; they stall progress, introduce confusion, and create indecision.

Let's break down the key reasons why traditional discovery is failing modern businesses.

> The real tragedy is not that organizations can't decide. It's that they already have the insight; they just can't see it clearly enough to act.

It's Too Slow for the Speed of Business

The most obvious and damaging flaw of traditional discovery is that it takes far too long for all parties involved. In an era where market conditions, customer expectations, and technology trends evolve in real time, a discovery process that drags on for months or even years can render its own findings obsolete before they are even implemented.

Most traditional discovery efforts involve a long sequence of stakeholder interviews, internal workshops, surveys, and consultant-led assessments. While these methods may have once provided value, they are now a primary cause of bottlenecks and frustration within organizations.

A typical discovery process might begin with a series of internal meetings where different teams are asked to articulate their needs. These discussions can quickly become repetitive, with the same conversations happening across multiple sessions. After that, consultants or internal research teams compile the insights, often taking weeks, if not months, to distill them into reports. By the time leadership receives the final recommendations, the business landscape has already shifted, rendering large portions of the findings outdated.

Even worse, slow discovery cycles prevent organizations from keeping up with external pressures. Customer preferences shift rapidly, new competitors emerge, and industry leaders set new standards at a pace that legacy businesses struggle to match. Taking six months or longer to determine what technology to implement or what strategy to pursue thrusts companies into a constant state of reaction rather than proactive innovation.

The businesses that thrive today are those that operate in real time, not on a six-month delay. They use automated insights, real-time analytics, and structured decision-making frameworks to assess needs and implement solutions without unnecessary delays. Those that cling to traditional discovery, however, remain stuck in cycles of indecision, unable to act quickly enough to remain competitive.

It's Highly Subjective and Fragmented

Another major flaw of traditional discovery is that it is highly dependent on subjective opinions rather than structured, data-driven insights. Because discovery processes typically involve multiple business units, each with its priorities and perspectives, the result is often a fragmented and conflicting view of what the organization actually needs.

Stakeholders bring their own biases, agendas, and assumptions to the table. An IT team might prioritize security and stability, while marketing wants personalization and agility. Customer service teams might advocate for solutions that improve agent workflows, while finance focuses on cost control. Without a structured way to consolidate and prioritize these varying viewpoints, traditional discovery amplifies misalignment rather than resolving it.

Compounding the problem is the fact that many organizations rely on outside consultants to interpret their business needs. These consultants often conduct interviews, collect stakeholder feedback, and produce lengthy reports filled with subjective insights, most often based on what employees believe they need rather than what real data suggests.

Instead of helping organizations make data-backed decisions, traditional discovery forces leadership teams to navigate conflicting opinions, making it difficult to determine the best course of action.

As a result, instead of creating clarity, the process often leads to more confusion, making decision-making even more difficult than before.

Modern organizations cannot afford to rely on subjective insights. The most successful companies use real-time data analytics, AI-driven sentiment analysis, and structured prioritization models to determine their actual business needs, eliminating the guesswork and ensuring that decisions are based on facts, not opinions.

It Fails to Drive Action

Perhaps the most frustrating and damaging issue with traditional discovery is that even after months of research and analysis, it often fails to drive meaningful action.

It is not uncommon for companies to invest significant time and resources into stakeholder interviews, consultant engagements, and internal assessments, only to receive a comprehensive report that ultimately sits on a shelf, never acted upon. Traditional discovery focuses too much on identifying problems and not enough on solving them, which is why so many reports end up on a shelf.

There are several reasons why traditional discovery fails to produce action:

- **Reports are often too broad and lack clear prioritization.** Leadership teams receive documents filled with vague recommendations rather than actionable steps.
- **Decision-makers get trapped in endless debates over the findings.** Instead of executing, teams spend weeks or

months reanalyzing the data and questioning the validity of the insights.

- **No structured framework exists to move from discovery to execution.** Even when organizations agree on priorities, they often lack a clear process to turn those insights into immediate action.

The result is paralysis. Instead of accelerating transformation, traditional discovery delays it. Initiatives that could have been implemented months ago remain stalled in review cycles while competitors move forward, capturing market share and customer loyalty.

In order to break free from this pattern, businesses must replace static, manual-driven discovery with a dynamic, continuous, and action-oriented model. Instead of spending months gathering and debating insights, organizations should:

- Use automated data collection tools to assess business needs in real time.
- Leverage structured decision-making frameworks to align stakeholders quickly and efficiently.
- Ensure that every discovery effort ends with clear, prioritized action items that they implement immediately.

The organizations that thrive do not spend months perfecting their plans; they execute, learn, and iterate in real-time.

Breaking Free from Traditional Discovery

Traditional discovery is fundamentally too slow, too subjective, and too ineffective to meet the demands of modern business. Companies that cling to outdated processes will continue to experience delays, misalignment, and decision paralysis. However, those that embrace faster, data-driven, and structured discovery frameworks will accelerate transformation and gain a competitive edge.

Organizations that break free from traditional discovery will:

- **Make faster, more confident decisions** based on real-time insights rather than outdated reports.
- **Achieve alignment across business units** without lengthy debates and conflicting priorities.
- **Turn discovery into action,** ensuring that every insight leads to meaningful progress.

> **In today's business landscape, speed is survival. Companies that continue to rely on outdated discovery methods risk falling further behind, while those that embrace a new model of decision-making and execution will define the future of their industries.**

The choice is clear: continue following broken discovery processes or break free and transform the way your organization makes decisions. The businesses that choose the latter will not only move faster—they will lead.

The Solution: Modern, Structured Discovery Frameworks

To overcome the failures of traditional discovery, organizations must adopt a new model—one built for speed, efficiency, and impact. The modern business landscape no longer allows months of manual data gathering, fragmented stakeholder interviews, and consultant-driven interpretations that are outdated before they are even implemented.

Organizations that want to stay ahead must replace these legacy processes with a structured, real-time discovery framework—one that enables fast, informed decision-making, seamless alignment, and immediate action.

A modern discovery framework is not just an incremental improvement over traditional methods, it is a fundamental shift in how businesses surface insights, prioritize initiatives, and drive execution. It eliminates the delays, misalignment, and subjectivity that plague legacy discovery and replaces them with data-driven intelligence, automation, and structured decision-making.

This new approach rests on four key pillars:

1. **Automating Data Collection Instead of Relying on Lengthy Interviews**

   One of the biggest inefficiencies of traditional discovery is the reliance on one-on-one stakeholder interviews and consultant-led workshops to gather business requirements. While these methods may have worked in the past, they are far too slow and inefficient for modern business environments. Organizations today cannot afford to spend months conducting interviews, manually transcribing responses, and waiting for consultants to compile findings.

A modern discovery framework eliminates this bottleneck by leveraging automation, digital assessments, and AI-powered data collection tools to gather input at scale.

- Instead of waiting for scheduled interviews, stakeholders can provide structured input asynchronously, ensuring that feedback is gathered in days, not weeks or months.
- AI and machine learning algorithms can analyze trends, identify recurring themes, and categorize responses in real-time, eliminating the need for manual interpretation.
- Organizations can access insights instantly rather than waiting for lengthy consultant reports.

This automation speeds up the discovery process and increases accuracy by removing human bias from data collection. It ensures that every stakeholder's voice is captured without unnecessary delays or distortions caused by intermediaries.

2. Surfacing Priorities Instantly Across All Business Units

One of the biggest challenges with traditional discovery is that different business units have competing priorities and fragmented viewpoints. Marketing may want personalization and agility, IT may prioritize security and scalability, finance may focus on cost control, and customer service may push for operational efficiency.

These conflicting perspectives often lead to misalignment and stalled decision-making.

A modern discovery framework solves this problem by providing a structured, data-driven approach to identifying and ranking priorities across the organization.

- Real-time stakeholder dashboards allow leadership to see where different departments align and where they diverge, instantly surfacing areas of consensus and conflict.
- Weighted scoring models ensure that business priorities are ranked based on strategic impact, feasibility, and customer experience outcomes rather than subjective opinions.
- AI-powered decision-support tools highlight potential trade-offs, allowing leaders to resolve conflicts quickly and effectively rather than getting trapped in endless discussions.

By providing instant visibility into business priorities, this framework ensures that organizations are not just collecting input, but actively using it to make decisions faster and more effectively.

3. Using Real-Time Analytics Instead of Subjective Interpretations

In traditional discovery, most business decisions are based on opinion-driven analysis rather than hard data. Stakeholders often advocate for solutions based on their personal experiences, gut feelings, or departmental goals without real-time evidence to support their recommendations.

Consultants, in turn, interpret these inputs, often filtering them through their own frameworks and perspectives, which may not align with the business's actual needs.

A modern discovery framework eliminates subjectivity by guiding decision-making through real-time analytics, AI-driven insights, and structured data models.

- Predictive analytics tools can assess customer trends, operational bottlenecks, and financial impact in real-time, ensuring that decisions are based on facts rather than assumptions.
- Dynamic scoring models rank potential solutions based on historical performance, industry benchmarks, and business objectives, providing a clear, evidence-backed roadmap for execution.
- Real-time collaboration dashboards ensure that every stakeholder has access to the same data, reducing the risk of miscommunication and conflicting interpretations.

By shifting from opinion-based decision-making to analytics-driven insights, organizations can make faster, smarter, and more impactful choices that align with their business goals.

4. Delivering Clear, Actionable Insights That Drive Immediate Decisions

One of the most frustrating outcomes of traditional discovery is that, after months of meetings, interviews, and analysis, businesses often get massive reports without a clear path forward.

These reports, while comprehensive, lack actionable next steps, leading to indecision, further delays, and lost momentum.

A modern discovery framework ensures that every insight leads to immediate action by providing structured, prioritized, and executable recommendations.

- Instead of delivering static reports, organizations receive real-time, interactive decision roadmaps that outline specific steps, ownership, and timelines.
- AI-powered decision engines generate prescriptive recommendations, ensuring that teams know what to do next without the need for additional analysis.
- Execution plans are built into a structured, iterative framework, allowing organizations to implement changes quickly, measure impact, and continuously refine their approach.

By transforming discovery into an action-driven process, businesses can move from planning to execution in record time, ensuring that their insights do not sit unused but directly drive measurable improvements.

Breaking Free

The shift from traditional discovery to a modern, structured framework is not just a small improvement; it is a fundamental transformation in how businesses assess needs, prioritize initiatives, and execute strategies. Organizations that embrace this new model will outpace competitors, make smarter decisions, and accelerate CX innovation in ways that were previously impossible.

The companies that will lead their industries are those that:

- Replace slow, manual data collection with real-time, automated insights.
- Reveal what matters across teams, eliminating internal roadblocks.
- Use analytics and AI to make fact-based decisions, not opinion-based ones.
- Ensure that every discovery effort leads to immediate, structured action.

Those who fail to evolve will remain trapped in outdated, inefficient processes, watching as faster, more agile competitors move ahead. The choice is clear: continue with legacy discovery methods and risk stagnation or adopt a modern framework that will drive speed, precision, and transformation. Businesses that break free will not only move faster but also shape the future of their industries.

The 4-Step Framework for Modern Age Discovery

To achieve this transformation, organizations must follow a structured, four-step process:

Step 1: Define and Structure the Discovery Process

As we've covered in previous chapters, traditional discovery lacks clear structure, leading to confusion, inefficiency, and delays.

The modern approach begins with defining the discovery process upfront, answering critical questions before gathering input:

What are the business objectives? (Technology adoption? Customer experience transformation?)

Who are the key stakeholders? (IT, Marketing, Operations, Finance, Procurement, Customer Experience, Service and Support, etc.)

What data needs to be collected? (Pain points, priorities, budget considerations, needs, etc.)

What is the decision-making timeline? (A time-boxed approach prevents delays.)

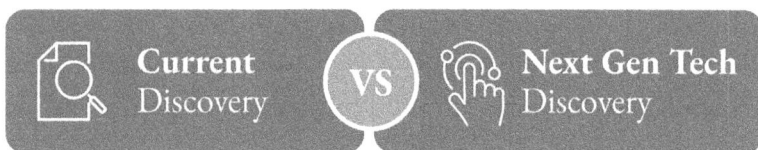

Instead of letting discovery spiral out of control, organizations must set clear boundaries and expectations with all stakeholders involved in the process from the start.

Step 2: Listen at Scale

The biggest problem with traditional discovery is manual information gathering. Instead of one-on-one interviews and consultant-led meetings, modern discovery automates data collection using structured journeys and technology-driven insights.

How?

Digital journeys & structured frameworks – All stakeholders provide input asynchronously, eliminating scheduling delays.

AI-driven analysis – Real-time scoring and prioritization replace manual interpretation.

Dynamic feedback loops – As responses come in, organizations see patterns emerge immediately instead of waiting for final reports.

This modern discovery approach removes bottlenecks, ensures faster insights, and eliminates bias from the process.

Step 3: Align Stakeholders in Days, Not Months

Alignment is the number one reason discovery processes fail.

Without a clear process, different business units and teams push their own agendas:

- Sales wants faster enablement and fewer roadblocks to closing deals.
- Customer Service demands tools that reduce effort and increase satisfaction.
- HR focuses on change readiness and employee retention.
- Product teams push for flexibility and iterative improvements.

The result? Conflicting priorities, endless debates, and decision paralysis. The modern approach solves this problem with structured alignment:

1. Unified dashboards present all stakeholder input side by side.
2. Instant prioritization frameworks surface where teams agree and disagree.
3. Automated trade-off analysis that objectively ranks initiatives based on business impact.

Structured alignment means that instead of months or even up to a year or more of alignment meetings, stakeholders can reach consensus in days and weeks. The business can take control of the discovery process and ensure that all teams are given the opportunity to provide feedback and score their priorities and needs.

Step 4: Move From Knowing to Doing

Traditional discovery often fails at the final step, turning insights into real decisions and actions. The modern approach ensures every discovery process ends in execution by:

Generating prioritized action plans based on stakeholder inputs and business goals.

Eliminating ambiguity with clear recommendations instead of vague reports.

Embedding continuous improvement mechanisms to keep discovery an ongoing process, not a one-time event.

By structuring insights into actionable next steps, organizations ensure that discovery actually leads to progress.

The Intelligence Was Always There

The old way of discovery is slow by design. Caution. Compliance.

But today? Discovery is speed. It's insight. It's alignment that scales.

The truth is that your organization already has the intelligence it needs to move faster and smarter.

The problem isn't access; it's activation.

That's what the modern discovery framework does: it surfaces clarity where there was clutter, gives voice to priorities, removes the guesswork, and makes it impossible to stay stuck.

In the next chapter, we'll show you how to turn these insights into business-wide consensus and execution.

This approach is how intelligent organizations decide. That is how you break free.

CHAPTER 6

Step 2 – Move as One: Unlocking Alignment Through Shared Intelligence

The Alignment Problem

The alignment problem isn't just about disagreement, it's about disconnection. True alignment is not consensus for consensus' sake; it's **shared intelligence**, a synchronized understanding of what matters most and why. It's the foundation that allows high-performing organizations to move as one—swiftly, confidently, and with purpose. Without it, even the most visionary strategies frequently die quietly in the boardroom, buried under layers of indecision and departmental friction.

Many organizations fall into this trap. Despite having advanced technology, smart people, and big ideas, they fail to move forward. Not because the ambition isn't there, but because of misalignment at the organization's core. Teams work in silos. Priorities clash. Meetings multiply while progress stalls. Projects lose momentum, and employees become discouraged as they watch high-impact opportunities dissolve in a sea of bureaucracy and internal debate.

The issue isn't a lack of will or intelligence; it's a lack of structure. Different teams see different slices of the picture. Without a unified framework to align those views and turn them into collective action, companies remain stuck.

That's where **truCX** comes in.

truCX was built specifically for executive leaders who are ready to break free from slow, fragmented decision-making. It's more than a platform; it's a force multiplier. truCX enables organizations to unlock alignment in days, not months, by providing a structured, repeatable framework for surfacing true business priorities, eliminating indecision, and activating cross-functional buy-in fast. It replaces gut-feel debates and endless meetings with data-backed clarity, real-time insights, and visible consensus across all stakeholders.

With truCX, alignment becomes a competitive advantage, not a barrier. It empowers leadership teams to move with speed and unity and to drive transformation with confidence. The future belongs to organizations that can act decisively. truCX is the platform that gets you there.

The Real Cost of Misalignment

Before diving into how to achieve alignment, it is crucial to understand why misalignment is one of the most damaging issues an organization can face. Many businesses assume that internal disagreements and competing priorities are just part of the process, but they fail to recognize the true cost of these inefficiencies. When leadership teams, business units, and stakeholders are not aligned, progress stalls, resources are wasted, opportunities are lost, and employee engagement declines. These consequences don't just slow down a company's growth; they actively push it backward while competitors move ahead.

Delayed Decisions Kill Momentum for Projects

One of the most immediate and visible consequences of misalignment is decision paralysis. When different teams within an organization fail to align on priorities, strategic decisions that should take weeks end up stretching into months or even years. Every department approaches the decision-making process with its own agenda, making it difficult to move forward.

For example, IT prioritizes items like scale, uptime, security, and system stability, ensuring that any new technology implementation does not introduce vulnerabilities and becomes a time suck for the IT department. Meanwhile, marketing focuses on customer engagement, campaigns, personalization, and agility, pushing for solutions that allow them to create dynamic experiences at scale. Finance, on the other hand, wants to control costs and expenses, scrutinizing every investment to maximize profitability or drive a return on investment with hard dollar savings. Then there's operations, which needs seamless integration and minimal disruption, ensuring that day-to-day processes remain stable.

With these competing priorities, reaching a consensus becomes nearly impossible. Instead of making a clear choice and moving forward, organizations become trapped in endless internal debates. Leaders and teams schedule a multitude of meetings and generate reports, yet discussions go in circles, and no one is willing to commit to a final decision. As time drags on, the opportunity for real change slips further away.

The impact of these delays is severe. Projects that could have transformed the business are put on hold. Revenue-driving initiatives are never executed. Customer experience and technology improvements that could have provided a competitive edge are deprioritized. While leadership teams continue debating, competitors are taking action, implementing solutions, and capturing market share.

Internal Conflict Leads to Wasted Time and Resources

Beyond delaying decisions, misalignment causes departments to work against each other rather than with each other. When teams do not share a unified strategy they end up pulling in different directions, wasting valuable time, effort, and financial resources.

Rather than collaborating toward a shared vision, teams push conflicting priorities. IT might work to lock down security measures, only for marketing to push for new technologies that require more flexibility. Finance may impose budget restrictions that prevent CX teams from rolling out enhancements that could significantly impact customer retention. Instead of a streamlined, coordinated effort to drive the business forward, each department fights for its own goals, resulting in disjointed execution and operational inefficiencies.

The cost of this misalignment is staggering. Employees spend hundreds of hours in meetings that lead nowhere, discussing issues that remain unresolved. Consultants and outside experts are brought in to provide guidance, leading to significant expenditures on research and strategy sessions, yet the business still fails to act. The result? More time lost, more money wasted, and zero tangible outcomes.

Missed Opportunities and Competitive Disadvantages

While one company is stuck debating its options, another is making bold moves and executing them. Misalignment doesn't just slow an organization down; it actively gives competitors the opportunity to seize market leadership while others remain stagnant.

Businesses that align quickly capture market share first. When an industry shift occurs, whether it's the rise of AI-powered CX, new automation tools, or changing customer preferences, the companies that act first define the new standard. Customers naturally flock to brands that deliver innovation faster and provide better experiences. By the time a misaligned company finally makes a decision, its competitors have already implemented and optimized their strategy, leaving little room for late adopters to catch up.

The cost of inaction compounds over time. A business that hesitates for six months may find itself a year behind by the time it catches up. Those that take years to align on a major initiative may find that by the time they are ready to launch, the market has already moved on. They are no longer just behind; they are obsolete. Instead of just gathering input, modern organizations instantly surface the intelligence within, pulling from every department.

Employee Frustration and Attrition

Beyond its external impact, misalignment also creates internal disillusionment. Employees want to work for dynamic, forward-thinking companies capable of executing big ideas. When they see decision-making delayed repeatedly, they begin to lose confidence in leadership and the company's ability to succeed.

The psychological toll of repeated delays is profound. Employees become disengaged, questioning why they should put in effort if their initiatives never get implemented. They grow frustrated, realizing that the same problems they discussed a year ago are still unresolved. Eventually, they start looking for opportunities elsewhere.

Top talent doesn't want to work for a company stuck in a perpetual cycle of indecision. They want to be part of an organization that is growing, evolving, and taking bold action. When leadership fails to align and make progress, employees begin to question their own future within the company. And when they leave, they take their institutional knowledge, expertise, and innovative thinking with them.

Organizations that struggle with alignment often experience higher employee turnover, forcing them to spend significant time and resources on recruiting and training new hires, only for those employees to experience the same frustrations and leave as well. Meanwhile, competitors that act decisively and align their teams attract the best and brightest talent, further widening the gap between leaders and laggards.

The Cost of Misalignment is Too High to Ignore

Misalignment is more than just an internal challenge; it is a critical business risk that affects speed, efficiency, competitiveness, and talent retention. Organizations that fail to align will experience delayed decisions, wasted resources, lost opportunities, and an exodus of their most valuable employees.

The good news is that alignment is not an unsolvable problem. Businesses that adopt a structured, data-driven approach to decision-making and stakeholder alignment can eliminate delays, reduce friction, and create momentum that drives real progress. By shifting from fragmented, opinion-driven debates to structured, objective prioritization, organizations can break free from the costly cycle of misalignment and start executing with speed and precision.

The companies that succeed in today's fast-moving world are not necessarily the biggest or the most well-funded; they are the ones that align quickly, make bold decisions, and move forward without hesitation.

For those who fail to recognize the cost of misalignment, the future is uncertain. But for those who take action to solve it, the opportunity to lead is limitless.

The 3 Moves to Shared Momentum

Traditional alignment efforts fail because they rely on long, unstructured meetings, consultant-led interviews, and a lack of clear processes.

Our modern alignment framework solves this by focusing on three key steps:

1. **Capture Stakeholder Priorities at Scale** – Identify the true business needs and priorities across all departments and teams.
2. **Create Instant Clarity on Conflicting Priorities** – Surface areas of alignment and misalignment through data-driven insights and charts.
3. **Turn Alignment into Actionable Decisions** – Build a clear, time-boxed plan to move forward quickly, speeding up the vendor alignment and selection process.

Let's break down each step.

Step 1: Listen to the System

Why Most Businesses Fail at This Step.

What is the biggest mistake organizations make? They assume they know what their teams need without actually asking.

Most companies rely on:

- One-on-one interviews that take months, based on schedule misalignment and manual effort
- Consultants interpreting stakeholder needs (often inaccurately, flawed discovery)
- Lengthy, unstructured meetings where louder voices dominate.

This leads to:

- Incomplete or biased information about what the business prioritizes and needs.
- Misrepresenting team priorities because only a handful of people get heard.
- Wasting months gathering data manually instead of only a few days using modern tools and methods.

The Solution: A Structured, Fast-Track Discovery Process
Instead of manual interviews and meetings, modern alignment uses structured assessments and real-time analytics to gather stakeholder input instantly and at scale.

How truCX Works:

1. All stakeholders participate in a structured digital journey. Instead of waiting for meetings, stakeholders provide input asynchronously on their own time, but it is still deadline-driven.
2. AI-driven analysis categorizes priorities and feedback, while business intelligence analyzes responses in real time, ranking priorities and requirements based on their business impact.
3. Key themes and areas of misalignment surface instantly—no more waiting months for consultant reports.
   - Speeding up input collection from months to days.
   - Eliminating subjective consultant interpretations.
   - Capturing every stakeholder's voice.

Step 2: Reveal the Map

The Problem: Conflicting Agendas Kill Progress

Even when businesses gather stakeholder input, they don't always know how to resolve conflicting priorities. They often fail to act because:

- Sales and marketing have their own interests in the project.
- Stakeholders are often missed in the discovery process, further delaying the process of driving change and projects.
- Seniority drives the majority of opinions.

The Solution: Use Decision-Making Frameworks That Surface Priorities Visually

Instead of relying on endless discussions and subjective debates, modern alignment uses real-time prioritization dashboards that:

1. Show where teams agree and disagree, no more guessing.
2. Rank priorities based on business impact – Aligns decisions with company goals.
3. Highlight trade-offs and solutions instantly – Instead of debating, teams get clear resolution paths.
   - Turning misalignment into structured, objective discussions.
   - Giving leadership a real-time view of decision impact.
   - Eliminating drawn-out debates with clear next steps.

Step 3: Lock in the Move

The Problem: Many Organizations Reach a Consensus But Never Execute

Even when companies align on priorities, they often fail to act because:

- No one owns the next steps.
- Teams revisit the decision multiple times.
- Bureaucracy slows implementation.

The Solution: A Time-Boxed Execution Framework

Alignment must immediately lead to execution. This happens through:

1. A clear decision mandate – The final decision is documented and owned by leadership.
2. Time-boxed execution deadlines – No room for revisiting old discussions.
3. Ongoing alignment check-ins – Ensures execution stays on track.
   - Preventing alignment from being a theoretical exercise.
   - Ensuring decisions translate into action fast.
   - Building a culture of momentum and execution.

The Key Takeaway: Alignment Should Take Days, Not Months

Organizations don't need months of internal debates to align their teams. They need a structured framework that collects input instantly, resolves conflicts objectively, and turns alignment into execution immediately.

By following this 3-step process, businesses can:

- Unlock alignment in days, not months
- Ensure every stakeholder is heard without slowing down
- Use data to drive structured decision-making, not opinions
- Turn consensus into immediate execution

Move as One or Fall Behind

Alignment is not about compromise. It's about momentum.

It's not about everyone agreeing. It's about everyone seeing clearly.

When intelligence is shared, speed follows.

When priorities are visible, execution begins.

The companies that move as one will lead.

The rest will keep debating while the market moves on.

In the next chapter, we'll show you how to turn alignment into continuous improvement so you never stall again.

Clarity. Action. Movement. That's how smart organizations break free.

CHAPTER 7

Step 3 – Evolving at the Speed of Intelligence

Why Technology Innovation Must Be Ongoing

Innovation isn't a one-time decision; it's a continuous discipline.

Too many companies approach technology and customer experience (CX) transformation as a one-time event, a project to be completed rather than a mindset to be cultivated.

They invest in new technology, a revamped customer journey, or an AI-driven contact center and assume that they've finished their work. They basically repeat the same design and mimic the programming from the previous solution. They celebrate the launch, announce the transformation, and expect long-term success from a single initiative.

But in today's fast-moving business landscape, this one-and-done mentality is a recipe for failure.

- Customer expectations are constantly evolving. What worked last year may feel outdated today.
- Technology is advancing faster than ever. A cutting-edge solution today could be obsolete in months.
- Competitors are continuously improving. If you're not evolving, they will—and your customers will follow them.

The organizations that thrive in this new era aren't the ones with the best tools. They're the ones with the best reflexes. They listen in real time, adapt without waiting, and build systems that evolve faster than the challenges around them.

Technology doesn't transform companies. Intelligence does. And intelligence is continuous.

This chapter introduces a structured, repeatable process that allows companies to:

- Stop treating technology and CX improvements as one-time projects.
- Embed continuous innovation into the company's DNA.
- Use real-time feedback and data to refine technology and CX strategy constantly.

Customer experience is never "done." It is either improving or falling behind.

The Cost of Stagnation: Why One-Time Technology Projects Often Fail

These companies didn't fail because they lacked tools.

They failed because they treated a transformation like a finish line, not a feedback loop.

Before we break down the continuous improvement framework, let's examine why so many "big tech initiatives" fail when treated as a single event rather than an ongoing strategy.

1. Customer Needs Change Faster Than Static CX Programs

Companies that invest once and stop evolving eventually see their CX efforts decay.

- A retailer rolls out a new omnichannel shopping experience but fails to iterate, and customer complaints about mobility usage surge within a year.
- A telecom company implements a chatbot for customer service but never refines its responses based on real customer feedback. As a result, the chatbot becomes frustrating instead of helpful.
- A bank upgrades its call center technology but ignores new AI and self-service advancements, and customers defect to competitors utilizing smarter automation.

2. Technology Moves Too Fast for One-Time Fixes

The pace of technological change is outpacing traditional business timelines.

- AI-driven chatbots evolve monthly—but many companies fail to update them, sometimes for years.
- Self-service portals become outdated if they don't continuously improve with customer needs.
- Personalization algorithms require constant refinement—a set-it-and-forget-it approach ensures they become ineffective.

3. Competitors Are Always Innovating

If your business is standing still, your competitors are passing you.

- Amazon updates its CX experience constantly, testing and refining every part of the customer journey.
- Tesla treats its vehicles as evolving products, deploying software updates that improve the customer experience years after purchase.
- Apple refines its retail experience continuously, integrating new technology and adapting to customer expectations.

Improvement isn't a project. It's a posture. The most advanced organizations treat their internal systems like living organisms, always listening, always adapting, always learning.

The 3-Step Framework for Continuous Innovation in AI, Unified Communications, CX, and Contact Center Technologies for Internal Stakeholders

The Problem with Traditional Technology Improvement Models

Most organizations rely on outdated, rigid processes to evaluate and implement CX, AI, and contact center technology improvements for their internal teams. The common approach is to conduct an annual review, gather feedback, analyze pain points, and roll out changes—but only once a year.

This model is fundamentally broken.

Technology evolves every month, if not every week, and internal teams—from IT and operations to contact center managers and frontline employees—can't afford to wait months or years for critical improvements. When internal users struggle with outdated tools, slow processes, and inefficient workflows, the entire business suffers.

For organizations to stay competitive and empower their internal teams, they need a continuous innovation framework—one that ensures CX, AI, and contact center solutions evolve at the speed of business, not the speed of bureaucracy.

The New Model for Continuous Internal Innovation

This chapter outlines a 3-step framework that businesses can adopt to ensure that internal teams—IT, operations, contact center leaders, and frontline employees—always have the tools and support they need to succeed:

1. **Listen Before it Breaks** – Continuously listen to employees, track system performance, and identify inefficiencies.
2. **Refine in Motion** – Deliver small, ongoing improvements instead of waiting for large-scale upgrades.
3. **Make Testing the Culture** – Empower teams to test, refine, and optimize workflows and technology continuously.

By adopting this approach, businesses can:

- Reduce internal frustration caused by outdated systems and slow improvements.
- Ensure IT and operations teams stay ahead of technology trends instead of reacting too late.
- Optimize workforce productivity by eliminating inefficiencies before they escalate.

Step 1: Listen Before It Breaks

Why Traditional Internal Feedback Models Fail

Most organizations rely on delayed, disconnected feedback loops, leaving internal teams stuck with inefficient tools and processes for far too long.

Common outdated methods include:

✗ Annual employee surveys – By the time results are reviewed, priorities have shifted.
✗ Manual help desk tickets – Issues pile up, and resolutions take weeks or months.
✗ Reactive system audits – IT and operations teams only address problems after they disrupt productivity.

The result? Frustrated employees, misaligned priorities, and a reactive IT and operations strategy that constantly plays catch-up.

The Solution: Continuous, Real-Time Listening for Internal Users

Instead of waiting for internal frustrations to boil over, organizations must proactively collect real-time feedback and performance data from internal teams.

☑ AI-driven monitoring of system performance – Detects slowdowns, inefficiencies, and usability issues before employees report them.
☑ Live employee feedback loops – Gather insights from internal users immediately after they interact with a system rather than waiting for quarterly reviews.
☑ Cross-team collaboration platforms – Enables IT, operations, and frontline teams to flag issues and propose improvements in real-time.

A real-time feedback loop ensures that IT and operations teams can identify and resolve inefficiencies before they impact productivity rather than reacting after the damage is done.

Step 2: Refine in Motion

Why Organizations Struggle to Act on Internal Technology Issues

Even after identifying problems, many businesses fail to implement improvements quickly due to:

- ✗ Slow approval processes that delay needed updates.
- ✗ Fear of disrupting existing workflows.
- ✗ Departments working in silos, causing misalignment and inefficiency.

This hesitation leads to widespread inefficiencies—while technology advances, internal teams are stuck waiting for upgrades, process improvements, and system optimizations that should have happened months ago.

The Solution: A Structured, Agile Iteration Model for Internal Innovation

Instead of waiting for large-scale system overhauls, businesses must adopt an agile, iterative approach to internal technology improvements.

The 3-Part Iteration Model for Internal Teams

1. **Identify small, high-impact improvements** – Instead of waiting for a complete system upgrade, roll out quick enhancements that improve usability and efficiency immediately.

2. **Test and measure rapidly** – Use A/B testing, sandbox environments, and pilot rollouts to ensure new changes improve internal workflows before full deployment.

3. **Scale what works and discard what doesn't** – Expand successful innovations quickly, while ineffective solutions should be refined or phased out without delay.

   ☑ Prevents massive system failures caused by outdated, neglected technology.

   ☑ Reduces resistance to change by introducing improvements incrementally.

   ☑ Ensures internal teams always have the best tools available to maximize efficiency.

The most successful organizations don't wait for technology to become obsolete before upgrading—they continuously refine and optimize their internal systems, keeping their workforce at peak productivity.

Step 3: Make Testing the Culture

The Problem: Corporate Resistance to Change

Many businesses struggle to adopt a continuous improvement mindset internally because of the following:

✗ Fear of disrupting existing processes.

✗ Leaders who prefer large, traditional rollouts over agile, ongoing improvements.

✗ Employees who are hesitant to suggest changes due to bureaucratic barriers.

When businesses punish failure instead of treating it as a learning opportunity, internal teams stop innovating, and businesses fall behind.

The Solution: An Experimentation-Driven Culture for Internal Innovation

High-performing organizations don't wait for perfection; they create environments where continuous testing, learning, and adaptation are standard practice.

How?

- Encourage small, low-risk experiments – Pilot new technologies and workflows with a small group before scaling them organization-wide.
- Empower employees to propose process improvements – Frontline teams use technology daily, and their feedback should directly shape system optimizations.
- Reward internal innovation – Recognize and incentivize teams that proactively improve internal workflows, AI integrations, and CX technologies.

By fostering an internal culture of experimentation, businesses create a workforce that embraces change instead of resisting it, leading to faster adoption of AI, smarter CX strategies, and optimized contact center operations.

"Rich is the definition of a business disruptor. His expertise in consulting and technology adoption has helped leaders like myself rethink the way we approach change. He doesn't just talk about speed; he shows you exactly how to achieve it. If you're looking to get ahead of the competition, this book is the answer."
— Missy Porth, AVP, Worksite Capabilities, Enterprise Insurance Company

Final Takeaway: Intelligence Doesn't Pause. Neither Should You.

The era of "set it and forget it" is over.

Organizations that wait "to evolve" fall behind, quietly, then suddenly.

The future belongs to the companies that evolve continuously.

That listen relentlessly.

That empowers their teams not just to execute, but to improve the system itself.

That's how you activate the intelligence within. Not once. Always.

Are you ready to empower your internal teams with **truCX?**

CHAPTER 8

The Transformation:
When Intelligence Leads,
Everything Changes

The Moment Everything Changes

Every company hits a moment of reckoning.

The systems stop working, the meetings go in circles, and the old playbook feels heavier than the opportunity ahead.

The question is no longer if you need to change. It's: **Are you built to move?**

This chapter is about what happens when the answer is yes.

Some organizations stay stuck, trapped in slow decision-making, internal misalignment, and CX strategies that fail to evolve. They remain comfortable but stagnant, watching competitors surpass them while customers drift away.

But the organizations that choose to break free experience something radically different:

- They move with speed and confidence, making decisions in weeks instead of years.
- They align their entire organization, eliminating delays caused by silos and conflicting priorities.
- They embrace continuous improvement, ensuring they are constantly innovating and meeting evolving customer expectations.

And the impact?

- Increased revenue from faster, customer-centric decision-making.
- Higher customer satisfaction as technology and CX initiatives drive real, measurable change.
- Greater agility to pivot and adapt to market shifts before competitors.
- More engaged employees who feel empowered to drive transformation.

When you activate the intelligence within, you unlock something more than alignment. You unlock acceleration.

Breaking Free from Stagnation

The tragedy is that most companies aren't lacking ideas. They're drowning in them.

They lack **shared intelligence and a system for acting on it**, which keeps them stuck.

Before diving into the transformation stories, it's important to understand why so many organizations struggle to break free in the first place.

1. Fear of Change

Many companies operate under a mindset of:

"We've always done it this way."
"Change is risky, what if we make the wrong decision?"
"Let's wait until we have all the information before moving forward."

But in today's business landscape, standing still is more dangerous than making the wrong move. Companies that hesitate fall behind, quickly and quietly.

2. Overdependence on Outside Experts

Too often, organizations wait for consultants or vendors to define their problems, delaying progress and outsourcing clarity.

"Let's bring someone in to tell us what to do."
"We'll move faster once we get the report."
"We need outside validation before we align internally."

But real transformation can't be outsourced. Breakthroughs happen when teams trust their own insights and activate shared intelligence from within.

3. Misplaced Focus on Tools Over Truth

In the rush to modernize, many businesses chase technology instead of clarity.

"What tool should we buy?"
"This new platform will fix everything."
"If we implement it fast, results will follow."

But without alignment and purpose, even the best tech becomes shelfware. The smartest organizations don't lead with tools, they lead with truth.

The Breakthrough: Real-World Stories of Transformation

Now, let's explore three powerful stories of businesses that broke free, embraced a new way of working, and unlocked massive improvements in customer experience, agility, and profitability.

What does it look like when internal intelligence replaces internal friction?

Story #1: From 12 Months to 90 Days — When Momentum Takes Over

The Problem: A Slow, Bureaucratic Decision-Making Process amongst 25 key stakeholders

A leading healthcare BPO struggled with CX transformation because every decision required approval from multiple teams - including IT, security, development, human resources, operations, and customer service.

- A new digital agent interface initiative took over a year to approve due to conflicting priorities and endless meetings.
- Employees grew frustrated, waiting for improvements that never materialized.
- Momentum for the project slowed as the anticipated technology migration away from stagnant and older platforms seemed unlikely.

The Breakthrough: A New Decision-Making Framework and Company-Wide Contact Center and CX Alignment

By adopting **truCX** as a structured decision-making model, they transformed their process:

- Automated internal discovery eliminated months of consultant interviews.
- A real-time prioritization framework surfaced the most urgent needs immediately.
- Data-driven analytics provided data-backed insights to align leadership quickly.

The Outcome: Faster Decisions, Happier Employees, Executive Alignment

- Decision-making timelines went from 12 months to just 90 days.
- CX and technology initiatives went live 5x faster, improving customer retention.
- Adding new features and capabilities is now much faster and easier.

By using a structured alignment process, the company:

- Conducted real-time journeys that gathered input from all teams.
- Used dashboards to surface common priorities and trade-offs.
- Implemented a clear roadmap for CX transformation with buy-in from all departments.

Key Takeaway: By eliminating internal bottlenecks, organizations can move at market speed instead of being held back by bureaucratic inertia.

Story #2: When Alignment Powers Progress

The Problem: Disconnected Departments & Conflicting Priorities

A mid-size utility provider was facing mounting pressure to modernize how it served customers in an increasingly digital world—but internal misalignment was stalling progress.

- IT was laser-focused on system reliability and regulatory compliance, deprioritizing self-service upgrades and digital channels.
- Customer service and CX teams pushed for personalized, seamless interactions but lacked the influence to shift priorities.
- Finance leaders were hesitant to approve cloud migrations or invest in modern platforms due to concerns about cost volatility.

These disconnects between departments caused:

- Rising call volumes due to poor digital self-service.
- Growing customer dissatisfaction over long wait times and limited support options.
- Lost trust and customer attrition as competitors embraced smarter, more proactive service models.

The Breakthrough: Aligning the Internal Intelligence of the Teams
Through a deliberate, organization-wide alignment strategy, the utility company was able to shift course:

- Ran cross-functional technology journeys and frameworks to capture pain points and goals from every department.
- Leveraged AI-driven insights and business intelligence to identify shared priorities and key capabilities.
- Developed and rolled out a unified roadmap for customer experience transformation, with every function at the table.

Key Takeaway: When everyone rallies around improvement, the impact is transformational.

Alignment doesn't just smooth internal operations; it accelerates innovation, drives adoption, and secures long-term success.

Story #3: Always Evolving — Why Loyalty Loves Progress

The Problem: A Stagnant CX Strategy

A fast-growing SaaS company had seen early success, but as competitors entered the market, customer retention began to decline.

- They implemented a CX strategy two years before but never refined it.
- Customer expectations evolved, but their support model remained static.
- They collected product feedback but rarely acted on it.

The company assumed its initial CX success would last forever, but it was a one-time snapshot of a plan and lacked continuous improvement, so it fell behind.

The Breakthrough: Embedding Continuous Technology Innovation

By shifting to a continuous technology improvement model, they:

- Launched real-time journeys as projects became relevant, reducing time spent on research by up to 40%.
- Created a trends and comparisons framework, surfacing insights around improvements within months after after Go Live projects.
- Embedded technology innovation into company culture, rewarding employees for improving customer experience initiatives and participation in company projects.

Key Takeaway: Technology transformation is never finished. Companies that continuously evolve outperform those that remain static.

What It Means to Operate With Intelligence and What It Delivers

When you break free, it's not just your decisions that get faster. It's your entire system of growth.

- You stop guessing and start knowing.
- You stop rehashing and start releasing.
- You stop waiting and start leading.

The transformation isn't a future state. It's a new operating rhythm.

And once you experience it? You'll never go back to the old way again.

**The intelligent organization isn't an idea.
It's an advantage.**

The question is, are you ready to operate at that level?

**Break free. Move fast. Think together.
Decide forward.**

CHAPTER 9

Speed Is What Intelligence Feels Like in Motion

Why Speed is the Ultimate Business Advantage

Speed is not a shortcut.

It's not recklessness—it's what happens when an organization **knows itself well enough to move with clarity**.

Speed isn't about going faster just to keep up. It's about **accelerating with intention**, fueled by the intelligence already inside your business.

In today's business world, speed is everything. Companies that move quickly set the standard for innovation, capture market share, and dominate their industries. Speed is the defining factor between winning and losing, between being the disruptor and being disrupted.

Organizations that hesitate while waiting for the perfect moment, overanalyzing decisions, and operating with bureaucratic inefficiencies ultimately find themselves left behind. The marketplace does not wait for companies to catch up, and customers do not pause their expectations to give slow-moving businesses time to improve.

> **The organizations that operate with speed aren't just ahead. They're aligned, informed, and unshackled.**

Speed is not just about making decisions quickly for the sake of efficiency. It is about achieving a level of agility that allows businesses to seize opportunities before their competitors, adjust to market shifts in real-time, and continuously innovate.

Organizations that embrace fast, well-informed decision-making consistently outperform those that rely on traditional, drawn-out processes. They win more customers because they are the first to deliver the experiences that modern consumers demand. They attract top talent because high performers want to work for companies that take action rather than getting stuck in analysis paralysis. They innovate at scale, constantly refining their offerings while competitors remain bogged down by outdated ways of thinking.

Despite this reality, many businesses still cling to slow, bureaucratic decision-making processes. They operate under the false belief that taking more time will result in better outcomes, that endless internal discussions will eventually lead to the perfect strategy, or that waiting until they've mitigated all possible risks is the safest approach. This is a lie.

The truth is that indecision is far more dangerous than making the wrong decision. A company that makes a decision, even if imperfect, can adjust, refine, and move forward. A company that remains frozen in uncertainty never progresses.

"The Intelligence Within doesn't just challenge how organizations think—it rewires how they move. In an era of AI acceleration, this book delivers the missing blueprint: how to harness discovery as a system, not a stall. It's bold, brilliant, and long overdue."
— Geoffrey A. Best, AI Strategist & Bestselling Author of the 42 Rules trilogy for Using, Planning, and Managing AI in Your Contact Center

---

The cost of indecision is often invisible until it is too late.

- The companies that stall aren't starved for information; they're bloated with unstructured opinions.
- While they spin in unproductive cycles, intelligent organizations decide, act, and learn in a cycle that wins.
- While executives and teams spend months deliberating, competitors are already executing, adapting, and gaining an insurmountable lead.
- Customers grow frustrated with the lack of progress and turn to companies that are actively improving their experience.
- Talented employees, eager to contribute to something dynamic and forward-thinking, leave for organizations that embrace momentum.

The worst part is that many slow-moving companies do not realize the full extent of the damage until they are too far behind to recover.

This chapter will prove why speed is the ultimate competitive advantage. It will demonstrate how companies that embrace fast, data-driven decision-making gain an edge that is nearly impossible for competitors to replicate. More importantly, it will provide a roadmap for organizations that are ready to break free from sluggish processes and take control of their future.

The good news is that businesses do not have to figure this out alone. Many organizations recognize the need for speed but struggle with execution. They face internal resistance, conflicting priorities, and legacy systems that slow down progress. However, with the right frameworks, tools, and guidance, any organization can transform its approach and start making decisions at the pace required to thrive in today's economy.

Here's where the right partner becomes invaluable. Organizations that choose to work with experts in rapid decision-making and customer experience innovation can bypass the common obstacles that slow companies down. Instead of wasting time trying to reinvent the wheel, they can leverage proven methodologies that accelerate their transformation.

The companies that will lead the future are the ones that commit to speed, alignment, and continuous innovation. They recognize that the biggest risk is not taking a calculated leap forward but standing still while the world moves ahead. The time to act is now. The businesses that break free today will be the industry leaders of tomorrow.

Organizations that commit to fast, intelligent decision-making consistently leave their competitors behind.

- They earn customer loyalty by acting on insight before others even recognize the opportunity.
- They draw elite talent—people who want to build, not wait.
- They outpace disruption by iterating faster than legacy businesses can respond

Still, too many companies confuse caution with strategy. They rely on drawn-out reviews, endless approvals, and outdated governance models—thinking time will solve what only clarity can.

But here's the truth:
Hesitation is the real risk.

Every day spent overthinking is a day your competition is executing. In a market defined by speed, delay isn't safer—it's lethal.

This chapter reveals why velocity with insight outperforms slow consensus, and how the smartest organizations are building decision systems that create clarity, drive alignment, and fuel unstoppable momentum.

The good news? You don't have to figure it out alone. We are the force multiplier you need to break free.

> *"Rich is a person with the highest level of integrity, outstanding business knowledge, and expert insights in the voice, contact center, and CX space. He cuts through the clutter to get to the heart of the issue, gives incredible advice, and is willing to share his vast knowledge to help you and your team be better."*
> — Jeffrey Berger, CIO, Jacob Stern & Sons

The Companies That Move Fast, Win

Speed isn't just a nice-to-have—it's the defining trait of the world's most successful companies.

The organizations that lead their industries are obsessed with moving faster than their competitors. They don't wait for perfect conditions; they take action, adjust, and refine as they go.

Let's look at some of the world's most dominant companies and how their speed-first approach has made them unbeatable.

Amazon: Speed as a Growth Strategy

Amazon is the undisputed king of speed.

- It launched Prime's two-day shipping in 2005, forcing every competitor to either adapt or become irrelevant.
- It constantly experiments and iterates, rolling out thousands of small innovations every year rather than waiting for one big transformation.
- Its supply chain, AI recommendations, and customer service improvements are all designed to move at a pace its competitors can't match.

Amazon doesn't wait until every detail is perfect—it moves quickly, gathers data, and improves while others are still debating.

Tesla: The Fastest Innovator in the Automotive Industry
Tesla didn't just change the auto industry—it reinvented it.

- Traditional car companies spend 5+ years developing a new model.
- Tesla continuously updates vehicles with software improvements in real-time.
- It innovates at a speed legacy automakers can't keep up with, rolling out new features before the competition even realizes they're necessary.

Netflix: Rapid Adaptation Creates Market Domination
Netflix moved fast and broke the entertainment industry.

- It transitioned from DVD rentals to streaming faster than anyone expected, leaving Blockbuster scrambling.
- It pioneered original content at scale, making quick decisions on what works instead of long approval cycles.
- While competitors are still trying to figure out streaming, Netflix is already optimizing AI-driven content personalization.

The common theme?
These companies don't wait. They move. And because of that, they win. Now, let's talk about why speed isn't just for tech giants; it's a competitive advantage for every industry.

Why Slow Companies Are Losing More Than Ever

The companies that still believe in slow, careful decision-making are losing customers, talent, and revenue at an alarming rate.

Here's why:

1. Customers Expect Instant Improvements

- Customers today demand rapid innovation—they won't wait months (or years) for you to catch up.
- If they see better experiences elsewhere, they switch. Earning loyalty happens through constant evolution, not one-time fixes.
- Companies that wait too long to innovate find themselves irrelevant overnight.

2. Talent Flocks to Companies That Take Action

- The best employees don't want to work for slow-moving companies.
- Top talent thrives in fast, innovative environments where decisions happen quickly.
- If your company is known for bureaucratic red tape, endless meetings, and slow execution, you'll lose your best people to companies that move fast and make things happen.

3. Competitors Who Move Faster Will Outperform You

- If a competitor launches a better product, improves their CX, or adopts new technology faster than you, they capture market share before you even start.
- The longer you take to decide, the more ground you lose.

"Speed is the new competitive advantage, and no one understands that better than Rich. His consulting expertise has helped businesses rethink discovery, accelerate decision-making, and adopt technology at record speed. If you want to future-proof your company and lead with confidence, this book is essential reading."
— Shailesh Goswami, Chief Executive Officer, Foyr

The bottom line? If your business isn't constantly making fast, data-driven decisions, you're already falling behind.

Now, let's talk about how you can fix this before it's too late.

Breaking Free: The Speed-Driven Business Model

We've helped organizations just like yours go from slow, stagnant, and struggling to keep up → to → fast, agile, and industry-leading.

The difference? They embraced the Speed-Driven Business Model.

This model contains three principles:

1. Let The Signal Lead – No more waiting months for research—use real-time insights to make decisions instantly.
2. Unlock the Brain – Cut through the red tape and tap into the "tribal knowledge" known as internal intelligence.
3. Stay In Motion – Move quickly, refine as you go, and stay ahead of your competitors.

Now, let's break it down step by step.

Step 1: Let The Signal Lead

Slow decision-making happens when companies rely on opinions instead of data.

Our model replaces outdated decision-making processes with a structured, real-time data framework.

- Instead of holding endless stakeholder meetings, businesses use real-time analytics to surface the best choices instantly.
- AI-powered insights rank priorities objectively, eliminating the need for months of internal debates.
- Leaders can see business needs in real time instead of waiting for consultant reports that are outdated before being read.

Momentum Moments:
A large healthcare BPO used this approach to reduce technology evaluation timelines from 14 months to 6 weeks, giving them a massive advantage over competitors who were still debating options.

Step 2: Unlock The Brain

One of the biggest obstacles to speed is internal roadblocks.
Our model helps organizations cut through red tape and make decisions 10x faster.

- Streamlining decision-making so approvals happen in days, not months.
- Eliminating siloed department conflicts by aligning teams through structured prioritization.
- Removing low-value meetings that slow down execution.

Momentum Moments:
A utility company implemented our bureaucracy-busting frameworks and reduced data gathering to less than 30 days to drive their core technology requirements.

Step 3: Stay In Motion

Speed isn't just about making decisions quickly; it's about constantly improving.

Companies that embrace speed don't wait for perfect plans - they act, gather feedback, and refine continuously.

- Launch new initiatives quickly, then optimize them based on real-world data.
- Use A/B testing, customer feedback, and rapid iteration to improve CX on the fly.
- Make continuous improvement part of company culture, so you're always ahead of the curve.

Momentum Moments:
A SaaS company that adopted this approach cut product research cycles by more than 40% by implementing a time-based approach to driving "real" business requirements.

The Future Doesn't Wait. Neither Should You.

Speed is no longer a "nice to have." It's the new baseline.

Organizations that lead don't wait for permission. They move. They listen to their internal signal. And they act before competitors even finish talking.

Here is what business agility really means:

- Decisions in days, not quarters.
- Technology data gathering weekly, not annually.
- Measuring momentum in weeks, not strategy decks.

Speed isn't the risk. It's the insurance policy.

And it starts with activating the intelligence within.

CHAPTER 10

The Future Isn't Given. It's Taken.

The Crossroads of Transformation

Every business stands at a decision point.

Not someday. Not next quarter. **Right now.**

The choice? Evolve—or evaporate.

Move boldly—or drift quietly into irrelevance.

This is not about transformation theory. It's about whether you're ready to lead or become a distant story from the past.

Every business eventually arrives at a crossroads where a crucial decision must be made. Do you continue operating as usual, following the same processes, relying on outdated methods, and hoping for the best?

This is not a theoretical decision. It defines the future of every organization. Those who adapt and move forward with confidence will dominate their industries, while those who hesitate, resist, or fail to act will struggle to remain relevant.

The world is changing faster than ever before. Technology is advancing at an exponential rate, customer expectations are constantly evolving, and market dynamics are shifting in unpredictable ways. The traditional playbook that businesses once relied upon is no longer effective.

> **The companies that will lead the next era of customer experience are not waiting for change to happen to them; they are driving change proactively, shaping the future on their terms.**

The companies that will lead the next era of customer experience are not waiting for change to happen to them; they are driving change proactively, shaping the future on their terms.

This final chapter is a call to action. It is an opportunity for business leaders to commit to breaking free from the old ways of working and step into a future where speed, alignment, and innovation are the cornerstones of success.

This is not just about staying competitive; it is about becoming a category leader, setting the pace for others to follow, and ensuring that customer experience is not just a function within the business but a strategic advantage that propels growth.

The Harsh Reality: Businesses That Hesitate Will Be Left Behind

History has shown time and time again that businesses that fail to adapt eventually become obsolete. There is no clearer example than the retail industry, where companies like Blockbuster and Sears once reigned supreme but are now cautionary tales of what happens when organizations refuse to evolve. These companies had every opportunity to innovate, embrace new technologies, and shift their strategies. Instead, they chose to stick with what had worked in the past, falsely assuming that their dominance would protect them from disruption.

In today's digital-first economy, this same reality is playing out across every industry. Customer expectations are no longer static; they evolve continuously based on the experiences delivered by market leaders. Customers do not compare businesses within the same industry; they compare every experience to the best they have ever had. If an organization does not consistently raise the bar, customers will find an alternative that does.

For those who hesitate, the cost of inaction is staggering. The inevitable outcome for those who wait is the loss of customers to competitors who are moving faster, the inability to attract top talent who want to work for forward-thinking organizations, and the eventual erosion of market share. Businesses that fail to move at the speed of customer expectations will find themselves trapped in a cycle of declining relevance, forced into reactive decisions rather than proactive innovation.

What the Future Looks Like for Businesses That Break Free

If you're reading this, you're already ahead. You know speed isn't chaos; it's clarity. You've seen how alignment turns noise into signal.

You've understood that intelligence isn't hiding; rather it's just been trapped in slow systems.

But knowing isn't the end. **Acting is.**

Organizations that embrace the future with boldness and determination will find themselves in a vastly different position. These businesses will not only survive the changing landscape but will thrive in it. They will set the standard for customer experience, leading their industries by constantly evolving, iterating, and delivering unparalleled value.

A future-driven organization does not view transformation as a one-time project but as a continuous journey. These companies do not wait for annual strategy reviews to determine their next steps; they operate in real-time, using data-driven insights to make decisions quickly and effectively. They recognize that customer experience is never "done," and because of this mindset, they consistently outperform competitors who are still following traditional decision-making models.

When businesses break free from outdated methods, decision-making accelerates. What once took months can happen in weeks or even days. Teams operate with alignment, eliminating the frustrating bottlenecks that slow progress. Employees feel empowered, knowing that their contributions directly influence the company's success rather than being buried in bureaucracy. Customers notice the difference, feeling a stronger connection to a brand that is always improving and innovating.

Financial performance follows this transformation. Revenue grows faster because customers stay longer, engage more deeply, and become brand advocates. Precise decisions and the elimination of operational inefficiencies increase profitability. Competitive differentiation becomes stronger as the organization becomes known for delivering exceptional experiences that no one else can match.

The Force Multiplier That Makes It Possible

Many business leaders understand the importance of transformation, but they struggle with where to start. They recognize the need for speed, agility, and continuous innovation, but the internal challenges of alignment, decision-making, and execution seem overwhelming. Here is where the right partner becomes a force multiplier.

Organizations that attempt to navigate transformation on their own often find themselves stuck in the same cycles of inefficiency that they were trying to escape. Without a structured approach, internal resistance can stall progress. Without the right frameworks, alignment can remain elusive. Without external expertise, teams may default to what is familiar, even if it is ineffective.

Working with a force multiplier means gaining access to a proven model that accelerates transformation without the typical roadblocks. It means having the tools, processes, and insights necessary to move quickly, align teams effortlessly, and embed continuous improvement into the company's culture. Rather than struggling to reinvent the wheel, businesses that partner with experts in CX innovation can focus on execution, seeing tangible results faster than they ever thought possible.

The Path to Becoming a Market Leader

Organizations that commit to breaking free and embracing the future of customer experience are not just making incremental improvements; they are making a fundamental shift in how they operate. They are choosing to prioritize customer-centricity at a level that competitors cannot match. They are choosing to move at a pace that others cannot keep up with. They are choosing to create an ecosystem where innovation is not just encouraged but expected.

The path forward is clear. It begins with eliminating slow, outdated decision-making processes and replacing them with a structured framework for speed and agility. It requires aligning teams around a shared vision so that every department is working toward the same goals rather than competing for priorities. It demands an unwavering commitment to continuous CX improvement, ensuring that the business is always evolving to meet and exceed customer expectations.

For those who take this path, the rewards are immense: the ability to attract and retain customers who become lifelong advocates, the competitive edge that comes from always being one step ahead of the market, the financial growth that comes from increased efficiency and smarter decision-making, and the cultural transformation that turns employees into innovators who drive progress from within.

Proof in Motion: From Talk to Global Standard

"Every organization talks about digital transformation, but few know how to do it without getting stuck in bureaucracy and inefficiency. Rich has cracked the code on how to move fast, cut through friction, and get technology implemented without the usual headaches. His insights are invaluable for any executive serious about accelerating success. His recommendations have led to a global standard for us. Truly a business partner in every sense."

— Ken Wierman, VP & Chief Information Officer,
(recently retired)

The Breaking Point: Will You Seize Control or Be Left Behind?

Right now, at this very moment, you stand at a crossroads. What you have in your hands isn't just another business book; it's a warning. The strategies you've read aren't hypothetical; they are the proven playbook of companies that refuse to die in mediocrity.

Some will read this book and file it away.

Others will turn it into a movement.

If you want to win in the era of real-time technology decision-making, here's the truth:

You don't need more meetings. You don't need more demos.

You don't need another consultant deck.

You need to **move**.

Make speed your culture.

Make intelligence your engine.

Make alignment your advantage.

The future isn't something you observe. It's something you build.

The Intelligence Within was never missing. You just hadn't set it free until now.

CONCLUSION

The Future Is Built From Within

Taking Action is Critical

Every business leader faces a choice: stay in place or step into motion.

Not someday. **Now.**

You've seen what happens when organizations cling to the old way, slow, siloed, reactive.

You've also seen what's possible when they break free:

- Decisions in days and weeks
- Alignment in real-time
- Innovation that doesn't pause

And it all begins with one truth: **The intelligence you need is already inside your business. You just haven't activated it— until now.**

What a Future-Built Organization Looks Like

Imagine running a business where momentum is your default setting.

- CX is no longer an initiative. It's an instinct.
- AI and automation don't replace people, they elevate them.
- Your contact center becomes a crystal ball, seeing what's coming before your customers even ask.
- Decision-making becomes a rhythm, not a ritual.

This is what happens when you operate with speed and clarity when you stop waiting and start leading, and when your culture stops asking for permission and starts building the future.

It's What Your Bigger, Better Future Looks Like

What Happens If You Don't

But let's be honest, there's another pathOne where you hesitate while others accelerate.

Where the best employees leave, the best customers defect, and the best ideas stay stuck in slide decks, where relevance quietly fades until it's gone.

Organizations that delay don't maintain their position. They lose it.

And in a world where expectations shift every quarter, the cost of hesitation is exponential.

Your Defining Moment

You are not at the end of a book.

You are at the beginning of a decision.

You've seen the frameworks.

You've heard the stories.

You know what works.

Now it's your move.

Will you stay in the debate?

Or move into action?

Will you default to what's comfortable?

Or commit to what's necessary? Because the companies that win next won't be the ones that talk about change.

They'll be the ones who operate like it's already here.

One Final Thought

The intelligence within you is ready. The market is moving.

The future belongs to the bold.

Break free—and lead.

What to Do Next

You've read the insights. You've seen the blueprint. You understand the urgency.

Now, it's time to act.

Step 1: Decide That You're Ready to Break Free

Transformation begins with a decision. If you recognize that your business can no longer afford slow decision-making, internal misalignment, and outdated CX strategies, then commit to moving forward right now. The companies that win are the ones that take decisive action.

Step 2: Get in Touch With Us

You don't have to navigate this journey alone. We are the force multiplier that will help you implement the strategies you've just read about—faster, smarter, and with immediate impact. The next step is simple: reach out. Let's discuss your challenges, your goals, and how we can help you accelerate success.

Step 3: Execute with Speed and Precision

Once we agree on your organization's needs, we move fast. There is no lengthy sales cycle and no wasted time. Together, we'll deploy a structured, data-driven approach to transform how your company makes decisions, aligns teams, and continuously innovates its customer experience.

Step 4: Lead Your Industry, Not Follow It

Companies that act now will define the future of their industries. Those that hesitate will be forced to react to change instead of driving it. The choice is clear: lead boldly, move quickly, and build a competitive advantage that no one can match.

The Future Won't Wait, And Neither Should You

The time to act is now. The longer you wait, the harder it will be to catch up. The best companies don't sit on the sidelines. They step forward, take control, and make bold moves.

So, what will you do?

Contact us today. Become a freedom fighter, the future belongs to those who break free.

FREE TRIAL

ABOUT THE AUTHOR

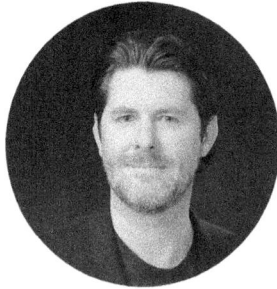

Richard Tarity is a serial entrepreneur, innovator, and Founder and CEO of truCX, the first-ever platform built to help businesses take control of customer experience (CX) and technology discovery. Designed to accelerate decision-making in the complex world of contact centers, unified communications, AI, and CX, truCX reflects Richard's mission: to simplify the complex and empower organizations to move boldly.

For more than 26 years, Richard has been behind the scenes and often out in front, building technology companies from the ground up. He's a builder in every sense of the word. His work blends strategic insight with a human-centered view of technology, rooted in a deep fascination with how people emotionally connect with the tools they use. He believes the best technology doesn't just work; it resonates.

His ventures have been recognized by INC 500/5000, Deloitte Fast 50, CRN Fast 100, and the Philadelphia 100. He was named a Philadelphia Business Journal 40 Under 40 honoree for his contributions to innovation and business leadership and in 2017 received the SmartCEO's Future 50 award presented by Comcast Business.

Richard is passionate about transforming ideas into meaningful impact. He helps leaders challenge and unlearn the status quo. His work is dedicated to creating solutions that empower individuals and organizations to unlock their fullest potential and shape the future.

EXERCISES AND APPENDICES

The exercises and appendices should serve as practical tools that reinforce the book's core message, **breaking free from outdated decision-making processes and accelerating the intelligence within.** These should not just be theoretical but actionable, helping leaders apply the principles immediately. Below are **five powerful exercises and three appendices** that will add tremendous value to your organization.

EXERCISES

Exercise 1: The Decision Bottleneck Audit

Purpose: Identify where decision-making slows down in your organization and uncover the real reasons behind the delays.

Instructions:

1. **List the last five major decisions your organization made** (e.g., technology selection, process changes, platform migrations, CX improvements).
2. For each decision, answer the following:
   o **How long did it take from discussion to execution?**
   o **What were the main reasons for delays?** (Stakeholder conflicts, lack of clarity, waiting on approvals, lack of requirements, etc.)
   o **Who were the key people involved in the decision? Were the right people involved from the onset? If not, why?**
   o **How much did hesitation or delay cost the business?** (Lost revenue, missed opportunities, operational inefficiencies.)

3. **Identify patterns**—where do delays consistently occur? People? Departments? Teams?

4. **Create a decision acceleration plan**—for each bottleneck, write down one action your team can take to move faster in the future.

Outcome:

Leaders will gain clarity on what's slowing them down and create an actionable plan to eliminate delays. truCX can help you break free and move with speed and clarity.

Exercise 2: The Speed vs. Risk Matrix

Purpose: Help organizations determine which decisions require deep analysis vs. which ones should be made quickly and iteratively.

Instructions:

1. **Draw a 2x2 matrix** with:
   o **Speed (Fast vs. Slow) on the X-axis**
   o **Impact/Risk (Low vs. High) on the Y-axis**
2. **Plot your company's recent decisions** in the four quadrants:
   o **Low Risk / High Speed** (Quick decisions that can be made without hesitation)
   o **Low Risk / Slow Speed** (Unnecessary delays—should be accelerated)
   o **High Risk / High Speed** (Where structured frameworks and expert insights help drive confident execution)
   o **High Risk / Slow Speed** (Decisions requiring careful deliberation)
3. **Adjust future decision-making** by prioritizing **high-speed, low-risk decisions** and finding ways to accelerate **high-risk, high-speed** decisions through structured frameworks.

Outcome:

This exercise helps eliminate unnecessary slowdowns while ensuring critical decisions are made with precision. truCX ensures teams can accelerate decision-making when required and also provide deeper data-driven requirements when you need to move through the change process with careful decision-making.

Exercise 3: The Alignment Scorecard

Purpose: Help teams assess how aligned they are and where gaps in priority or communication exist.

Instructions:

1. **Gather key decision-makers** from different departments (IT, Finance, Marketing, Sales, CX, Operations).
2. **Individually, have each team member score** the following statements on a scale of 1-5 (1 = Strongly Disagree, 5 = Strongly Agree):
   o We have a clear and shared definition of success.
   o Our priorities align across departments.
   o We make decisions efficiently without unnecessary delays.
   o We trust data more than opinions when making decisions.
   o Our organization acts decisively on CX initiatives.
3. **Compare scores across departments**—where are the biggest gaps?
4. **Facilitate a discussion** to resolve major misalignments and create an action plan for faster, more unified decision-making.

Outcome:
That process creates immediate visibility into alignment gaps, allowing companies to resolve conflicts before they slow execution. truCX is a platform designed for all departments, teams, and stakeholders, so your organization can gain consensus as needed. And the best part—if you accidentally miss someone upfront, you can easily invite them to participate and quickly gather all their priorities and data and add to your overall insights.

Exercise 4: The "No More Waiting" Action Plan

Purpose: Help businesses create a clear roadmap to **eliminate hesitation and accelerate execution**.

Instructions:

1. **Write down one major business decision stuck in review, approval, or endless discussion.**
2. **Identify the core reasons** for the delay. What's preventing execution? (e.g., Lack of data? Internal misalignment? Fear of risk?)
3. **Define the worst-case scenario** of moving forward now— how bad would it really be?
4. **List 3 immediate actions** that could get this initiative moving in the next **seven days and unstuck**.
5. **Assign ownership**—who is responsible for making sure this happens?

Outcome:
This exercise forces teams to push past indecision and take immediate action on stalled initiatives. truCX gives organizations the ability to get projects and initiatives unstuck by providing exceptional insights. These insights are backed by sophisticated analytics that reveal the "why" behind business challenges and clearly articulate the justifications needed to drive alignment, secure funding, and accelerate execution.

Exercise 5: The "Break Free" Strategy Map

Purpose: Help organizations **visualize their transformation from slow, outdated processes to fast, strategic execution**.

Instructions:

1. **Divide a blank page into three columns:**
   o **Current State (What's Broken?)**
   o **Breaking Free (New Strategy/Approach)**
   o **Future State (Business Impact After Change)**

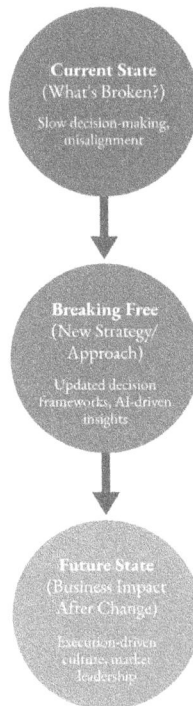

2. **Fill in each section:**
   o Identify 3-5 **inefficiencies or roadblocks** in current decision-making.
   o Write **new strategies or frameworks** you will adopt to accelerate progress.
   o Define the **expected impact** in terms of speed, efficiency, and CX success.
3. **Use this strategy map** in leadership discussions to drive accountability and execution.

Outcome:
A clear, visual transformation plan that ensures businesses are moving toward faster, smarter decision-making. truCX is the industry's first optimization platform, accelerating decision-making across many technology categories.

APPENDICES

Appendix A: The Rapid Decision-Making Framework

Overview:
This appendix provides **step-by-step diagrams** for making complex decisions in **days and weeks rather than months**.

Framework Includes:

- The **5 Key Questions** to ask before any major decision

Question	Why It Matters
What is the core business objective this decision supports?	Ensures the decision is tied to strategic goals and not just reactive.
What is the financial, operational, and CX Impact if we act—or don't act?	Defines urgency and risk factors by quantifying business impact.
Who are the key stakeholders, and how do their priorities align?	Prevents misalignment and internal roadblocks before they happen.
What data do we have to support this decision, and what data is missing?	Encourages data-driven decision-making rather than relying on opinions.

What is the minimum viable action we can take immediately to avoid delays?	Shifts focus from perfect planning to immediate execution with interactive improvements.

- The **Decision Prioritization Matrix** (how to categorize decisions based on urgency and risk)

HIGH URGENCY

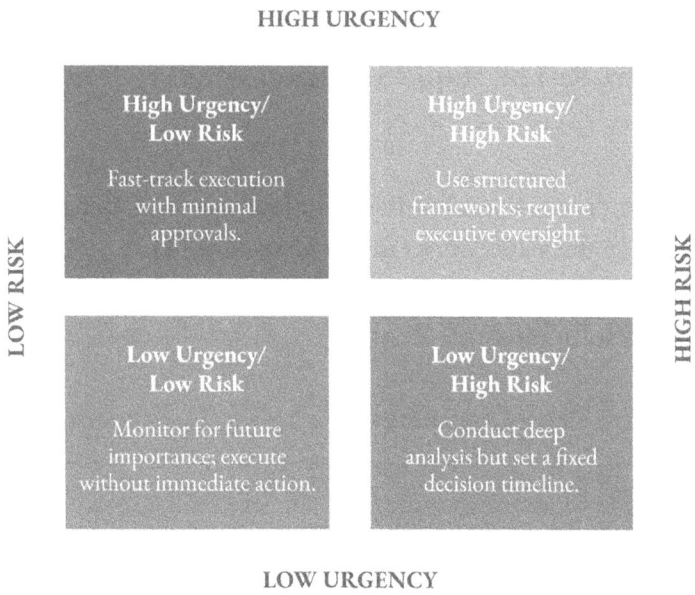

LOW RISK

High Urgency/ Low Risk

Fast-track execution with minimal approvals.

High Urgency/ High Risk

Use structured frameworks; require executive oversight.

Low Urgency/ Low Risk

Monitor for future importance; execute without immediate action.

Low Urgency/ High Risk

Conduct deep analysis but set a fixed decision timeline.

HIGH RISK

LOW URGENCY

- A **Quick-Action Playbook** for executing decisions immediately. A step-by-step execution guide to prevent over-analysis and accelerate decision-making with confidence.

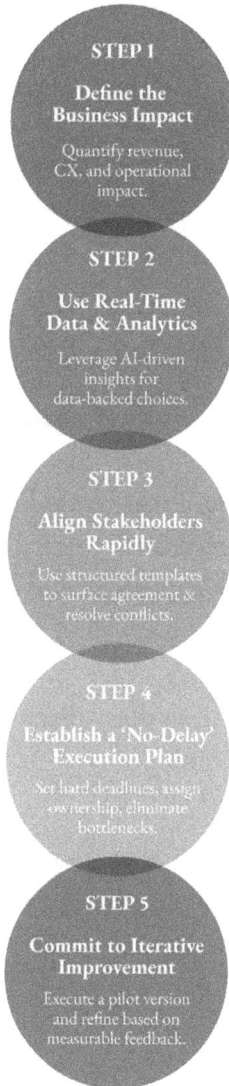

STEP 1

Define the Business Impact

Quantify revenue, CX, and operational impact.

STEP 2

Use Real-Time Data & Analytics

Leverage AI-driven insights for data-backed choices.

STEP 3

Align Stakeholders Rapidly

Use structured templates to surface agreement & resolve conflicts.

STEP 4

Establish a 'No-Delay' Execution Plan

Set hard deadlines, assign ownership, eliminate bottlenecks.

STEP 5

Commit to Iterative Improvement

Execute a pilot version and refine based on measurable feedback.

How This Helps:

It empowers leaders to stop over-analyzing and start executing with confidence.

Appendix B: The Alignment Accelerator Checklist

Overview:

A **checklist-style guide** that organizations can use **before** making a major business or technology decision to ensure alignment across all stakeholders.

Checklist Includes:

- Have all key stakeholders **agreed on the problem we are solving?**
- Is there a **structured way to rank priorities?**
- Have we **eliminated unnecessary approval delays?**
- Do we have **clear next steps and execution plans?**

How This Helps:
It prevents **misalignment, endless discussions, and last-minute roadblocks** that stall execution.

Appendix C: Breaking Free—The 90-Day Action Plan

Overview:

A structured **90-day roadmap** that helps organizations **implement everything from this book in a phased, high-impact way.**

Plan Includes:

- **Week 1-4:** Audit decision-making bottlenecks and align leadership
- **Week 5-8:** Implement structured discovery and decision-making frameworks
- **Week 9-12:** Measure impact, refine processes, and embed continuous improvement culture

How This Helps:
Ensures that businesses don't just read about breaking free—they execute and see measurable results within 90 days.

You're now ready to Break Free and Unleash the Intelligence Within!